KU-431-127

Progress in Pathology

VOLUME 4

Edited by

Nigel Kirkham MD FRCPath
Consultant Histopathologist and Cytopathologist,
Royal Sussex County Hospital, Brighton, UK

Nicholas R. Lemoine MD PhD MRCPath
Acting Director, Imperial Cancer Research Fund Molecular Oncology Unit,
Imperial College School of Medicine, Hammersmith Hospital, London, UK

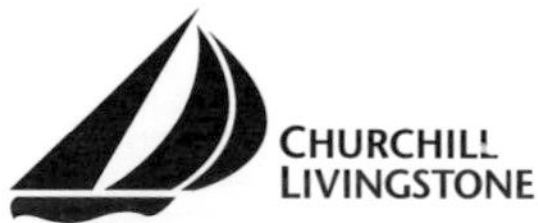

EDINBURGH LONDON NEW YORK PHILADELPHIA SAN FRANCISCO SYDNEY TORONTO 1998

CHURCHILL LIVINGSTONE
A Division of Harcourt Brace & Co. Ltd

Robert Stevenson House, 1–3 Baxter's Place, Leith Walk, Edinburgh EH1 3AF, UK

© Harcourt Brace & Co. Ltd 1998

All rights reserved. No part of this publication may be reproduced, stored in a retrieval system, or transmitted in any form or by any means, electronic, mechanical, photocopying, recording or otherwise, without the prior permission of the publishers (Churchill Livingstone, Robert Stevenson House, 1-3 Baxter's Place, Leith Walk, Edinburgh, EH1 3AF) or a licence permitting restricted copying in the United Kingdom issued by the Copyright Licensing Agency Ltd, 90 Tottenham Court Road, London, W1P 9HE.

First published 1998

ISBN 0443-06032-0

British Library Cataloguing in Publication Data
A catalogue record for this book is available from the British Library

Library of Congress Cataloging in Publication Data
A catalog record for this book is available from the Library of Congress

Medical knowledge is constantly changing. As new information becomes available, changes in treatment, procedures, equipment and the use of drugs become necessary. The authors and publisher have, as far as possible, taken care to ensure that the information given in this text is accurate and up-to-date. However, readers are strongly advised to confirm that the information, especially with regard to drug usage, complies with current legislation and standards of practice.

Produced by BA & GM Haddock
Printed in Singapore

The publisher's policy is to use **paper manufactured from sustainable forests**

Contents

Dedication

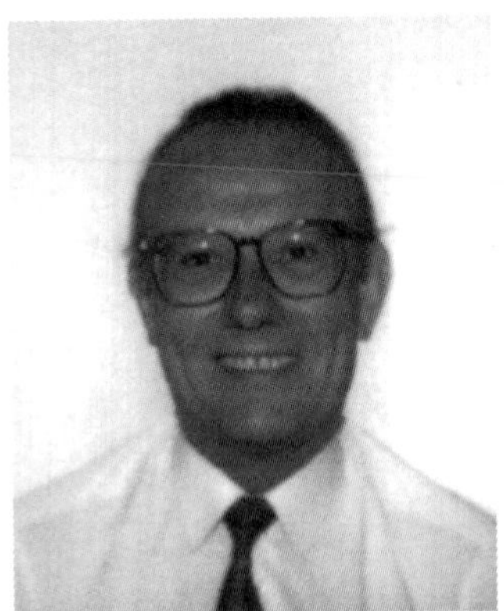

This volume of *Progress in Pathology* is dedicated to the memory of **Dr David Springall** who was a lecturer in histochemistry at the Royal Postgraduate Medical School (now the Imperial College School of Medicine) until his tragic death after a cerebral haemorrhage at the beginning of 1997. He had intended to contribute an article in this volume on his specialist field, the role of the nitric oxide synthetase system in pulmonary vascular disease.

The Editors offer their condolences to his family and colleagues by whom he is greatly missed.

Preface

Another year has passed and so it is time for a further volume in this series. Pathology is advancing on two main fronts at the present time. Continuing developments in molecular pathology, whether by the introduction of new methods or by the refinement and wider application of existing technology, have led to a variety of insights into the mechanisms behind many diseases. Some of this knowledge is maturing to the point where it is starting to find a place in diagnostic practice. We ignore this progress at our peril. In Volume 3, Mapstone and Quirk told us that 'changes in society are occurring more and more rapidly. The changes which have happened in the last 25 years will be easily outstripped by those in the next 25. The combination of advances in information technology, molecular biology and automation together with political changes in health care delivery make the future challenging to us all.'

In the present Volume, we have several contributions that consider the place of molecular pathology in our practice. Human prion disease research has been very much in the news this year, all the way from new variant CJD to the award of the Nobel prize. Further chapters look at developments in our understanding of the telomeres, of Hodgkin's disease and of prostatic cancer.

The second front has been partly determined by the wind of political change blowing through pathology. The widespread development of guidelines and minimum data sets have led to the need for pathologists to demonstrate a greater degree of uniformity in diagnosis and in the provision of reports full of staging and prognostic information. We have several chapters dealing with some of the main tumour areas, careful reading of which should help in achieving better standards.

We trust that you will enjoy reading this book and look forward to meeting you again shortly.

Brighton N.K.
London N.R.L.
1998

Contributors

A. E. Bishop PhD
Department of Histochemistry, Imperial College School of Medicine, Hammersmith Hospital, London, UK

C. S. Foster MD PhD FRCPath
Professor and Director of Anatomic Pathology, Department of Cellular and Molecular Pathology, University of Liverpool, Liverpool, UK

Pierluigi Gambetti MD
Division of Neuropathology, Institute of Pathology, Case Western Reserve University, Cleveland, Ohio, USA

Bernardino Ghetti MD
Department of Pathology, Indiana University Medical Center, Indianapolis, Indiana, USA

W. J. Gullick BSc PhD FRCPath
Professor, ICRF Molecular Oncology Unit, Imperial College School of Medicine,Hammersmith Hospital, London, UK

P. S. Hasleton MD FRCPath
Department of Pathology and Regional Cardiothoracic Centre, South Manchester University Hospitals NHS Trust, Wythenshawe Hospital, Manchester, UK

Y. Ke PhD
Department of Cellular and Molecular Pathology, University of Liverpool, Liverpool, UK

Nigel Kirkham MD FRCPath
Consultant Histopathologist and Cytopathologist, Royal Sussex County Hospital, Brighton, UK

El-Nasir Lalani BSc MBChB MRCPath PhD
Imperial College School of Medicine, Hammersmith Hospital, London, UK

Nicholas R. Lemoine MD PhD MRCPath
Acting Director, Imperial Cancer Research Fund Molecular Oncology Unit, Imperial College School of Medicine, Hammersmith Hospital, London, UK

K. E. Leverton BSc PhD
ICRF Molecular Oncology Unit, Imperial College School of Medicine, Hammersmith Hospital, London, UK

Piero Parchi MD
Division of Neuropathology, Institute of Pathology, Case Western Reserve University, Cleveland, Ohio, USA

Pedro Piccardo MD
Department of Pathology, Indiana University Medical Center, Indianapolis, Indiana, USA

Sandra Perlikowski MSc
Research Assistant, Ontario Cancer Institute, Princess Margaret Hospital, 610 University Avenue, Toronto, Ontario, Canada M5G 2M9

J.M. Polak DSc MD FRCPath
Professor and Head, Department of Histochemistry, Imperial College School of Medicine, Hammersmith Hospital, London, UK

Philip Quirke BM PhD FRCPath
Professor and Honorary Consultant, Division of Clinical Sciences, School of Medicine, University of Leeds; and Head, Department of Histopathology and Molecular Pathology, Institute of Pathology, Leeds General Infirmary, Leeds, UK

Terence P. Rollason BSc FRCPath
Consultant Histopathologist, Department of Pathology, Birmingham Women's Hospital, Edgbaston, Birmingham B15 2TJ, UK

H.M. Romanska PhD
Department of Histochemistry, Imperial College School of Medicine, Hammersmith Hospital, London and Department of Paediatric Surgery, Institute of Child Health, London, UK

Jeremy A. Squire PhD
Director, Cancer Cytogenetics Laboratory, Ontario Cancer Institute, Princess Margaret Hospital, Toronto, Ontario, Canada

L. Spitz PhD
Department of Paediatric Surgery, Institute of Child Health, London, UK

Gordon W.H. Stamp MBChB FRCPath
Imperial College School of Medicine, Hammersmith Hospital, London, UK

Freda K. Stevenson DPhil FRCPath
Consultant Immunologist and Professor of Immunology, Molecular Immunology Group, Tenovus Laboratory, Southampton University Hospitals, Southampton, UK

Andrew Stubbs PhD
Post Doctoral Fellow, Royal Postgraduate Medical School, Hammersmith Hospital, London, UK

Dennis H. Wright MD FRCPath
Emeritus Professor of Pathology, Department of Pathology, Southampton University Hospitals, Southampton, UK

David Wynford-Thomas PhD MB
Professor, Department of Pathology, University of Wales College of Medicine, Cardiff, UK

1

Molecular cytogenetics in modern pathology

Jeremy A. Squire   Sandra Perlikowski

INTRODUCTION

In recent years, advances in the analysis of chromosomes and genes have occurred rapidly, and have played a central role in the development of a conceptual understanding of human genetic diseases and cancer. Cytogenetics is no longer limited to the morphological analysis of chromosomal aberrations, but now has a fundamental role in the molecular identification of gene sequences involved in cancer and subtle rearrangements in human genetic diseases.[1] This recent evolution of cytogenetics into the much more colourful discipline of 'molecular cytogenetics' is due largely to the impressive progress in the genome project that has provided a diversity of DNA probes to improve the repertoire of genes available for the study of specific chromosomal changes in human cells. It has become possible to identify and isolate specific disease genes, and then use them as probes for prenatal diagnosis, dysmorphology and as tumour-specific markers. The use of gene probes in cytogenetics is called 'molecular cytogenetics' and the key analytical technique of this discipline is fluorescence *in situ* hybridization (FISH). Many new specific FISH tests can assay for subtle chromosomal changes that would have been impossible to detect by conventional G-banded analysis. This chapter will review contemporary molecular cytogenetic methodology and highlight the role of FISH in cancer and its ability to improve our understanding of the pathobiology of diseases in which chromosomal rearrangements are involved.

Jeremy A. Squire PhD, Director, Cancer Cytogenetics Laboratory, Room 9-721, Ontario Cancer Institute, Princess Margaret Hospital, 610 University Avenue, Toronto, Ontario, Canada M5G 2M9

Sandra Perlikowski MSc, Research Assistant, Ontario Cancer Institute, Princess Margaret Hospital, 610 University Avenue, Toronto, Ontario, Canada M5G 2M9

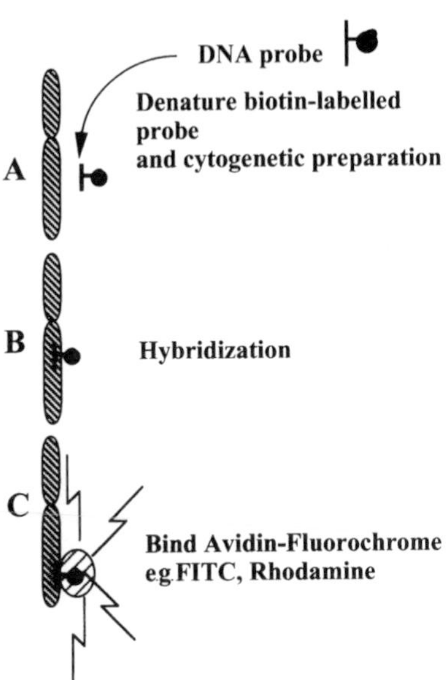

Fig. 1 Schematic depiction of FISH method. DNA probes, specific for a gene, chromosome segment, or a `paint', are labelled, usually by incorporation of biotin and/or digoxigenin. (**A**) DNA probe and target chromosomal DNA are made single stranded by heat denaturation. (**B**) DNA probe is added to the target DNA on slides and is sealed under glass cover slips with rubber cement and incubated for several hours. The DNA probe will re-anneal to the denatured piece of DNA at its precise location on the chromosome. (**C**) The unbound probe is washed off using dilutions of a warm buffered saline salt solution, and the hybridized sequences are detected using avidin, which binds strongly to biotin, and/or antibodies to digoxigenin, coupled to fluorescein isothiocyanate (FITC), rhodamine, or an equivalent fluorochrome. The sites of hybridization are clearly visualized as fluorescent points of light where the probe is bound to the chromosomal DNA (hatched area).

FLUORESCENCE *IN SITU* HYBRIDIZATION (FISH) TECHNIQUE

OVERVIEW OF THE TECHNIQUE

The ability of single-stranded complementary nucleic acids to hybridize, or renature, is fundamental to molecular genetic analysis. When a double-stranded DNA probe is heated, the complementary strands separate (denature) to form single-stranded DNA. Given suitable conditions, the separated complementary regions of DNA can join together to reform a double-stranded molecule. This renaturation process is highly faithful, and when extensive hybridization has occurred, the resulting DNA duplex is very stable. DNA strands that are not highly complementary will not hybridize to one another, or interfere with complementary strand hybridization. The extraordinary specificity and sensitivity of the hybridization process is controlled by very precise experimental conditions and meticulous care to detail is required for all *in situ* procedures.[2]

Early *in situ* methods employed isotopic labelling that were labour intensive, lengthy in signal detection times, and used routinely by only a relatively small group of cytogeneticists. The newer FISH methods take full advantage of the specificity of hybridization, but couple this capability with the excellent signal detection properties of epifluorescence microscopy.

To perform FISH, slides are prepared from cells that grow in suspension culture, such as lymphocytes and lymphoblasts, or from sections of solid tissue. Probes utilized for FISH can include segments of DNA specific for regions associated with cancer or genetic diseases. These probes are either generated in research laboratories or can be purchased commercially. DNA probes are labelled, usually by incorporation of haptens such as biotin or digoxigenin, and are then hybridized to metaphase chromosomes (Fig. 1). The DNA probe will re-anneal to the denatured piece of DNA at its precise location on the chromosome. After washing off the unbound probe, the sites of hybridization are clearly visualized as fluorescent points of light when the fluorochrome becomes bound to the hapten on each chromosome.[2] As the target DNA within the chromosome or nucleus remains intact, information is obtained directly about the positions of probes in relation to chromosome bands thus 'mapping' the probe (see example, Fig. 2A). Chromosomal aberrations can, therefore, be defined using combinations of different coloured probes which delineate particular chromosomes or chromosomal regions associated with genetic diseases or cancer breakpoints.

TYPES OF PROBES USED FOR FISH

The most frequently used probes in molecular cytogenetics are the chromosome-specific (usually centromere-specific) probes which allow the

Table 1 DNA probes commonly used for molecular cytogenetic analysis, their signal intensity, and some of their applications

Type	Intensity	Applications
Centromere probes	Strong	Most commonly used probes. Ideal for detecting whole chromosome trisomies (Fig. 4A) and monosomies (Figs 2C & 4B) and determining the sex of cells for transplantation studies (Fig. 2B)
Telomere probes	Moderate	Ideal for determining whether small reciprocal translocations near chromosome ends have taken place
Chromosome paints	Strong—moderate	Useful for identifying small marker chromosomes or aberrations where insufficient banding is present for identity determination
Translocation junction probes	Moderate	Useful for detecting the presence of diagnostic chromosome translocations in interphase nuclei (see Figs 2D & 4D,E)
Microdeletion probes	Moderate	Ideal for determining whether submicroscopic deletions have taken place (see Fig. 4F)
Probes to detect gene amplification	Strong	For detecting the presence of prognostic oncogene increases in copy number (amplification) in interphase nuclei (see Figs 2E—G & 4C)

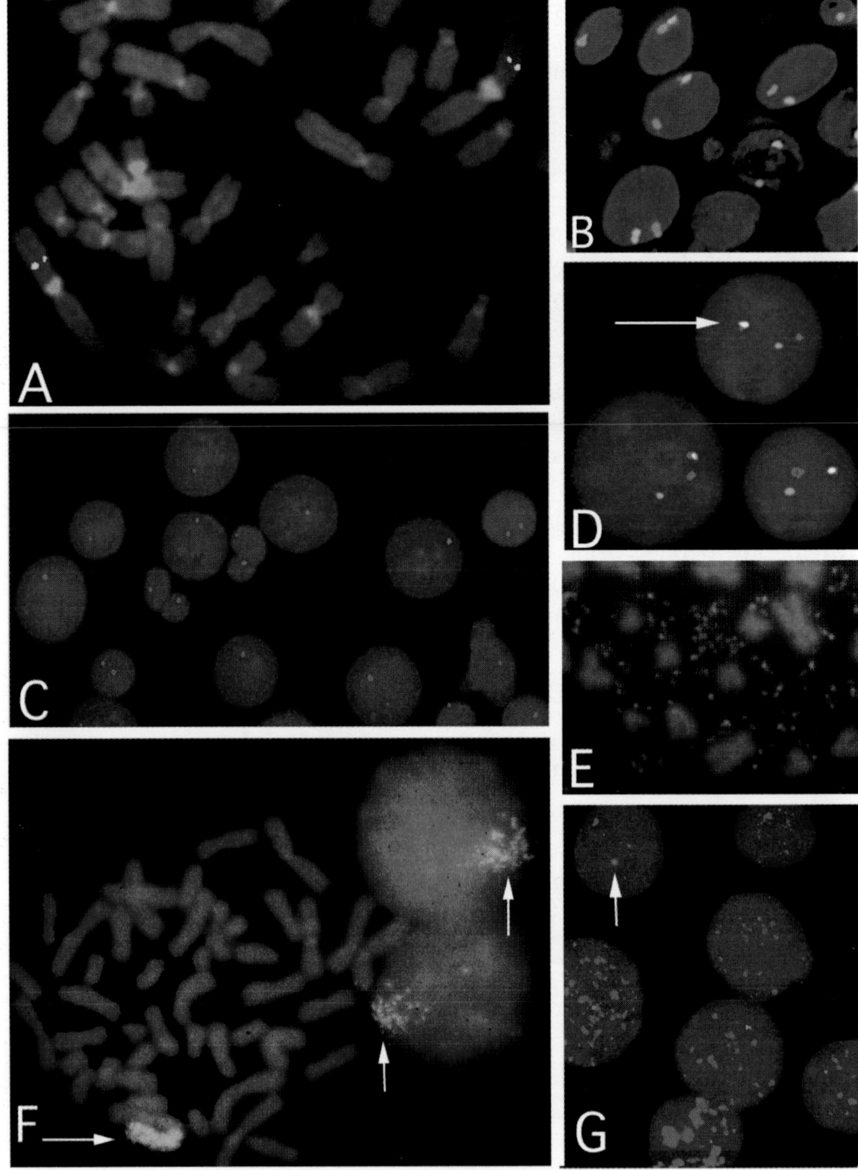

Fig. 2 Diversity of molecular cytogenetic methods. (*see opposite page for details*)

overall chromosome number or the sex chromosome constitution to be determined. This latter application is useful for monitoring intersex bone marrow engraftment (Fig. 2B). Some single copy gene probes, such as cosmids or PACs (P1 artificial chromosome probes), contain large stretches of human genomic DNA and make excellent probes for FISH analysis (Table 1). Chromosome paint probes are derived from an entire human chromosome and will label any chromosomal material originating from the chromosome used to generate the 'paint'. One disadvantage of such large genomic probes is that they are very likely to contain simple repetitive sequences interspersed with

Fig. 2 Diversity of molecular cytogenetic methods. (**A**) Example of FISH mapping of a single copy genomic probe to chromosome 1. This is a DAPI (blue counterstain) banded normal metaphase preparation showing the location of positive signals (yellow signals) obtained with a cosmid probe containing an insert size of 40 kb of DNA from a gene on chromosome 1. A positive FISH signal is present on each chromatid of both pairs of chromosome 1 at band 1q25. (**B**) FISH analysis using paraffin sectioned material[44] to determine the sex identity of cells using sex-chromosome specific probes. The green signal represents the Y chromosome while the pink signal will identify the X chromosome indicating that the cells in this sample is from a male. This technique is helpful in monitoring intersex transplantation. (**C**) Monosomy 13 detected in DAPI stained interphase nuclei of a multiple myeloma bone marrow aspirate using FISH with a single copy genomic probe that maps close to band 13q14. Some nuclei have two pink signals per nucleus indicating that the monosomy may be a secondary clone or that normal bone marrow cells were present in the aspirate. (**D**) Detection of a Philadelphia chromosome in interphase nuclei of CML. All nuclei contain one green signal (BCR), one pink signal (ABL), and an intermediate fusion signal (Ph1) (arrow). (**E**) Double minute (dmin) chromosomes can be detected using a *MYCN* single copy cosmid probe as areas of yellow FISH signal (FITC) against a propidium iodide (red) counterstain in and around the neuroblastoma metaphase chromosomes. (**F**) Detection of a homogeneously staining region (hsr) (arrows) present in a metaphase cell preparation from a retinoblastoma cell line using the *MYCN* probe. (**G**) *MYCN* amplification in neuroblastoma detected by FISH with a *MYCN* cosmid (pink) and a deletion of the short arm of chromosome 1 with a genomic probe that maps to the commonly deleted region at band 1p36. The signal (pale green) from the remaining normal chromosome 1 is arrowed in the upper left nucleus.

unique sequences and, therefore, the probes will require suppression with unlabelled human DNA enriched for the repetitive component (called 'Cot-1 DNA'). Generally, any large genomic probes, such as yeast artificial chromosomes (YACs), PACs, cosmids, paints and those probes with repetitive sequences, should be pre-annealed in the presence of Cot-1 DNA for 1—3 h to prevent non-specific hybridization. Two or three experiments may be required to establish the optimal conditions for these probes. Simple repetitive, i.e. alpha-satellite and telomeric probes, and most cDNA probes, do not usually require suppression with Cot-1 DNA.

MOLECULAR CYTOGENETICS OF MICRODELETION SYNDROMES

One of the most important contributions of molecular cytogenetic technology to clinical genetics has been the improved resolution in detecting subtle or submicroscopic chromosomal abnormalities. One chromosome band using the best banding conditions will contain 3×10^6 base pairs (3 Mb) of DNA so there could be greater than 100 genes deleted before detection is possible by conventional karyotype analysis. Such rearrangements have been detected by FISH in parents of children with Miller-Dieker syndrome[3] and Wolf-Hirschhorn syndrome[4] (Table 2). In many microdeletion syndromes, the chromosome anomalies first recognized were due to large alterations, such as an unbalanced translocation in the case of DiGeorge syndrome,[5] visible deletions in the case of Prader-Willi syndrome,[6] or a ring chromosome, in Miller-Dieker syndrome.[7] In some syndromes, the phenotype may correlate with the size of the deletion. For example, large deletions of Xp21 may eliminate the genes associated with Duchenne muscular dystrophy, chronic granulomatous disease, McLeod syndrome, retinitis pigmentosa, mental retardation, glycerol kinase deficiency, and adrenal hypoplasia congenita,

Table 2 Some of the microdeletion syndromes detectable by FISH

Syndrome	Band
Wolf-Hirschhorn[4]	4p16.3
Williams[39]	7q11.2
WAGR*[40]	11p13
Prader-Willi/Angelman[41]	15q11-13
Rubinstein-Taybi[42]	16p13.3
Miller-Dieker/lissencephaly[3]	17p13.3
DiGeorge/Velo-Cardio-Facial syndrome[43]	22q11.21—22q11.23

*WAGR = Wilms tumour, aniridia, genital anomalies, growth retardation.

resulting in a very complex phenotype.[8] Any one of these deficiencies may also occur as an individual disease.

To identify a submicroscopic deletion, one probe is usually directed against DNA sequences contained completely within the consensus deleted region for the syndrome. The other probe will hybridize to DNA sequences located outside this critical region and is used to identify the chromosome of interest and serve as a positive control for the hybridization conditions (Fig. 4F). Commercial probes are often cocktails of several overlapping cosmids and produce strong hybridization signals suitable for use in the clinical laboratory. The control probe and the microdeletion probe should be at least 3—5 Mb apart and detectable using a two-colour FISH protocol. Some of the FISH methodologies, such as chromatin or fiber FISH,[2] which can map the position of probes below the level of resolution of a chromosome band have proved useful in determining gene order and location relative to the critical deleted region when designing FISH microdeletion assays for the clinical laboratory.

FISH ANALYSIS OF INTERPHASE NUCLEI

A major difficulty in tumour cytogenetics is the inability to obtain chromosome spreads from many types of tumours. FISH, however, can also be performed on interphase nuclei from tumour biopsies or cultured tumour cells which enables cytogenetic aberrations to be visualized without the need for obtaining good quality chromosome preparations. This procedure is called 'interphase cytogenetics'. Another major advantage of interphase FISH is that it can be performed on relatively small samples, such as bone marrow aspirates, which may not have been feasible using standard molecular techniques. Numerical chromosome aberrations can be detected using specific centromere probes which give two signals from normal nuclei but only one signal when there is one copy of the chromosome (monosomy; Figs 2C & 4B) or three signals when there is an extra copy (trisomy; Fig. 4A).

The use of interphase FISH analysis for prenatal diagnosis allows for a rapid result to be obtained directly from uncultured amniotic fluid. Aneuploidies of chromosomes X, Y, 21, 18, and 13 account for the majority of chromosomal abnormalities leading to a prenatal diagnosis of human fetal aneusomy,[1] all of which, in theory, could be detected by interphase FISH studies. An interphase FISH result can be obtained within 24–48 h, while a

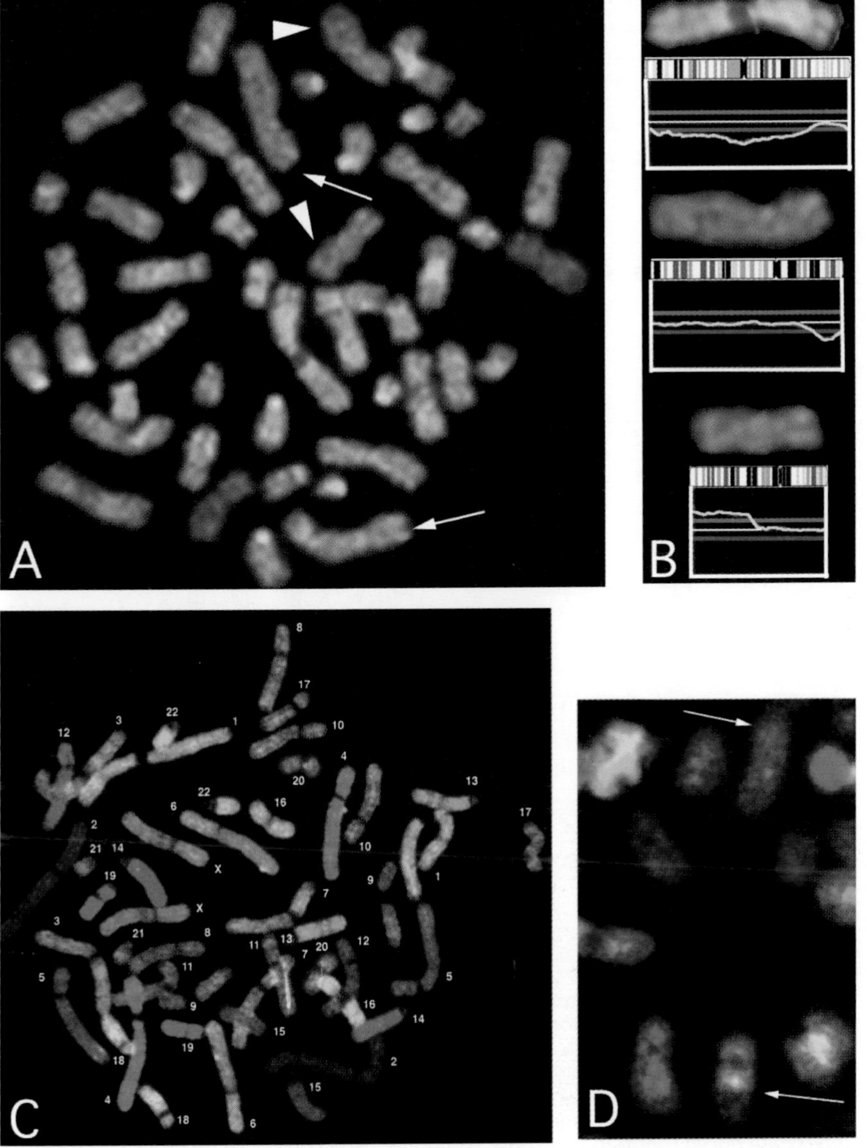

Fig. 3 New molecular cytogenetic methods. (**A**) Comparative genomic hybridization of a neuroblastoma cell line to demonstrate detection of chromosomal gains (green fluorescence), e.g. the distal part of the short arm of chromosome 2 (long arrow), and chromosomal losses (red fluorescence), e.g. chromosome 6q (arrow head). (**B**) The CGH analysis profile from a neuroblastoma cell line. Chromosome 1 shows an overall gain of DNA indicated by an increase in the level of green signal (top panel) In this cell line most of chromosome 1 was trisomic. Chromosome 2 has a strong green signal at band 2p24 due to amplification (50 copies/cell) of *MYCN* in the cell line (middle panel). The long arm of chromosome 6 shows a loss (deletion) of DNA and a shift towards the red signal (bottom panel). (**C**) Spectral karyotype analysis of normal blood lymphocytes. Each chromosome pair will have a unique colour to aid in its identification. (**D**) Specific details of a spectral karyotype analysis of a rhabdomyosarcoma cell line to demonstrate the presence of two translocations. The arrows indicate translocation breakpoint junctions.

complete karyotypic analysis usually takes 7—10 days. One disadvantage of relying on interphase FISH analysis is that it can only detect numerical chromosomal abnormalities. Metaphase studies are required to exclude the presence of structural changes that result in fetal aneuploidy. An advantage of interphase cytogenetics is in the analysis of constitutional mosaicism where it is possible to rapidly obtain estimates of the relative contribution of each chromosomal type in the mosaic.[9]

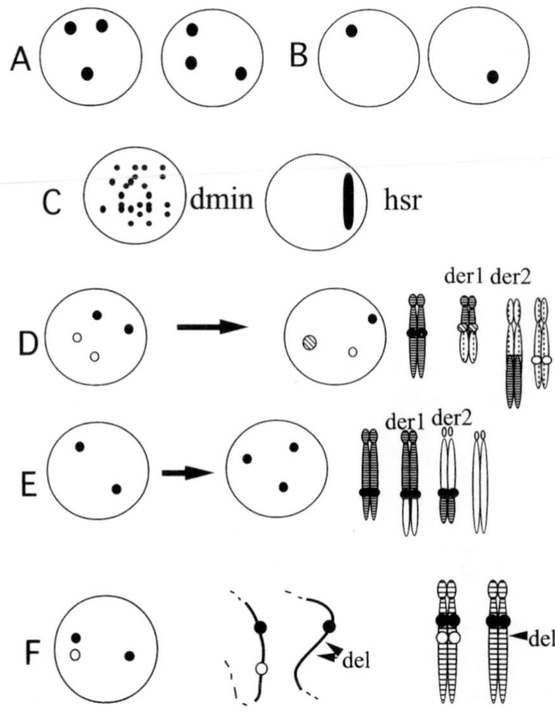

Fig. 4 Schematic depictions to illustrate the interpretation of FISH signals in different applications of molecular cytogenetic analysis (**A**) Trisomy detection in interphase nuclei (signals are solid). (**B**) Monosomy detection in interphase nuclei (remaining signal is solid). (**C**) Gene amplification by double minute chromosomes (dmin) in interphase nuclei (left) in which the additional genes will produce large numbers of signals per nucleus; gene amplification by homogeneously staining regions (hsr) in interphase nuclei (right) in which the additional gene copies can be detected as a large block of signal. (**D**) Detection of a specific reciprocal translocation in interphase nuclei and a schematic depiction of the signal pattern on metaphase chromosomes with the translocation. All normal nuclei contain two black signals and two white signals. The probes flank one of the derivative (der) chromosomes of the reciprocal translocation (in this example derivative 1) and generate an intermediate coloured signal (hatched). (**E**) Detection of a reciprocal translocation in interphase nuclei where only one gene is consistently involved (e.g. *MLL*). All normal nuclei contain two black *MLL* signals. The probe straddles the common breakpoint for the reciprocal translocation so that both derivative chromosomes will have *MLL* sequences and will generate a net number of three signals per nucleus. (**F**) Identification of a submicroscopic deletion. The test probe (white) is within the consensus deleted region. The control probe (solid) is located outside this critical region and is used to identify the chromosome of interest and demonstrates that the hybridization conditions were optimal. The centre of the panel shows the configuration of the deleted and non deleted chromosome. The two probes will typically be 2—3 Mb apart and the FISH signals will still be slightly separate on metaphase chromosome analysis.

Chromosome deletions need not be detected by metaphase FISH analysis only. They can also be detected at interphase by using probes from the deleted region and counting the number of signals per nucleus. Similarly, translocations can be detected by interphase FISH as well. If the 2 probes used for FISH are labelled with 2 different fluorochromes and are close to specific translocation breakpoints on different chromosomes, they will appear joined as a result of the translocation generating a 'colour fusion' signal (Figs 2D & 4D). These procedures are particularly useful in cancer cytogenetics for rapid detection of aberrations such as the *BCR-ABL* rearrangement in chronic myeloid leukemia (see below), thus providing immediate and directly quantitative diagnostic information.

MOLECULAR CYTOGENETICS OF HAEMATOLOGICAL MALIGNANCIES

CHRONIC MYELOGENOUS LEUKEMIA (CML)

Consistent and in some cases highly specific chromosome aberrations have been found in hematological malignancies and solid tumours (Table 3) as reviewed in Heim and Mitelman.[10] Chronic myelogenous leukemia (CML) was the first malignancy in which a reproducible chromosomal abnormality was described. In almost all patients with CML, the leukemic cells contain a unique small chromosome, called the Philadelphia chromosome (commonly abbreviated Ph[1] or simply Ph) which Rowley (1973)[11] showed to result from a reciprocal translocation between chromosomes 22 and 9. This rearrangement causes an in-frame fusion between the *BCR* and *ABL* oncogenes and presents an ideal substrate for two colour FISH analysis. During periods of CML remission, when malignant cells are undetectable, all of the dividing myeloid cells (i.e. erythrocytes, granulocytes and megakaryocytes) are diploid, with the Ph chromosome translocation being the only detectable karyotypic abnormality. Two colour FISH detection of the Ph chromosome in interphase nuclei (Fig. 2D) can be used to determine if residual disease following treatment is still present.[12] FISH can be conveniently performed on aspirates and cytology preparations when residual disease is suspected in any of the leukemic disorders where a consistent translocation has been identified.[10] When CML patients enter the blast crisis phase, other chromosome abnormalities frequently appear. Among the most common changes are the appearance of a second Ph chromosome, an isochromosome of the long arm of chromosome 17 or an extra copy of chromosome 8. Such changes in karyotype are a grave prognostic sign, and can be identified relatively easy by direct FISH analysis of interphase nuclei in a patient's bone marrow aspirate.

ACUTE LYMPHOCYTIC AND MYELOID LEUKEMIA (ALL/AML)

Certain types of acute lymphocytic and myeloid leukemias have translocations that alter the function of MLL, a leukemia-specific transcription factor encoded by a gene mapping to chromosome band 11q23. The oncogenic rearrangements

Table 3 Common types of chromosomal abnormalities in leukemias and solid tumours detectable by interphase FISH

Malignancy	Chromosomal aberrations	Molecular lesion	Interphase FISH
Acute leukemias	Reciprocal translocations	Fusion oncoprotein	Detection of fusion by two-colour FISH
AML-M4Eo	inv(16)(p13q22)	*MYH11—CBFB* fusion	Disruption of contiguous signal
Therapy-related AML	–5/del(5q), –7/del(7q)	Unknown tumour suppressor genes	One signal in nuclei
Acute leukemias	Translocations at 11q23	*MLL* and various partner genes	Disruption of signal generates 3 signals/nucleus
CML blast crisis	(9;22)(q34;q11), +8, +Ph[1], +19, or i(17q)	*BCR—ABL*	Fusion signal, + additional signals for trisomies
ALL with good prognosis	Hyperdiploidy	Unknown	Additional signals for trisomies
Small cell lung carcinoma	del(3)(p14-23)	Unknown tumour suppressor genes	One signal in nuclei
Neuroblastoma (poor prognosis)	del(1)(p32),	Unknown tumour suppressor genes	One signal in nuclei
	dmins	*MYCN* amplified	Multiple signals
Breast carcinoma (poor prognosis)	Amplification	*ERBB2*	Multiple signals

always have breakpoints within band 11q23 causing *MLL* to be juxtaposed in-frame with one of 20 different partner genes, including *AF4* at 4q21, *AF9* at 9p21 and *ENL* at 19p13.[13] Since a specific molecular assay is not possible for a gene that rearranges to different target chromosomal locations, a single FISH assay has been developed,[14] where disruption of the *MLL* gene by any translocation will cause interphase nuclei to contain three signals instead of the normal two since the *MLL* gene spans the translocation breakpoint region (see Fig. 4E).

CHRONIC LYMPHOCYTIC LEUKEMIA (CLL)

Chronic lymphocytic leukemia (CLL) is the most common form of leukemia in Caucasians and the identification of a high-risk population requiring a more aggressive therapy would be useful. Recent evidence has suggested that trisomy 12 is an independent predictor of poor outcome, however, because of the low proliferation rate, adequate karyotypic analysis may be difficult. FISH, therefore, appears to be the method of choice for the detection of trisomy 12 and other selected cytogenetic abnormalities in chronic lymphocytic leukemia.[15]

DIFFICULTIES IN PERFORMING CHROMOSOMAL STUDIES

It has proven difficult to obtain comprehensive information about chromosomal abnormalities in solid tumours. The major reason has been the difficulty in obtaining suitable cellular preparations for chromosome analysis. In contrast to leukemias, which grow naturally as single-cell suspensions or are easily disrupted into single cells, the cells in solid tumours are held together by tight junctions. Disruption of tumours into a single-cell suspension suitable for karyotype analysis often results in cell death. When chromosomes are obtained, their morphology is usually poor and they may be grossly rearranged.[10] Furthermore, solid tumours are often contaminated with a significant portion of normal infiltrating stromal cells, so that representative karyotypes can be difficult to obtain.

The use of molecular cytogenetic techniques in the analysis of solid tumours has shown that there are distinct aberrations in different categories of solid tumours, resulting in increased diagnostic accuracy and a greater understanding of tumour pathogenesis.[16–20] Some tumours can also be assigned to good or bad prognostic categories according to their cytogenetic profiles and the ability to perform interphase FISH analysis has helped in the characterization of some of the consistent aberrations associated with solid tumours.

DETECTING TRANSLOCATIONS IN SARCOMAS

Sarcomas include soft tissue tumours that often have characteristic chromosome translocations that result in the formation of chimaeric genes encoding transcription factors.[21] As in leukemias and lymphomas, the chimaeric transcription factor often retains the DNA binding domain from one of the translocated genes and the transcriptional transactivating domain from the other. Other sarcomas show recurrent chromosome aberrations preferentially affecting particular chromosomal regions. For example, Ewing sarcoma which usually occurs in children, can be diagnosed using morphology and immunohistochemical markers, but precise classification is often difficult. The majority of Ewing sarcomas and the related tumour, peripheral neuroepithelioma have a recurring t(11;22)(q24;q12)[22] translocation. In these tumours, the *EWS* gene from chromosome 22q12, is fused in-frame with a member of the ETS family of transcription factors, *FLI1*, on chromosome 11q24.[23] The original mapping of this rearrangement and its subsequent detection in interphase nuclei (Fig. 4D) have depended largely on a combination of FISH mapping, interphase analysis and molecular genetic cloning.[24] Recently, a variant, the t(7;22)(p22;q12), has been described in a case of Ewing sarcoma.[25] In this case, *EWS* is fused to the human equivalent of the murine ETS gene *Er81*, termed *ETV1* (for Ewing translocation variant 1).[26] When molecular diagnostic methods based on PCR fail to detect a *EWS-FLII* transcript, the FISH analysis for one of the variant EWS translocations is advisable.

GENE AMPLIFICATION IN SOLID TUMOURS

In addition to translocations and deletions, cells in solid tumours often show increases in genetic material, associated with overexpression of oncogenes. Solid tumours frequently have large numbers of chromosomes, often approaching a tetraploid number, and increases in specific chromosomes or in portions of a chromosome are also detected. Cells from many tumours show double minutes (dmins) or homogeneously staining regions (hsr), which are both indicative of gene amplification. Some of the gene amplifications studied in detail, include the oncogenes *MYCN*, *ERBB2*, *GLI*, *HST1*, *INT2*, *MDM2*, a number of which are cell cycle control genes.

In neuroblastoma, the *MYCN* oncogene is frequently amplified, presenting cytologically as dmins (Figs 2E & 4C,left) or a hsr (Figs 2F & 4C,right) and together with deletion of the short arm of chromosome 1 confers a poor outcome when present (see Fig. 2G).[27] Copy numbers greater than 10 are considered to indicate a poorer prognosis but molecular methods, such as the polymerase chain reaction (PCR) and Southern blotting, analyze a mixture of cells and, therefore, can provide only an average copy number result for a particular tumour. FISH analysis of neuroblastoma offers the advantage over the other methods in that it can detect tumours with small numbers of amplified cells which would otherwise be missed[28] and in cases of low (3—10) copies of *MYCN*, can distinguish small numbers of amplified cells (poor prognosis) from triploid tumours (good prognosis).[29] Similar studies of *ERBB2* oncogene copy numbers in human breast cancer have shown a similar correlation of relapse and survival with the presence of amplification.[30]

RECENT ADVANCES IN MOLECULAR CYTOGENETIC TECHNOLOGY

COMPARATIVE GENOMIC HYBRIDIZATION (CGH)

Molecular cytogenetics has shown that gene amplification is common in solid tumours. The acquisition of additional chromosomal regions and increased gene copy number is likely to confer a strong selective advantage to some tumours and the further characterization of amplified genes may give useful prognostic information about various solid tumours. However, when the gene or genes that are amplified are unknown, it is not possible to determine whether gene amplification is present. Fortunately, a new screening method called comparative genomic hybridization (CGH) has been developed that allows investigators to produce a detailed map of the differences between chromosomes in different cells without any prior knowledge concerning the regions that are amplified (see Pinkel[31] for review). This method detects gains (amplifications) or losses (deletions) of segments of DNA.[32]

In typical CGH experiments, DNA from malignant and normal cells, such as fibroblasts, is labelled with two different fluorochromes and then hybridized simultaneously to **normal** chromosome metaphase spreads. Tumour DNA is labelled with biotin and detected with fluorescein (green fluorescence); the control DNA is labelled with digoxigenin and detected with rhodamine (red fluorescence). Regions of loss or gain of DNA sequences in the tumour, such as deletions, duplications, or amplifications, are seen as changes in the ratio of the intensities of the two fluorochromes along the target chromosomes (Fig. 5). An amplified sequence will generate increased green fluorescence (Fig. 3A,B top and middle panel), whereas a deletion will shift the red/green ratio towards red (Fig. 3B bottom panel). For low copy number amplifications and hemizygous deletions, this change in the fluorescence ratio is often difficult to distinguish by eye and requires specialized image analysis software. One disadvantage of CGH is that it can only detect large blocks (5 Mb) of over- or under-represented chromosomal DNA; balanced rearrangements, such as inversions or translocations, escape detection. CGH has gained wide acceptance as a new and promising approach for understanding the cytogenetic changes in solid tumours,[33] particularly for characterizing the complex aberrations and aneuploidies in carcinomas.[34] The ability to associate tumour aggressiveness with a specific chromosomal aneuploidy should improve tumour prognosis beyond that possible from measurements of total nuclear DNA content alone.

Although the CGH apparatus is expensive and may not be currently accessible to all laboratories, CGH is easily integrated into the clinical laboratory setting. It is also possible to use CGH to screen for DNA copy number changes in archival formalin-fixed paraffin-embedded tumour samples. In these studies, tumours are examined using an inverted microscope, and areas of interest are microdissected with a sterile needle from

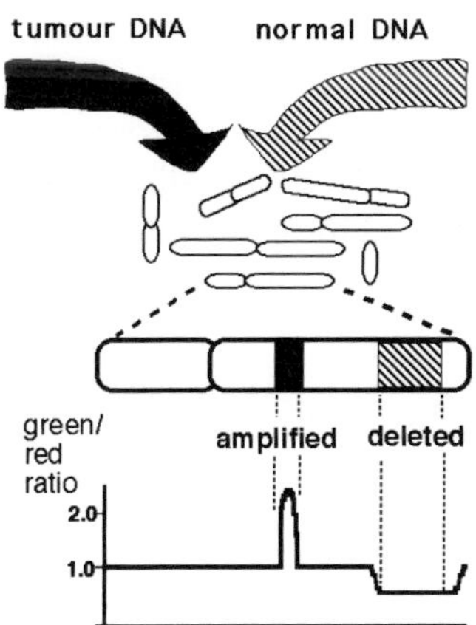

Fig. 5 Schematic depiction of comparative genomic hybridization technique. Tumour DNA is labelled with a green fluorochrome (black arrow) and normal reference DNA is labelled with a red fluorochrome (hatched arrow) and an equal mixture of each is hybridized to normal human metaphase chromosomes. Unlabelled repetitive human DNA (Cot-1) is included to suppress binding of labelled DNA to repetitive elements. Regions of DNA gain are seen as an increase fluorescence intensity on the target chromosomes (shown in black); regions of DNA loss are seen as increased fluorescence intensity (shown as hatched). Regions on the chromosome that are stained equally for both green and red indicate equal copy number for tumour and reference DNA. A ratio of 1.0 indicates no copy-number change. High green to red ratio (>1.0) indicates a DNA gain, and low green to red ratio (<1.0) indicates a DNA deletion.

specific areas of the tissue section.[45] DNA is extracted from microdissected cells, and the method of whole genome amplification, termed primer extension preamplification is performed to increase the amount of DNA for CGH.[2] After the microdissected DNA has been amplified by PCR, it is fluorescently labelled, and examined by CGH to determine DNA copy number changes and correlate genetic aberrations with clinical outcome.[35] The study of genetic progression from premalignant to fully malignant lesions, or comparison of the genetic aberrations seen in primary tumours and their metastases would also be feasible. CGH has the potential to investigate the accumulation of chromosome aberrations as a measure of genetic stability[36] as well as providing a promising approach to screen for and aid in understanding the basis for the complex cytogenetic changes seen in human malignancies.

SPECTRAL KARYOTYPING (SKY)

Recently, a universal chromosome painting technique called spectral karyotyping (SKY) has been developed. SKY is based on the concept that the diagnostic potential of FISH would be greatly improved if it was possible to analyze the entire genome simultaneously on the basis of the differential display of all human chromosomes.[37,38] Spectral imaging combines the use of Fourier spectroscopy, charge-couple (CCD) imaging and optical microscopy to simultaneously measure the sample emission spectra for each human chromosome after FISH. Using combinations of 23 different coloured paints as a 'cocktail probe', subtle differences in fluorochrome labelling profiles after hybridization with this cocktail allows the computer to assign a unique colour to each chromosome pair. In this way, extremely complex rearrangements in the karyotype can be identified by the pattern of colour distribution along the abnormal chromosome (Fig. 3C). In contrast to CGH, subtle karyotype rearrangements that are not dependent on copy number change can be detected easily, so that small translocations will lead to a transition from one colour to another at the position of the breakpoint (Fig. 3D). CGH and SKY in combination will likely provide a much more detailed description of the highly abnormal karyotypes often present in advanced solid tumours. This approach also adds to the power of clinical cytogenetic analysis of constitutional chromosomal aberrations by facilitating the identification of subtle structural rearrangements or small marker chromosomes that may contain an aneuploidy with potential pathological consequences.

SUMMARY

The level of understanding of any scientific phenomenon depends on the capabilities and sophistication of the technology available for its investigation. In recent years, advances in the analysis of chromosomes and genes have occurred rapidly, and have played a central role in the development of a conceptual understanding of cancer and human genetic diseases. Molecular cytogenetics represents a new analytical approach, that combines elements of conventional cytogenetics and molecular biology methodologies with sensitive computerized imaging. A diversity of new molecular cytogenetic methods have helped to characterize the genetic processes that underlie the chromosomal changes seen in cancer cells and have provided a greater resolution of some of the human microdeletion syndromes. This progress has resulted in the development of specific FISH-based tests to assay rapidly for genetic change in tumours in the clinical laboratory. Novel molecular cytogenetic technologies such as CGH and SKY are providing both a more comprehensive and detailed description of the molecular rearrangements and karyotype abnormalities present in solid tumours. As more genes are identified whose structure and/or function is modified in these tumours, there are likely to be more opportunities to identify unique targets in human tumours for therapeutic intervention and newly emerging molecular cytogenetic approaches will be helpful in monitoring the success of modern therapies in the next millenium.

ACKNOWLEDGEMENTS

We would like to thank Dr Barbara Beatty for critically reading this manuscript as well as Jane Bayani, Derek Bouman, Teresa Scheidl, Teresa Selander and Zong Mei Zhang for providing the images for Figures 2 and 3 and Ajay Pandita for assistance with image analysis. We also extend our gratitude to Dr Thomas Reid for allowing us to use some of the spectral analysis images captured in his laboratory.

We acknowledge the use of Vysis probes in Figure 2 and thank them for their support in defraying the cost of colour photography.

This work was supported by the National Cancer Institute of Canada with support from the Canadian Cancer Society, and the Canadian Genome Analysis and Technologies (CGAT) Program.

REFERENCES

1. Verma RS, Babu A (eds). Human Chromosomes. New York: McGraw-Hill, 1995; 184–231, 364–373
2. Dracopoli N, Haines JC, Korf BR et al (eds). Current Protocols in Molecular Genetics. New York: Wiley, 1996 [CD version]
3. Kuwano A, Ledbetter SA, Dobyns WB et al. Detection of deletions and cryptic translocations in Miller-Dieker syndrome by in situ hybridization. Am J Hum Genet 1991; 49: 707–714
4. Altherr MR, Bengtsson U, Elder FFB et al. Molecular confirmation of Wolf-Hirschhorn syndrome with a subtle translocation of chromosome 4. Am J Hum Genet 1991; 49: 1235–1242
5. de la Chapelle A, Herva R, Koivisto M et al. A deletion in chromosome 22 can cause DiGeorge syndrome. Hum Genet 1981; 57: 253–256
6. Ledbetter DH, Riccardi VM, Airhart SD et al. Deletions of chromosome 15 as a cause of the Prader-Willi syndrome. N Engl J Med 1981; 304: 325–329
7. Stratton RF, Dobyns WB, Greenberg F et al. Interstitial deletion of (17)(p11.2p11.2): report of six additional patients with a new chromosome deletion syndrome. Am J Med Genet 1986; 24: 421–432
8. Ballabio A, Parenti G, Tippett P et al. X-linked ichthyosis due to steroid sulphatase deficiency associated with Kallmann syndrome (hypogonadotropic hypogonadism and anosmia): linkage relationships with Xg and cloned DNA sequences from the distal short arm of the X chromosome. Hum Genet 1986; 72: 237–240

9. van Opstal D, van Hemel JO, Eussen BH et al. A chromosome 21-specific cosmid cocktail for the detection of chromosome 21 aberrations in interphase nuclei. Prenat Diagn 1995; 15: 705–711
10. Heim S, Mitelman F (eds). Cancer Cytogenetics, 2nd edn. New York: Wiley, 1995
11. Rowley JD. A new consistent chromosomal abnormality in chronic myelogenous leukaemia identified by quinacrine fluorescence Giemsa staining. Nature 1973; 243: 290–293
12. Raimondi SC. Current status of cytogenetic research in childhood acute lymphoblastic leukemia. Blood 1993; 81: 2237–2251
13. Rubnitz JE, Behm FG, Downing JR. 11q23 rearrangements in acute leukemia. Leukemia 1996; 10: 74–82
14. Martinez-Climent JA, Thirman MJ, Espinosa R et al. Detection of 11q23/MLL rearrangements in infant leukemias with fluorescence in situ hybridization and molecular analysis. Leukemia 1995; 9: 1299–1304
15. Rowley JD, Aster JC, Sklar J. The clinical applications of new DNA diagnostic technology on the management of cancer patients. JAMA 1993; 270: 2331–2337
16. Ilson DH, Motzer RJ, Rodriguez E et al. Genetic analysis in the diagnosis of neoplasms of unknown primary tumor site. Semin Oncol 1993; 20: 229–237
17. Mertens F, Mandahl N, Mitelman F et al. Cytogenetic analysis in the examination of solid tumors in children. Pediatr Hematol Oncol 1994; 11: 361–377
18. Pandis N, Bardi G, Heim S. Interrelationship between methodological choices and conceptual models in solid tumor cytogenetics. Cancer Genet Cytogenet 1994; 76: 77–84
19. Rodriguez E, Sreekantaiah C, Chaganti RSK. Genetic changes in epithelial solid neoplasia. Cancer Res 1994; 54: 3398–3406
20. Sreekantaiah C, Ladanyi M, Rodriguez E et al. Chromosomal aberrations in soft tissue tumors relevance to diagnosis, classification, and molecular mechanism. Am J Pathol 1994; 144: 1121–1134
21. Sorensen PHB, Triche TJ. Gene fusions encoding chimaeric transcription factors in solid tumours. Semin Cancer Biol 1996; 7: 3–14
22. Turc-Carel C, Aurias A, Mugneret F et al. Chromosomes in Ewing's sarcoma. I. An evaluation of 85 cases of remarkable consistency of t(11;22)(q24;q12). Cancer Genet Cytogenet 1988; 32: 229–238
23. Delattre O, Zucman J, Ploustagel B et al. Gene fusion with an ETS DNA binding domain caused by chromosome translocation in human cancers. Nature 1992; 359: 162–165
24. Delattre O, Zucman J, Melot T et al. The Ewing family of tumors – a subgroup of small-round-cell tumors defined by specific chimeric transcripts. N Engl J Med 1994; 331: 294–299
25. Squire J, Zielenska M, Thorner P et al. Variant translocations of chromosome 22 in Ewing's sarcoma. Gene Chromosom Cancer 1993; 8: 190–194
26. Jeon IS, Davis JN, Braun BS et al. A variant Ewing's sarcoma translocation (7;22) fuses the EWS gene to the ETS gene ETV1. Oncogene 1995; 10: 1229—1234
27. Brodeur GM. Molecular basis for heterogeneity in human neuroblastomas [Review]. Eur J Cancer 1995; 4: 505–510
28. Shapiro DN, Valentine MB, Rowe ST et al. Detection of N-myc gene amplification by fluorescence in-situ hybridization: diagnostic utility for neuroblastoma. Am J Pathol 1993; 142: 1339–1346
29. Squire J, Thorner P, Marrano P et al. Identification of MYCN copy number heterogeneity by direct FISH analysis of neuroblastoma preparations. Mol Diagn 1996; 1: 81–89
30. Slamon DJ, Clark GM, Wong SG et al. Human breast cancer: correlation of relapse and survival with amplification of the HER-2/neu oncogene. Science 1987; 235: 177–182
31. Pinkel D. Visualizing tumour amplification [news; comment]. Nature Genet 1994; 8: 107
32. Kallioniemi A, Kallioniemi O-P, Sudar D et al. Comparative genomic hybridization for molecular cytogenetic analysis of solid tumors. Science 1992; 258: 818–821
33. Bryndorf T, Kirchhoff M, Rose H et al. Comparative genomic hybridization in clinical cytogenetics. Am J Hum Genet 1995; 57: 1211–1220
34. Visakorpi T, Hyytinen E, Koivisto P et al. In-vivo amplification of the androgen receptor gene and progression of human prostate-cancer. Nature Genet 1995; 9: 401–406
35. Wiltshire RN, Duray P, Bittner ML et al. Direct visualization of the clonal progression of primary cutaneous melanoma: application of tissue microdissection and comparative genomic hybridization. Cancer Res 1995; 55: 3954–3957

36. Gray JW, Pinkel D, Brown JM. Fluorescence *in situ* hybridization in cancer and radiation biology. Radiat Res 1994; 137: 275–289
37. Marx J. New methods for expanding the chromosomal paint kit [news; comment]. Science 1996; 273: 430
38. Schrock E, du Manoir S, Veldman T et al. Multicolor spectral karyotyping of human chromosomes [see comments]. Comparative genomic hybridization in clinical cytogenetics. Science 1996; 273: 494–497
39. Ewart AK, Morris CA, Atkinson D et al. Hemizygosity at elastin locus in a developmental disorder, Williams syndrome. Nature Genet 1993; 5: 11–16
40. Drechsler M, Meijers-Heijboer EJ, Schneider S et al. Molecular analysis of aniridia patients for deletions involving the Wilms' tumor gene. Hum Genet 1994; 94: 331–338
41. Kuwano A, Mutirangura A, Dittrich B et al. Molecular dissection of the Prader-Willi/Angelman syndrome region (15q11-13) by YAC cloning and FISH analysis. Hum Mol Genet 1992; 1: 417–425
42. Breuning MH, Dauwerse HG, Fugazza G et al. Rubinstein-Taybi syndrome caused by submicroscopic deletions within 16p13.3. Am J Hum Genet 1993; 52: 249—254
43. Lindsay EA, Halford S, Wadey R et al. Molecular cytogenetic characterization of the DiGeorge syndrome region using fluorescence in situ hybridization. Genomics 1993; 17: 403—407
44. Leong P, Thorner P, Yeger H et al. Detection of MYCN amplification and deletions of chromosome 1p in neuroblastoma by in situ hybridization using routine histologic sections. Lab Invest 1993; 69: 43–50
45. Isola J, DeVries S, Chu L et al. Analysis of changes in DNA sequence copy number by comparative genomic hybridization in archival paraffin-embedded tumor samples. Am J Pathol 1994; 145: 1301–1308

2

Neural cell adhesion molecule (NCAM): a role in the development and function of the human gut

H.M. Romanska A.E. Bishop L. Spitz J.M. Polak

Effective motility of the bowel depends on the formation of efficient neuromuscular coupling and consequent interaction. Little is known, however, about how these processes of nerve–muscle recognition and communication are conducted and controlled. Development, maintenance and function of the neuromuscular junction have been studied mainly in skeletal and cardiac muscle and it has been found that one of the major factors involved in the interaction between nerves and myofibres is a cell-surface glycoprotein, neural cell adhesion molecule (NCAM).[1–6] Although the autonomic neuromuscular junction differs from that in striated muscle, it can be assumed that the system controlling interaction between nerves and muscle cells is similar in all types of muscle. The work described in this chapter aimed to provide evidence that NCAM is involved in the differentiation and function of the neuromuscular system of the human gut. This hypothesis is supported here by data on the immunohistochemical localization of NCAM expression in the musculature of human developing normal and abnormal bowel as well as in in vitro differentiating enteric myocytes. The findings presented are discussed in the context of their relevance to the pathogenesis of dysmotility disorders of the human gut and their potential clinical applications.

H.M. Romanska, Department of Histochemistry, Imperial College School of Medicine, Hammersmith Hospital, Du Cane Road, London W12 0NN, and Department of Paediatric Surgery, Institute of Child Health, Guilford Street, London WC1N 1EH, UK

A.E. Bishop, Department of Histochemistry, Imperial College School of Medicine, Hammersmith Hospital, Du Cane Road, London W12 0NN, UK

L. Spitz, Department of Paediatric Surgery, Institute of Child Health, Guilford Street, London WC1N 1EH, UK

J.M. Polak, Department of Histochemistry, Imperial College School of Medicine, Hammersmith Hospital, Du Cane Road, London W12 0NN, UK

NCAM

Neural cell adhesion molecule (NCAM) is one of the best characterized membrane molecules associated with the function of the neuromuscular junction and implicated in the interaction between nerves and muscle cells. The discovery of the NCAM family resulted from an extensive search for molecules thought to be involved in the formation of the central nervous system (CNS) and, in particular, in the molecular mechanisms by which neurons select their target cells in order to produce specific connections within the complex networks of the CNS. Three independent groups of scientists led by: (i) Gerald Edelman in New York; (ii) Elizabeth Bock in Copenhagen; and (iii) Christo Gordis in Marseille had initiated investigations aimed at elucidating this intriguing neurobiological puzzle. Using different experimental approaches and animal models, they identified NCAM,[7] known also as D2 protein[8] or BSP-2 (brain cell surface protein),[9] as a candidate mediator for the recognition processes within the CNS. These pioneering studies created the foundation for further extensive research into NCAM, its molecular structure, biochemistry and function both in the nervous system and non-neural tissues.

NCAM is the best known and most prevalent member of a group of Ca^{2+}-independent adhesion molecules and belongs to the immunoglobulin superfamily.[10] It is encoded by a single gene containing 19 exons which has been mapped to human chromosome 11. Several forms of mRNA, the number of which varies according to species, result from alternative splicing and are translated into 3 principal NCAMs with molecular masses of approximately 180 kDa (NCAM 180 or large domain), 140 kDa (NCAM 140 or small domain) and 120 kDa (NCAM 120 or small surface domain).[11,12] Different tissues can process NCAM molecules in specific ways. It has been discovered recently that muscle NCAM mRNA contains an additional exon situated between exons 12 and 13 (muscle specific domain/msd), not present in brain, and encodes a sequence of 37 amino acids which is unique to this tissue.[13–15] The observed diversity of NCAM isoforms (up to 20–30 forms)[16,17] is due not only to the alternative processing at the mRNA level but also to post-translational modifications, which include phosphorylation, sulphation and glycosylation.[18] Glycosylation has been particularly well studied since it has been postulated that large amounts of polysialic acid (PSA) can decisively affect NCAM function and markedly influence the adhesive binding properties of the molecule.[19,20] Other post-translational modifications affecting the external domain are manifested by the subsets of NCAM which contain a carbohydrate hapten, HNK-1, consisting of 3′-sulphated glucuronic acid.[21] The HNK-1 carbohydrate, first identified on human natural killer cells, has been detected also on other adhesion molecules such as L1 and it has been suggested that this carbohydrate may be a ligand in cell adhesion.[22]

Thus, although NCAM polypeptides have been broadly categorized into three main size classes, due to post-translational modifications, NCAM molecules of the same class are not identical and display a considerable degree of variation.

A physiological function of NCAM is to stabilize intercellular contacts. Very early appearance of NCAM has been reported in all three germ layers of embryonic tissues.[23] During embryogenesis, a period characterized by the intense activity of cell sorting and organizing into complex tissue structures, NCAM expression is maintained or suppressed permanently or temporarily according to the current requirements of the developing region of the embryo. In addition to up- and down-regulation of expression of various NCAM isoforms, post-translational processing and, in particular, glycosylation, seem to be designed especially to meet the requirements of embryonic development. The covalently attached PSA is present in the largest amounts (30 g/100 g protein) in NCAM from embryonic tissues and decreases to 30% of that value in most adult tissues. This negatively charged carbohydrate is believed not to be directly involved in binding but can influence binding indirectly so that embryonic forms of NCAM bind at slower rates than adult forms. It has been suggested that the PSA moiety regulates cell–cell apposition and creates a 'protective zone' around the cell at the time of its extensive differentiation.[3] Until recently, it had been agreed generally that all NCAM isoforms undergo the 'embryonic to adult' transition. Data from studies of explant cultures of mouse and chick tissues challenge this concept and suggest that this conversion is due to *de novo* synthesis of NCAM with lower sialic acid content.[24,25]

In skeletal and cardiac muscle, myogenesis is associated with sequential expression of specific isoforms of NCAM proteins and mRNA, as well as with dramatic changes in the distribution and level of expression of NCAM.[4,5,26,27] NCAM is present on the entire surface of embryonic myotubes but, as development proceeds, this expression gradually fades and the adult topographical distribution is restricted to the neuromuscular junctions.[1] Changes in the normal pattern of NCAM expression in the myofibres have been observed in a variety of muscular disorders. Re-expression of NCAM over the entire sarcolemma occurs after experimental denervation and in response to injury of muscle and/or nerve.[26,28] High levels of NCAM immunoreactivity have been seen on skeletal muscle in certain myopathies and in acute denervation syndromes, particularly those associated with regenerating fibres, and in paralysed muscle.[29–32]

There is no information available regarding the pattern of NCAM expression during morphogenesis of the human gastrointestinal tract or aberrations of this pattern induced by disruption of normal developmental processes.

NEUROMUSCULAR SYSTEM OF THE GUT

Normal development and subsequent function of the gut are dependent on coherent interactions between its neural and non-neural components. Intestinal motility is regulated by automatism of the smooth muscle and its modification under the influence of the autonomic innervation. The enteric nervous system is characterized by a remarkable diversity and abundance of neurons, the growth, plasticity and survival of which depend upon the complex interaction of many diverse factors involved in communication between cells.[33] It has been shown that target cells, such as smooth muscle, decisively influence the course of development of autonomic neurons both in vivo and in vitro and that, interestingly, smooth muscle from aganglionic bowel impairs neuronal development in culture.[34]

In contrast to skeletal muscle, neuromuscular interaction and transmission in smooth muscle are poorly understood. Elaborate neuromuscular junctions, similar to those in skeletal muscle, are not present in smooth muscle and the anatomical relation between nerve fibres and smooth muscle cells varies in different organs.[35–37] The essential feature of the model of the autonomic neuromuscular junction, as proposed by Burnstock,[36] is that transmitter is released *en passage* from axonal varicosities during conduction of an impulse. An electrical activation is spread within the muscle bundle through gap junctions connecting individual muscle cells. Frequently, a transmitted impulse is modulated pre- and postjunctionally by a variety of locally released agents.

Smooth muscle development and differentiation have been monitored closely during vertebrate embryogenesis, however, most investigators have centred on the *de novo* formation of blood vessels and comparatively little attention has been paid to the morphogenesis of visceral smooth muscle. Little is known also about the ontogeny of the musculature of the human bowel in general and about the molecules that regulate the differentiation and innervation of human smooth muscle cells, in particular.

NCAM DURING DEVELOPMENT OF THE GUT

Although it has been agreed that, in both man and animals, NCAM expression in skeletal and cardiac myofibres is developmentally regulated,[3–6] there is still controversy regarding expression of NCAM in smooth muscle cells. Previous immunocytochemical studies have revealed that, in rat and mouse, the smooth muscle of developing bowel transiently expresses NCAM.[38–40] No NCAM immunoreactivity could, however, be detected in the rudimentary gut of the chicken embryo.[23] Whether this apparent discrepancy is due to differences in species or antisera used is difficult to judge. However, if NCAM is indeed present in the developing smooth muscle cells and the level of its expression is modulated by the state of muscle differentiation and innervation, it is likely that it serves functions similar to those in skeletal and cardiac muscle. Support for this hypothesis is provided by the study of NCAM expression in neural and non-neural components of the human developing large bowel. The temporal and spatial patterns of NCAM immunoreactivity have been characterized using immunocytochemistry for major NCAM isoforms (pan-NCAM) and the 'embryonic' polysialylated form of NCAM (PSA-NCAM).[41]

NCAM IN ENTERIC NERVES

Within the developing neural complex of the gut wall, in both neuronal cell bodies and fibres, NCAM is expressed continuously from the early stages of embryonic life. Immunoreactivity for NCAM appears to develop in a similar and consistent pattern and follows the well documented transmural gradient of colonization of enteric nerves.[42,43] In contrast to the continuously expressed isoforms (pan-NCAM), PSA-NCAM is expressed in an age-dependent manner. During the course of differentiation, polysialylated forms of NCAM disappear from maturing nerves and, in the infant bowel, PSA-NCAM expression becomes significantly decreased in both nerve cell bodies and fibres. This observation is in agreement with the findings that, during the development of the central and peripheral nervous systems, except for a few areas where the level of PSA remains invariably high throughout life, NCAM generally shifts from a PSA-rich to a PSA-poor form.[17]

NCAM IN DIFFERENTIATING ENTERIC SMOOTH MUSCLE

The differentiation of intestinal musculature proceeds in a specific order. Muscularis propria, the first muscular layer to emerge from the thick mesenchyme, at 11 weeks, divides into circular and longitudinal layers and

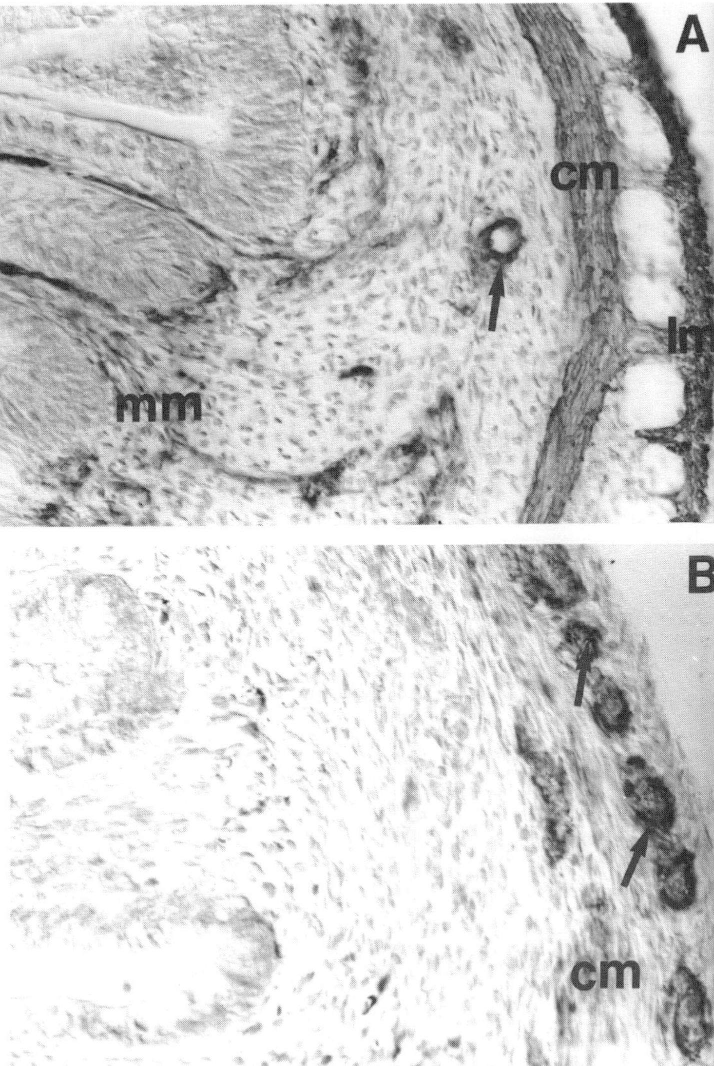

Fig. 1 Human large bowel at 15 weeks gestation (×300). (**A**) Immunostaining for α-SMA shows the differentiation of the muscularis propria into longitudinal (lm) and circular (cm) layers. Note weak α-SMA immunoreactivity in the area of the presumptive muscularis mucosae (mm). Immunoreactivity for α-SMA can also be seen in vascular smooth muscle (arrow). (**B**) NCAM in intestinal neuronal cell bodies and fibres (arrows), in myofibres of the circular muscle layer (cm) and in scattered nerves in the submucosa.

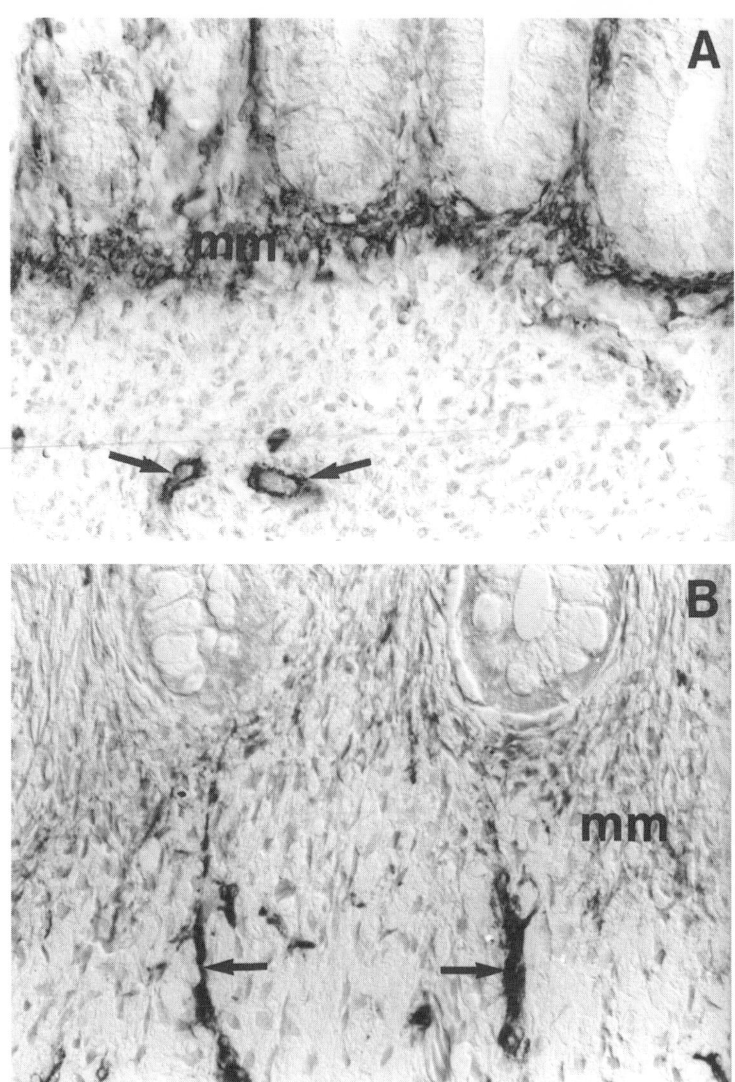

Fig. 2 Muscularis mucosae of the fetal large bowel at 20 weeks gestation (×400). (**A**) Immunoreactivity for α-SMA in muscle cells of the muscularis mucosae (mm). Note also α-SMA expression in vascular smooth muscle in the mucosa and submucosa (arrows). (**B**) Immunoreactivity for muscle-specific NCAM in the submucosal nerve fibres (arrows) and smooth muscle of the muscularis mucosae (mm).

this is followed by the differentiation of the muscularis mucosae, first delineating at 15 weeks gestation (Fig. 1A). The differentiation of smooth muscle cells and the particular stages of it are marked by the sequential appearance of a specific set of smooth muscle-associated proteins, indicating a gradual differentiation of the mesenchymal cells into a smooth muscle phenotype. In enteric muscle, this sequence of expression was monitored in the muscularis mucosae, the last intestinal muscular layer to develop.[44] As in cardiac and vascular smooth muscle, α-smooth muscle actin is the earliest indicator of the maturing muscle cells. Its appearance is followed by calponin, desmin, smooth muscle myosin and h-caldesmon. The onset of NCAM expression takes place almost simultaneously with that of calponin at 17 weeks gestation. Its presence on enteric myocytes seems to accompany the process of muscle differentiation (Fig. 2B) and when maturation is completed, it can no longer be demonstrated on muscle cells.[41] This consecutive expression of NCAM and smooth muscle-specific proteins might reflect the influence of NCAM on the modulation of the phenotype of intestinal muscle cells. It is likely that, as in skeletal muscle where innervation is a major determinant of the phenotype of myofibres,[45] the appearance of NCAM in enteric myocytes signifies the start of muscle innervation that subsequently would lead to the synthesis of a range of muscle-specific proteins. Thus, it is conceivable that, by controlling innervation, NCAM also secondarily influences phenotypic and, consequently, functional maturity of enteric muscle.

Unlike vascular smooth muscle, where α-smooth muscle actin and myosin are expressed almost simultaneously,[46,47] in intestinal smooth muscle, the appearance of the presumptive actin regulatory protein calponin precedes the expression of the specific myosin. This suggests that the vascular and intestinal smooth muscle cells arise from different lineages and do not share a common precursor.

A characteristic feature of NCAM expression in the muscularis propria of the colon from the gestational age of 15 weeks onwards is a tendency to concentrate at the submucosal border of the circular muscle. A similar distribution of NCAM has been observed in normal infant bowel from children between 5–18 months of age.[48] The significance of such a distinctive distribution of NCAM in human colonic muscle is not known at present. A separate origin for the innermost layer of the circular muscle has been postulated,[49] but this suggestion cannot explain the persistence of NCAM expression in this area beyond the perinatal period. The results of a number of studies of the interstitial cells of Cajal (ICC) demonstrated that the submucosal border of the circular muscle is occupied by a dense network of these cells, the origin and role of which remain unclear.[50,51] However, it is generally agreed that ICC mediate the neural modulation of intestinal pacemaker activity and are mesenchymal in nature. A lack of intestinal pacemaker (*c-kit*) has been reported more recently in aganglionic bowel of patients with Hirschsprung's disease.[52] It has been suggested that interactions between *c-kit* and its ligand stem cell factor (SCF) are of great significance in the development of a component of the pacemaker system that is required for the generation of autonomic gut motility.[53] Thus, there may be a relationship between the distribution of smooth muscle cells expressing NCAM, the structure of the submucosal network of ICC and expression of *c-kit*/SCF in human colon.

In conclusion, NCAM is expressed by nerves and muscle of differentiating human large bowel and gastrointestinal smooth muscle displays a differentiation programme which contrasts with that of smooth muscle cells of vascular origin. Although the morphoregulatory activity and the nature of the biochemical changes induced in cells by NCAM remain unclear, the spatio-temporal pattern of expression of NCAM displayed in the course of gut development, in relation to that of smooth muscle-specific proteins in the developing human gut, strongly advocates the participation of NCAM in the molecular mechanisms underlying the morphogenesis of the human enteric musculature.

NCAM IN DISEASED LARGE BOWEL

If the role of NCAM in nerve–muscle interaction within the gastrointestinal tract is indeed similar to that played in striated muscle, alterations of the pattern of its expression in enteric muscle should be anticipated in abnormally innervated bowel. In other words, a neurogenic disorder of the bowel such as that in Hirschsprung's disease, could precipitate abnormal expression of NCAM in intestinal muscle cells.

Since the first histopathological description of aganglionic bowel[54,55] until recent years, the absence of ganglion cells and the presence of hypertrophied

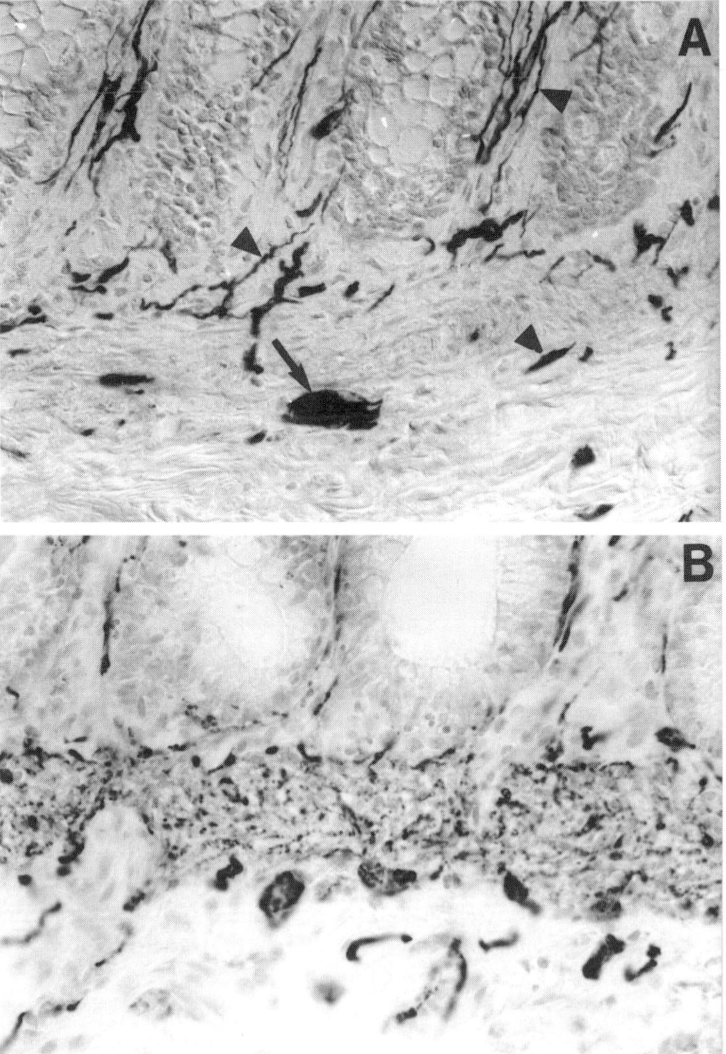

Fig. 3 NCAM in infant large bowel (×300). (**A**) Normal bowel from 5 month-old girl. NCAM expression is confined only to neural structures and can be seen in nerve fibres (arrowheads) and ganglion cell of the submucous plexus (arrow). (**B**) Distal aganglionic bowel from 6 month-old boy. NCAM is abnormally highly expressed in the muscle of the muscularis mucosae. Note the punctate distribution of NCAM immunoreactivity on muscle cells.

nerve trunks were considered to be the only abnormalities associated with Hirschsprung's disease. However, with the advent of immunocytochemical techniques, it has become possible to demonstrate that the diseased bowel displays also a variety of other anomalies, including the abnormal distribution of neuropeptides[56–62] and extracellular matrix proteins.[63–66] The disturbances of colonic motor activity in congenital aganglionosis are thought to result from an inefficient neural input in the distal segment of the large bowel, but the pathogenesis of this malformation of the enteric nervous system still remains speculative. It has been suggested that cell–cell communication within the human gastrointestinal tract during development and in adult life might be necessary for survival of the neurons.[34] Little is known about the nature of the neuromuscular disorder in Hirschsprung's disease. Immunohistochemical study of NCAM expression in surgical specimens from children operated on for Hirschsprung's disease showed that, in specimens of distal aganglionic bowel, abnormalities of enteric innervation were accompanied consistently by increased NCAM immunoreactivity in the muscle and particularly that of the muscularis mucosae (Fig. 3A,B).[48]

Interpretation of the reasons for increased NCAM in the muscle of aganglionic bowel is difficult, largely because the pathogenesis of Hirschsprung's disease, as well as the pathophysiology of intestinal smooth muscle deprived of normal neural control, still remain obscure. Plausible explanations that can be offered are based on the results of extensive investigations carried out during the past decade on NCAM expression in skeletal and cardiac muscle[26,28–32] and the assumption that the molecular basis of interaction between nerve and muscle cells is similar to that in striated muscle. Indeed, if NCAM in enteric smooth muscle participated in a mechanism of nerve-muscle adhesion, similarly to that in skeletal and cardiac muscle, mature smooth muscle would be expected to respond to disruption of its physiological, neurally-controlled equilibrium by increasing NCAM synthesis.

The reasons why abnormal NCAM expression in congenital aganglionosis is localized mainly to the muscularis mucosae are not clear either. Most studies on intestinal musculature are devoted to the external muscle and our knowledge of the ontogeny and physiology of the muscularis mucosae is very limited. Results of a study of NCAM expression in human fetal bowel demonstrated that the muscularis mucosae differentiated relatively late during development.[41] NCAM expression on muscle cells of the muscularis mucosae can be first revealed as late as 17 weeks gestation. It appears to be developmentally regulated and, after reaching its peak level, presumably in the second half of gestation or perinatally, it becomes gradually switched off from the muscle cells. If the primary events leading to aganglionosis occur after 17 weeks gestation, but before completion of differentiation and innervation of the muscularis mucosae, a prolonged expression of NCAM on muscle cells of this layer could be anticipated. On the other hand, if the increased NCAM immunoreactivity in the muscularis mucosae of the aganglionic bowel results from an arrest or disruption of the process of normal differentiation and innervation of this muscle layer, immature smooth muscle cells should preserve their fetal characteristics, including expression of PSA-NCAM. In the specimens of the aganglionic bowel studied, increased expression of pan-NCAM was noticed but not of PSA-NCAM (unpublished observation). It has been shown in diseased human skeletal muscle that expression of PSA-NCAM can be observed only in activated or regenerating myofibres,[32] but whether such an extrapolation from skeletal to smooth muscle can be justified is not known at present.

High NCAM expression in smooth muscle may, however, indicate that the muscle cells are still in a proliferative state, as has been shown in experimental animals.[38] In patients with a normal submucous plexus but with depletion of neural elements from the myenteric plexus of the entire large and small bowel, extended myectomy of the circular and longitudinal muscles induces hypertrophy of the muscularis mucosae.[67] In Hirschsprung's disease, it is possible that attempts to compensate for the motility problems in the affected bowel result in some hypertrophy of the muscularis mucosae, but that deficiencies in both plexuses render these efforts incomplete and ineffective.

The cause of Hirschsprung's disease is unclear. Although, according to the traditional concept, aganglionosis is caused by a failure of the neuroblasts to complete their migration, experiments using animal models of congenital aganglionosis indicated that nerve cells may reach the correct position but then fail to develop or survive.[68–70] This has led to the hypothesis of incompatibility with the extracellular microenvironment.[34] Considerable work has been devoted to analysis of the extracellular matrix in the bowel in rodents and humans and alterations in the microenvironment of fetal gut hampering proper development of its neuromuscular system have been implicated in the pathogenesis of the disease.[71] It can be assumed, therefore, that the impaired peristaltic activity in the affected bowel may result from incomplete differentiation of both nerves and muscle and increased NCAM expression reflects the degree of this immaturity.

There are several hereditary animal models of Hirschsprung's disease in the mouse, rat and the horse. Studies of the terminal portion of the bowel of the congenitally aganglionic *ls/ls* mouse demonstrated a striking overgrowth of the muscularis mucosae, particularly in the outer longitudinal layer, due primarily to hypertrophy of smooth muscle cells.[72] Further examination using electron microscopy revealed abnormalities of the ultrastructure of individual *ls/ls* smooth muscle cells of the muscularis mucosae such as an extensive thickening of the basal lamina, an atypical configuration with long, thin, extensions of cytoplasm and a greater than normal degree of development of organelles associated with synthesis of proteins.[72] The fact that anomalies of the enteric muscle of the aganglionic bowel in Hirschsprung's disease are localized mainly to the muscularis mucosae[48] is in agreement with observations in the *ls/ls* mouse. Whether these pathological changes of smooth muscle of the muscularis mucosae of the aganglionic bowel are a primary or secondary defect is not possible to determine. If primary, they might reflect an inherited abnormality of mesenchymal cells in this region of the gut. If secondary, the observed defects in the smooth muscle of the muscularis mucosae leading to its hypertrophy may be induced by abnormal innervation of aganglionic muscle and inefficient motility in this zone of the bowel.

Studies of NCAM expression in skeletal muscle showed that accumulation of NCAM on myofibres might be mediated by disorders of innervation as well as by inactivity of muscle.[73] Since functional disability of the enteric muscle manifesting in severe, intractable constipation is a major symptom in Hirschsprung's disease, it is conceivable that a clinical state of non-obstructive constipation *per se* can induce muscular NCAM expression. In order to explore this possibility, NCAM expression was studied in chronically constipated, but fully innervated, human adult large bowel.[74] Localization of immunoreactivity for NCAM in the gut from non-Hirschsprung's chronic constipation, revealed that the pattern of its distribution is entirely comparable to that seen in normal controls, giving strength to the initial postulate that increased expression of NCAM on intestinal muscle in congenital aganglionosis is induced by abnormalities of the intestinal innervation.

In conclusion, the observation that NCAM immunoreactivity is increased in the muscle of congenitally aganglionic bowel fits with the concept that this glycoprotein might be involved in the intercellular interactions of innervation and formation of efficient junctions between enteric nerves and myocytes. The postulate that NCAM occurrence in the muscle of the gut is regulated by neural impulses of an appropriate pattern is further supported by the observation that NCAM expression is unchanged in the muscle of bowel from constipated patients with no neurogenic disorders.

NCAM DURING IN VITRO ENTERIC MYOGENESIS

The previous paragraphs described the pattern of NCAM expression in the human normal and diseased large bowel. The physiological significance of these findings, however, remains unclear since our knowledge of the factors that regulate the differentiation and function of the neuromuscular system of the human gastrointestinal tract and of NCAM, in particular, is still very limited. Although the presence of NCAM in developing enteric smooth muscle has been demonstrated ex vivo in mouse,[39,40] rat[38] and man,[41] its function in the differentiation of the human enteric musculature has never been investigated. Evaluation of the involvement of NCAM in this process, therefore, called for an in vitro experimental system of enteric tissue, where myogenesis could be observed under the simplified conditions of culture. This is the very first report of such in vitro investigations.

Tissue culture was first invented at the beginning of the century as a means to investigate biological systems under conditions which were difficult to achieve in vivo.[75,76] The capacity to maintain living animal cells in vitro, outside the organism, opened a new area of research into inter- and intracellular relationships and the mechanisms that control cell behaviour. The adequacy of the in vitro system as a model of physiological function in vivo, however, has been questioned frequently. The cultured cells are free from the systemic variations which may arise during normal homeostasis or under the stress of an experimental situation, and their cellular metabolism is more stable than in vivo. It can be argued, though, that the lack of interactions characteristic of the intact tissue of origin and of compensatory mechanisms in the homeostatic milieu, prevent an in vitro system from being truly representative of the tissue from which the cultured cells were derived. Many specialized functions are expressed, however, in culture and, since its physicochemical environment can be controlled very precisely, as long as the limitations of the in vitro model are recognized and appreciated, it can provide a valuable investigative tool in various aspects of cell physiology.

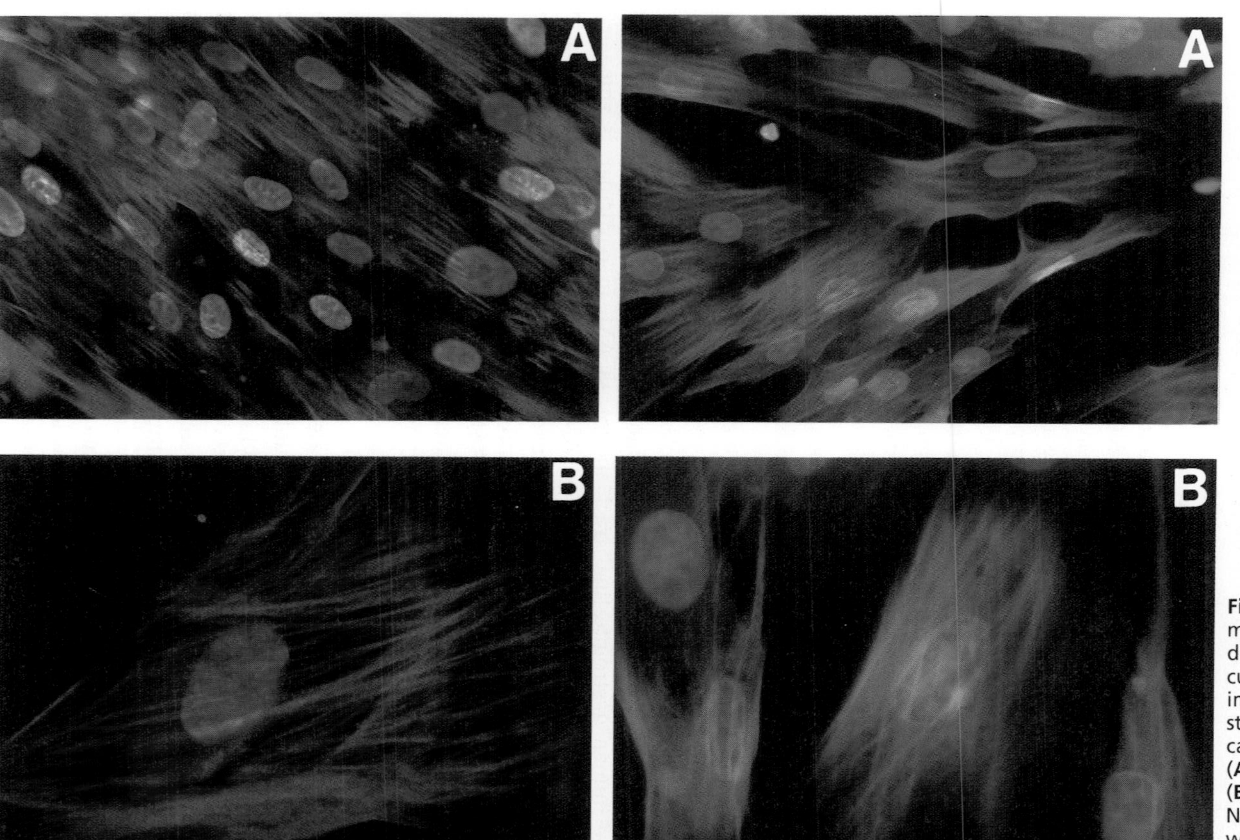

Fig. 4 Enteric muscle cells of differentiating culture immunostained for (α-SMA (red): (**A**) ×250; (**B**) ×1000. Nuclei stained with DAPI.

Fig. 5 Enteric muscle cells of differentiating culture immunostained for calponin (red): (**A**) ×250; (**B**) ×750. Nuclei stained with DAPI.

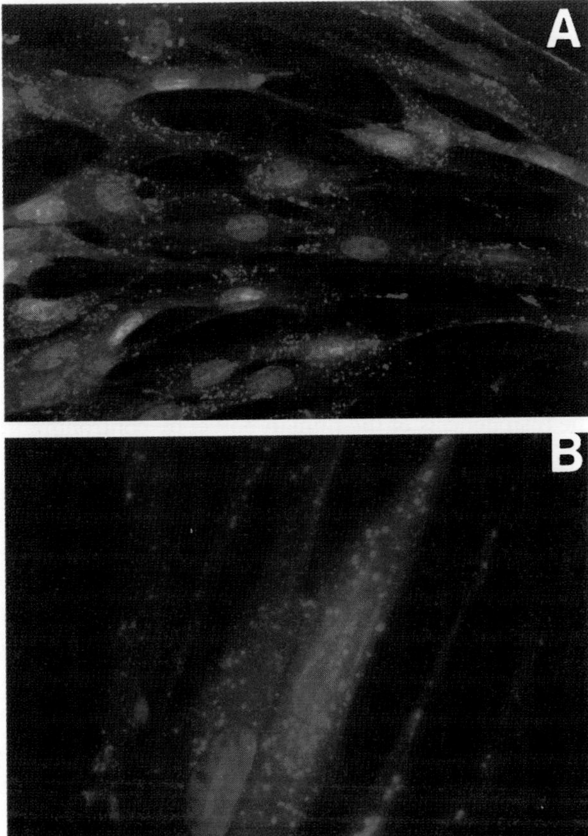

Fig. 6 Enteric muscle cells of differentiating culture immunostained for NCAM (red): (**A**) ×250; (**B**) ×1000. Note the punctate distribution of NCAM immunoreactivity in muscle cells. Nuclei stained with DAPI.

The differentiation of cells in terms of their expression of phenotypic properties characteristic of the functional mature cell in vivo, as well as maintenance of the specialized functions of the cell, are controlled by the in vitro environment.[77–79] The differentiation and behaviour of cultured cells are greatly influenced also by interactions with the substrate and with the neighbouring cells and, as occurs in vivo,[49] heterologous cell–cell interactions are believed to have a strong impact on the initiation and promotion of cell differentiation. A number of molecules that control cell–surface and cell–cell interactions as well as the whole life-time programme of cellular events, such as division, differentiation, movement, adhesion and death, has been identified during the last decade. These morphoregulatory molecules form a large family, of which NCAM is a well-recognized member, and are of critical importance during morphogenesis, providing the necessary link between differential gene expression and cellular driving forces.[80]

NCAM involvement in the in vitro differentiation of enteric myocytes was assessed in a primary culture system originated from human fetal gut. Studies of NCAM expression in relation to the phenotypic differentiation of cultured enteric muscle cells showed that the sequence of appearance of NCAM and muscle-specific proteins is similar during differentiation of smooth muscle cells both in vitro and in vivo (Figs 4–6). The onset of NCAM expression, as has been shown during in vivo differentiation,[41,44] coincided with that of calponin (unpublished observation) and this is in agreement with the finding that intensity of immunoreactivity for NCAM increases in well differentiated cultures of skeletal muscle.[27] As in muscle cells of human normal and aganglionic bowel,[48] NCAM was not continuously distributed on the cell surface but was present as discrete spots, which were particularly apparent at high power magnification. Although the significance of this punctate NCAM distribution is not clear, a similar pattern of immunoreactivity for NCAM was demonstrated by Akeson and co-workers in cultures of smooth muscle cell lines.[38]

On the basis of the morphological demonstration of NCAM expression in developing intestinal musculature, it has been suggested that NCAM might be involved in the histogenesis of the human bowel by controlling innervation.[41] It is essential, however, to remember that enteric myogenesis in vivo might not be identical to that taking place in vitro. Isolated intestinal smooth muscle cells are deprived of physiological neuronal input because not only have the external nerves been removed, but also the intrinsic ganglia, though still present in the primary culture, have lost most of the connections which normally exist within and between the intramural plexuses. Neuromuscular transmission has been shown to influence the development of skeletal myotubes.[81] However, since, not all smooth muscle cells are directly innervated by axons, unlike skeletal muscle, it is likely that signals other than neuronal ones trigger the cells to undergo differentiation. In skeletal muscle, NCAM has been implicated in a number functions, such as fusion, synaptogenesis and histogenesis[27] and it is possible that, in smooth muscle as well, apart from being involved in neuromuscular adhesion, it participates also in other developmental processes. The mechanisms that regulate the progression from myoblasts to terminally differentiated smooth muscle cells are mainly unknown. In skeletal muscle, synthesis of muscle-specific proteins is coordinately regulated during development.[82] It is tempting to speculate that smooth muscle differentiation is also controlled and determined by the activation of a 'master' gene, analogous to the skeletal muscle gene *MyoD*.[83] It can be assumed that NCAM may mediate not only cell-surface recognition and adhesion but also could be involved in the programme of gene activation that accompanies terminal myoblast differentiation. In our study, culture processing which led to differentiation of muscle cells, had a destructive effect on relatively labile intrinsic nerves. However, whether observed NCAM expression in cultured smooth muscle cells is due to the absence of nerves and indicates their susceptibility to innervation, or reflects NCAM participation in a nerve-independent programme of muscle differentiation, cannot be deduced from the morphological data presented.

NCAM involvement in neuromuscular interaction has been verified by the observation that NCAM-mediated adhesion is essential for the in vitro establishment of physical associations between autonomic nerves and skeletal myofibres.[84,85] The effect of neuromuscular interaction on myotube development in relation to regulation of expression of NCAM isoforms on muscle cells has been evaluated in perturbation experiments. It has been demonstrated that blocking of neuromuscular transmission during primary and secondary myogenesis in chick skeletal muscle results in striking changes in myotube organization due, most probably, to increased adhesiveness among muscle cells.[81] Since no switch in the expression of NCAM isoforms and up-regulation of (PSA), which normally occurs during myogenesis, could be detected in activity blocked muscle, it has been suggested that the expression of specific NCAM isoforms is dependent on functional innervation, lack of which leads to a developmental anomaly of muscle cells.[86]

It is possible that, in smooth muscle of the gut, NCAM plays a similar role in nerve–muscle communication. It has been demonstrated that target cells, such as smooth muscle, have a major impact on the developmental course of sympathetic neurons in vivo[87] and in vitro[88] suggesting that they guide, influence and then respond to their own innervation. In culture, nerve fibres appear to be able to distinguish between fibroblasts and smooth muscle cells within a short period after the initial contact. In experiments using explants of autonomic ganglia co-cultured with isolated smooth muscle cells, it was observed that associations between nerve fibres and fibroblast-like cells were transient, usually lasting no more than 1–2 h, whereas contacts between nerves and smooth muscle cells were maintained for extended periods of time.[89] The mechanism of recognition and preferential adhesion of nerves to smooth muscle cells is not known but it is likely that NCAM forms the molecular basis of these phenomena. Further functional investigations involving perturbation experiments in co-cultures of enteric myocytes and of autonomic nerves, are required to clarify this aspect of NCAM activity in the differentiating neuromuscular system of the human gut.

As was suggested earlier, a plausible explanation for increased NCAM expression in the aganglionic bowel is based on the assumption that NCAM might fulfil a function in the interplay between enteric nerve and myocyte similar to that played in striated muscle. To make this conjecture tenable, fully differentiated enteric smooth muscle cells, like striated myofibres, would have to be equipped with molecular mechanisms enabling re-synthesis of NCAM in response to denervation or other forms of physiological stress. Application of in vitro techniques allowed the exploration of this possibility and demonstrated that mature enteric myocytes, which when examined ex vivo did not express NCAM, do indeed exhibit the property of NCAM re-expression (unpublished observation). The question as to whether high immunoreactivity for NCAM in aganglionic bowel reflects prolonged expression or re-expression of the molecule remains open, however, as does that of what kind of 'accident' during morphogenic differentiation is responsible for this developmental abnormality. Although, on the basis of the morphological data presented in this chapter, it is not possible to deduce whether abnormal expression of NCAM is a primary or secondary feature of aganglionosis, the presented evidence provides support for the theory of the multifactorial origin of the disease. It seems that it is a common clinical misconception to consider Hirschsprung's disease as a single and uniform entity. Variations in the pattern of distribution of neural proteins and peptides, in particular, in surgical specimens from children operated on for Hirschsprung's disease[62] emphasize the heterogeneity of the condition. The demonstration that around 20% of colonic resections for Hirschsprung's disease fail to elicit a cure despite successful surgery,[90] argues for reconsideration of the criteria for the histological diagnosis of Hirschsprung's disease. Further investigation and long-term follow-up of patients with Hirschsprung's disease are required in order to assess the usefulness of immunocytochemistry for NCAM as a potential new diagnostic tool likely to improve the accuracy of diagnosis and success rate of therapeutic management.

SUMMARY

The evidence presented in this chapter supports the initial hypothesis and demonstrates that neural cell adhesion molecule (NCAM) is one of the factors participating in the differentiation of the neuromuscular system of the human gut. However, it should be realised that gastrointestinal development and function is a complex and highly integrated process involving a multistep series of inductive interactions and NCAM is but one of a diverse range of adhesion molecules with the potential to mediate morphogenic adhesion events. Investigations, both in vivo and in vitro, into the role of other cell adhesion molecules as well as receptor and non-receptor proteins (e.g. NGF, FGF), may enhance our knowledge of molecular mechanisms underlying the normal function of human gastrointestinal system as well as the pathophysiology of its neuromuscular disorders.

ACKNOWLEDGEMENTS

The authors wish to thank their colleagues Dr G. Moscoso, Miss V.M. Wright, Mr D.P. Drake and Mr E. Kiely for kindly supplying tissue samples and Dr G. Rougon for her generous donation of antibody to PSA-NCAM. This work was funded in part by The Sir Jules Thorn Charitable Trust.

REFERENCES

1. Rieger F, Grumet M, Edelman GM. N-CAM at the vertebrate neuromuscular junction. J Cell Biol 1985; 101: 285–293
2. Covault J, Sanes JR. Distribution of N-CAM in synaptic and extrasynaptic portions of developing and adult skeletal muscle. J Cell Biol 1986; 102: 716–730
3. Figarella-Branger D, Pellissier JF, Bianco N et al. Expression of various NCAM isoforms in human embryonic muscles: correlation with myosin heavy chain phenotypes. J Neuropathol Exp Neurol 1992; 51: 12–23
4. Moore SE, Walsh FS. Specific regulation of N-CAM/D2-CAM cell adhesion molecule during skeletal muscle development. EMBO J 1985; 4: 623–630
5. Gordon L, Wharton J, Moore SE et al. Myocardial localization and isoforms of neural cell adhesion molecule (N-CAM) in the developing and transplanted human heart. J Clin Invest 1990; 86: 1293–1330
6. Wharton J, Gordon L, Walsh FS et al. Neural cell adhesion molecule (N-CAM) expression during cardiac development in the rat. Brain Res 1990; 483: 170–176
7. Edelman GM. Cell adhesion molecules. Science 1983; 219: 450–457
8. Jørgensen OS, Bock E. Brain specific synaptosomal membrane proteins demonstrated by crossed immunoelectrophoresis. J Neurochem 1974; 23: 879–880
9. Hirn M, Pierres M, Deagostini-Bazin H et al. Monoclonal antibody against cell surface glycoprotein of neurons. Brain Res 1981; 214: 433–439
10. Cunningham BA. Cell adhesion molecules and the regulation of development. Am J Obstet Gynecol 1991; 164: 939–948
11. Rutishauser U, Goridis C. NCAM: the molecule and its genetics. Trends Genet 1986; 2: 72–76

12. Cunningham BA, Hemperley JJ, Murray BA et a]. Neural cell adhesion molecule: structure immunoglobulin-like domains, cell surface modulation, and alternative RNA splicing. Science 1987; 236: 799–806
13. Dickson G, Gower HJ, Barton CH et al. Human muscle neural cell adhesion molecule (N-CAM): identification of a muscle-specific sequence in the extracellular domain. Cell 1987; 50: 1119–1130
14. Thompson J, Dickson G, Moore SE et al. Alternative splicing of the neural cell adhesion molecule gene generates variant extracellular domain structure in skeletal muscle and brain. Genes Dev 1989; 3: 348–357
15. Walsh FS. The N-CAM gene is a complex transcriptional unit. Neurochem Int 1988; 12: 263–267
16. Santoni M-J, Barthels D, Vopper G et al. Differential exons usage involving an unusual splicing mechanism generated at least eight types of NCAM cDNA in mouse brain. EMBO J 1989; 8: 385–392
17. Doherty P, Fazelli MS, Walsh FS. The neural cell adhesion molecule and synaptic plasticity. J Neurobiol 1995; 26: 437–446
18. Lyles JM, Linnemann D, Bock E. Biosynthesis of the D2-cell adhesion molecule: post-translational modifications, intracellular transport, and developmental changes. J Cell Biol 1984; 99: 2082–2091
19. Sadoul R, Hirn M, Deagostini-Brazil H et al. Adult and embryonic mouse neural cell adhesion molecules have different binding properties. Nature 1983; 304: 349–351
20. Rutishauser U, Acheson A, Hall AK et al. The neural cells' adhesion molecule (NCAM) as a regulator of cell-cell interactions. Science 1988; 240: 53–57
21. Kruse J, Maihammer R, Wernecke H et al. Neural cell adhesion molecules and myelin-associated glycoprotein share a common carbohydrate moiety recognized by monoclonal antibodies L2 and HNK-1. Nature 1984; 311: 153–155
22. Kunemund V, Jungalwala FB, Fischer G et al . The L2/HNK-1 carbohydrate of neural cell adhesion molecules is involved in cell interactions. J Cell Biol 1988; 106; 213–223
23. Thiery JP, Duband JL, Rutishauer U et al. Cell adhesion molecules in early chicken embryogenesis. Proc Natl Acad Sci USA 1982; 79: 6737–6741
24. Friedlander DR, Brackenbury R, Edelman GM. Conversion of embryonic form to adult forms of NCAM in vitro: results from *de novo* synthesis of adult forms. J Cell Biol 1985; 101: 412–419
25. Nakayama J, Fukuda MN, Fredette B et al. Expression cloning of a human polysialyl-transferase that forms the polysialylated neural cell adhesion molecule present in embryonic brain. Proc Natl Acad Sci USA 1995; 92: 7031–7035
26. Covault J, Merlie JP, Goridis C et al. Molecular forms of N-CAM and its mRNA in developing and denervated skeletal muscle. J Cell Biol 1986; 102: 731–739
27. Moore SE, Thompson J, Kirkness V et al. Skeletal muscle neural cell adhesion molecule (N-CAM): changes in protein and mRNA species during myogenesis of muscle cell lines. J Cell Biol 1987; 105: 1377–1386
28. Danlloff JK, Levi G, Grumet M et al. Altered expression of neural cell adhesion molecules induced by nerve injury and repair. J Cell Biol 1986; 103: 929–945
29. Cashman NR, Covault J, Wollman RL et al. Neural cell adhesion molecule in normal, denervated, and myopathic human muscle. Ann Neurol 1987; 21: 481–489
30. Walsh FS, Moore S, Lake B. Cell adhesion molecule N-CAM is expressed by denervated myofibres in Werding-Hoffman and Kugelberg-Welander type of spinal muscular atrophies. J Neurol Neurosurg Psychiatry 1987; 50: 539–542
31. Walsh FS, Moore S, Dickson J. Expression of membrane antigens in myotonic dystrophy. J Neurol Neurosurg Psychiatry 1988; 51: 136–138
32. Figarella-Branger D, Nedelec J, Pellissier JF et al. Expression of various isoforms of neural cell adhesion molecules and their highly polysialylated counterparts in diseased human muscles. J Neurol Sci 1990; 98: 21–36
33. Saffrey MJ, Burnstock G. Growth factors and the development and plasticity of the enteric nervous system. J Auton Nerv Sys 1994; 49: 183–196
34. Langer JC, Betti P-A, Blennerhasserr MG. Smooth muscle from aganglionic bowel in Hirschsprung's disease impairs neuronal development in vitro. Cell Tissue Res 1994; 276: 181–186
35. Pick J. Fine structure of nerve terminals in human gut. Anat Rec 1967; 159: 131–146

36. Burnstock G. Autonomic neuromuscular junctions: current developments and future directions. J Anat 1986; 146: 1–30
37. Gabella G. The structural relations between nerve fibres and muscle cells in the urinary bladder of the rat. J Neurocytol 1995; 24: 159–187
38. Akeson RA, Wujek JR, Roe S et al. Smooth muscle cells transiently express NCAM. Mol Brain Res 1988; 4: 107–120
39. Thor G, Probstmeier R, Schachner M. Characterization of the cell adhesion molecules L1, N-CAM and J1 in the mouse intestine. EMBO J 1987; 6: 2581–2586
40. Lyons GE, Moore R, Yahara O et al. Expression of NCAM isoforms during skeletal myogenesis in the mouse embryo. Dev Dyn 1992; 194: 94–100
41. Romanska HM, Bishop AE, Moscoso G et al. NCAM expression in nerves and muscle of developing human large bowel. J Pediatr Gastroenterol Nutr 1996; 22: 351–358
42. Okamoto E, Ueda T. Embryogenesis of intramural ganglia of the gut and its relation to Hirschsprung's disease. J Pediatr Surg 1967; 2: 437–443
43. Tam PKH, Lister J. Developmental profile of neuron-specific enolase in human gut and its implications in Hirschsprung's disease. Gastroenterology 1986; 90: 1901–1906
44. Romanska HM, Moscoso G, Polak JM et al. Smooth muscle differentiation during human intestinal development. Basic Appl. Mycol 1996; 6: 13–19
45. Harris AJ, Fitzsimons RB, McEwan JC. Neural control of the sequence of expression of myosin chain isoforms in foetal mammalian muscles. Development 1989; 107: 751–769
46. Sawtell NM, Lessard JL. Cellular distribution of smooth muscle actins during mammalian embryogenesis: expression of the alpha-vascular but not gamma-enteric isoform in differentiating striated myocytes. J Cell Biol 1989; 109: 2929–2937
47. Zanellato AM, Borrione AC, Giuriato L et al. Myosin isoforms and cell heterogeneity in vascular smooth muscle. 1. Developing and adult bovine aorta. Dev Biol 1990; 141: 431–446
48. Romanska HM, Bishop AE, Brereton RJ et al. Increased expression of muscular NCAM in congenital aganglionosis. Gastroenterology 1993; 105: 1104–1109
49. Kedinger M, Simon-Assmann P, Bouziges F et al. Smooth muscle actin expression during rat gut development and induction in fetal skin fibroblastic cells associated with intestinal embryonic epithelium. Differentiation 1990; 43: 87–97
50. Faussone-Pellegrini MS, Cortesini C, Pantalone D. Neuromuscular structures specific to the submucosal border of the human colonic circular muscle layer. Can J Physiol Pharmacol 1990; 68: 1437–1446
51. Christensen J. A commentary on the morphological identification of the interstitial cells of Cajal in the gut. J Autonom Nerv Sys 1992; 37: 75–88
52. Yamataka A, Kato Y, Tibboel D et al. A lack of intestinal pacemaker (*c-kit*) in aganglionic bowel of patients with Hirschsprung's disease. J Pediatr Surg 1995; 30: 441–444
53. Maeda H, Yamagata A, Nishikawa S et al. Requirement of *c-kit* for development of intestinal pacemaker system. Development 1992; 116: 369–375
54. Whitehouse F, Kernohan JW. Myenteric plexus in congenital megacolon. Arch Intern Med 1948; 82: 75–111
55. Zuelzer WW, Wilson JL. Functional intestinal obstruction of congenital neurogenic basis in infancy. Am J Dis Child 1948; 75: 40–64
56. Bishop AE, Polak JM, Lake BD et al. Abnormalities of the colonic regulatory peptides in Hirschsprung's disease. Histopathology 1981; 5: 679–688
57. Taguchi T, Tanaka K, Ikeda K et al. Peptidergic innervation irregularities in Hirschsprung's disease. Virchows Arch [A] Pathol Anat Histopathol 1983; 401: 223–235
58. Larsson LT, Malmfors G, Sundler F. Defects in peptidergic innervation in Hirschsprung's disease. Pediatr Surg Int 1988; 3: 147–155
59. Larsson LT, Malmfors G, Ekblad E et al. NPY hyperinnervation in Hirschsprung's disease: both adrenergic and nonadrenergic fibres contribute. J Pediatr Surg 1991; 26: 1207–1214
60. Tsuto T, Okamura H, Fukui K et al. Immunohistochemical investigations of gut hormones in the colon of patients with Hirschsprung's disease. J Pediatr Surg 1985; 20: 266–270
61. Hamada Y, Bishop AE, Federici G et al. Increased neuropeptide Y-immunoreactive innervation of aganglionic bowel in Hirschsprung's disease. Virchows Arch [A] Pathol Anat Histopathol 1987; 411: 369–377

62. Romanska HM, Bishop AE, Brereton RJ et al. Immunocytochemistry for neuronal markers shows deficiencies in conventional histology in treatment of Hirschsprung's disease. J Pediatr Surg 1993; 28: 1059–1062
63. Parikh DH, Tam PKH, Lloud DA et al. Quantitative and qualitative analysis of the extracellular matrix protein, laminin, in Hirschsprung's disease. J Pediatr Surg 1992; 27: 991–996
64. Parikh DH, Tam PKH, van Velzen D et al. Abnormalities in the distribution of laminin and collagen type IV in Hirschsprung's disease. Gastroenterology 1992; 102: 1236–1241
65. Parikh DH, Tam PKH, van Velzen D et al. The extracellular matrix components, tenascin and fibronectin, in Hirschsprung's disease: an immunohistochemical study. J Pediatr Surg 1994; 29: 1302–1306
66. Parikh DH, Leibl M, Tam PKH et al. Abnormal expression and distribution of nidogen in Hirschsprung's disease. J Pediatr Surg 1995; 30: 1687–1693
67. Mishalany H, Olson A, Khan F et al. Deficient neurogenic innervation of the myenteric plexus involving the entire small and large bowel. J Pediatr Surg 1989; 24: 83–87
68. Webster W. Embryogenesis of the enteric ganglia in normal mice and in mice that develop congenital aganglionic megacolon: requirement for a permissive environment. J Embryol Exp Morphol 1973; 30: 573–585
69. Jacobs-Cohen RJ, Payette RF, Gershon MD et al. Inability of neural crest cells to colonize the presumptive aganglionic bowel of ls/ls mice: requirement for a permissive local microenvironment. J Comp Neurol 1987; 225: 425–428
70. Payette RF, Tennyson VM, Pomeranz HD et al. Accumulation of components of basal laminae: association with failure of neural crest cells to colonize the presumptive aganglionic bowel of ls/ls mice. Dev Biol 1988; 125: 341–360
71. Fujimoto T, Hata J, Yokoyama S et al. A study of the extracellular matrix protein in the migration pathway of neural crest cells in the gut: analysis in human embryos with special reference to the pathogenesis of Hirschsprung's disease. J Pediatr Surg 1989; 24: 550–556
72. Tennyson VM, Pham TD, Rothman TP et al. Abnormalities of smooth muscle, basal laminae, and nerves in the aganglionic segments of the bowel of lethal spotted mutant mice. Anat Rec 1986; 215: 267–281
73. Covault J, Sanes JR. Neural cell adhesion molecule (N-CAM) accumulates in denervated and paralysed skeletal muscle. Proc Natl Acad Sci USA 1985; 82: 4544–4548
74. Romanska HM, Bishop AE, Lee JCW et al. Idiopathic constipation does not induce NCAM expression on intestinal smooth muscle. Dig Dis Sci 1996; 41: 1298–1302
75. Harrison RG. Observations on the living developing nerve fiber. Proc Soc Exp Biol Med 1907; 4: 140–143
76. Carrel A. On the permanent life of tissues outside the organism. J Exp Med 1912; 15: 516–528
77. Florini JR, Magri KA. Effects of growth factors on myogenic differentiation. Am J Physiol 1989; 256: C701–C711
78. Goldman BI, Wurzel J. Effects of subcultivation and culture medium on differentiation of human fetal cardiac myocytes. In Vitro Cell Dev 1992; 28A: 109–119
79. Freshney RI. [Ed]. Biology of the cultured cell. In: Culture of Animal Cells. A Manual of Basic Technique, 3rd edn. New York: Willey–Liss, 1994; 9–16.
80. Edelman GM. Morphoregulation. Dev Dyn 1992; 193: 2–10
81. Fredette B, Rutishauser U, Landmesser L. Regulation and activity-dependence of N-cadherin, NCAM isoforms, and polysialic acid on chick myotubes during development. J Cell Biol 1993; 123: 1867–1888
82. Caplan AI, Fiszman MY, Eppenberger HM. Molecular and cell isoforms during development. Science 1983; 221: 921–927
83. Davis RL, Weintraub H, Lassar AB. Expression of a single transfected cDNA converts fibroblasts to myoblasts. Cell 1987; 51: 987–1000
84. Rutishauser U, Grumet M, Edelman GM. NCAM mediates initial interactions between spinal cord neurons and muscle cells in culture. J Cell Biol 1983; 97: 145–152
85. Grumet M, Rutishauser U, Edelman GM. Neural cell adhesion molecule is on embryonic muscle cells and mediates adhesion to nerve cells in vitro. Nature 1982; 295: 693–695
86. Fredette BJ, Landmesser LT. A reevaluation of the role of innervation in primary and secondary myogenesis in developing chick muscle. Dev Biol 1991; 143: 19–35

87. Jonakait GM, Black IB. Neurotransmitter phenotypic plasticity in the mammalian embryo. Curr Top Dev Biol 1986; 20: 165–175
88. Burton H, Bunge RP. The expression of cholinergic and adrenergic properties of autonomic neurons in tissue culture. In: Nelson PG, Lieberman M (Eds) Excitable Cells in Tissue Culture. New York: Plenum, 1981; 1–37
89. Burnstock G. Development of smooth muscle and its innervation. In: Bulbring E, Bracing AF, Jones AW, Tomita T. (Eds) Smooth Muscle: An Assessment of Current Knowledge. London: Arnold, 1981; 431–457
90. Tariq GM, Brereton RJ, Wright VM. Complications of endorectal pull-through for Hirschsprung's disease. J Pediatr Surg 1991; 26: 1202–1206

3

Human prion diseases

Piero Parchi   Pierluigi Gambetti   Pedro Piccardo   Bernardino Ghetti

Prion diseases, also called transmissible spongiform encephalopathies, are fatal neurodegenerative disorders that affect a wide variety of mammals. They have several characteristics that make them unique among neurodegenerative disorders. First, they all share a novel pathogenetic mechanism that may revolutionize established concepts of infectivity. Second, they are the only diseases that include sporadic, genetic, and transmitted forms. Third, in contrast to other major neurodegenerative diseases such as Alzheimer disease, amyotrophic lateral sclerosis and Huntington chorea, prion diseases display a large array of histopathological patterns.

In humans, prion diseases include Creutzfeldt-Jakob disease (CJD), Gerstmann-Sträussler-Scheinker syndrome (GSS), kuru, fatal familial insomnia (FFI) and prion protein cerebral amyloid angiopathy (PrP-CAA). CJD was originally described in 1920–21 by Creutzfeldt and Jakob as a rapidly progressive sporadic disease whereas GSS was reported in 1928 and 1936 as a slow, progressive, familial syndrome.[1–4] These two diseases were considered unrelated until the description of kuru by Gajdusek and Zigas in 1957.[5] Kuru afflicted the Fore Tribe of New Guinea and was strongly suspected to be acquired by ingestion during cannibalistic rituals.[5] William Hadlow, a veterinary pathologist, noted the similarity between the histopathologies of kuru and scrapie, a disease of sheep known to be transmissible since 1936, and recommended experiments to test the transmissibility of kuru.[6] The advise was promptly taken by Gajdusek, Gibbs and their collaborators who experimentally

Pierluigi Gambetti MD, Division of Neuropathology, Institute of Pathology, Case Western Reserve University, 2085 Adelbert Road, Cleveland, Ohio 44106, USA

Bernardino Ghetti MD, Department of Pathology, Med Sci A-142, Indiana University Medical Center, 635 Barnhill Drive, Indianapolis, Indiana 46202-5120, USA

Pedro Piccardo MD, Department of Pathology, Med Sci A-142, Indiana University Medical Center, 635 Barnhill Drive, Indianapolis, Indiana 46202-5120, USA

Piero Parchi MD, Division of Neuropathology, Institute of Pathology, Case Western Reserve University, 2085 Adelbert Road, Cleveland, Ohio 44106, USA

transmitted kuru, CJD and one subtype of GSS to primates.[7–9] In 1974, the iatrogenic form of CJD was established with the report of cases who acquired the disease by an infectious mechanism during a surgical manipulation.[10] In 1981, macromolecular structures named scrapie-associated fibrils (SAF) were identified by electron microscopy in scrapie-infected brain tissue, providing the first molecular link to the disease.[11]

The contemporary era of prion diseases was ushered in by the work of Prusiner and his colleagues who, in 1982, made the discovery that a single protease-resistant protein with a molecular weight of 27–30 kDa was consistently associated with purified fractions of brain extracts enriched for scrapie infectivity.[12] Prusiner tentatively identified the abnormal protein with the infectious agent and named it prion.[13] Unexpectedly, it was later found that the prion was an abnormal, protease-resistant isoform of a protein that is normally expressed in the brain.[14,15]

This review focuses on the histopathology of human prion diseases. However, to understand these diseases it is necessary to briefly review the biology and the pathology of the prion protein, and its role in the pathogenesis and transmission of prion diseases.

THE NORMAL PRION PROTEIN

The normal prion protein (PrP^C) is a membrane glycoprotein that is encoded in humans by a gene (*PRNP*) located in the short arm of chromosome 20.[16] After

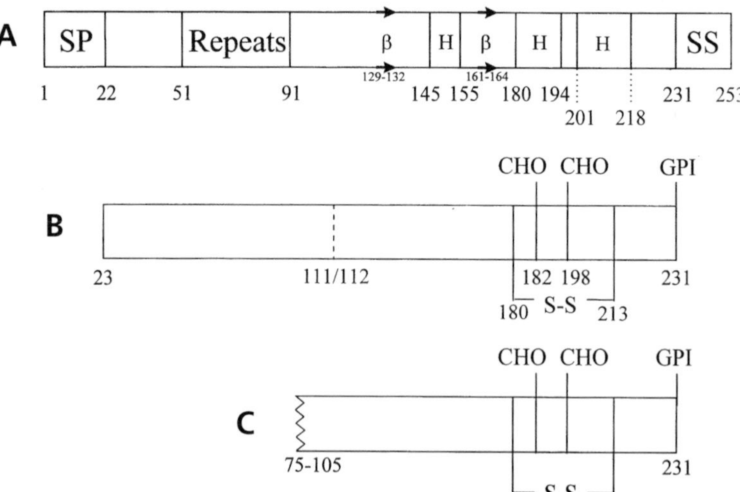

Fig. 1 Human prion protein. (**A**) Translational product. SP, signal peptide; repeats, octopeptide repeats; H, α helix domains (adapted from Riek et al[167]); β, β sheet domains (adapted from Riek et al[167]); SS, hydrophobic signal sequence for the anchor. (**B**) Post-translational product including the 23–231 full length form and the 111/112–231 truncated form; 111/112 indicates the site of cleavage of the full length form following re-internalization to the endosomal compartment. This form is then reinserted at the plasma membrane. CHO, glycosylation sites; S–S, disulfide bonds; GPI, glycosylphosphotidyl inositol anchor. (**C**) Protease resistant form (PrP^{res}) which has a ragged N-terminal edge presumably between the 75–105 residues following treatment with exogenous proteases.

being synthesized in the endoplasmic reticulum (ER), PrP^C undergoes a series of co-translational and post-translational modifications that include the attachment of a glycosylphosphotidyl inositol (GPI) anchor[17] and the non-obligatory addition of one or two N-linked oligosaccharide chains (Fig. 1).[18,19] The oligosaccharide chains are then modified in the ER and Golgi to become either high-mannose complex or hybrid glycans.[18,19] The differential glycosylation leads to the formation of three PrP^C glycoforms with distinct electrophoretic mobility: (i) the fully glycosylated form that is thought to contain two glycan chains, one complex and one hybrid; (ii) an intermediate form with only one complex chain; and (iii) a unglycosylated form.[18,20,21] Ultimately, most of the PrP^C is anchored to the cell surface by the GPI anchor. Cycling of PrP^C between the plasma membrane and the endosomal compartment has been demonstrated in culture cells.[22] During this process, PrP^C undergoes endoproteolytic cleavage and N-terminally truncated forms are generated. In human brain, a cleavage at amino acid residue 111 or 112 generates the major product of PrP^C proteolytic processing (Fig. 1).[20]

The physiological function of PrP^C in the CNS has not been established. Available evidence indicates that: (i) PrP^C is transported by fast axonal transport;[23] (ii) plays a role in GABA-receptor-mediated synaptic inhibition and long term potentiation;[24,25] and (iii) is involved in circadian rhythms and sleep regulation.[26]

CONVERSION OF PRP^C INTO PROTEASE-RESISTANT PRP (PRP^{res}): THE PATHOGENESIS OF PRION DISEASES

While there is unanimous consent that PrP is essential for the pathogenesis of prion diseases, the exact nature of the infectious agent causing these disorders is still the subject of great controversy. In addition to the virus theory that follows a more conventional way of thinking, the protein-only hypothesis or prion hypothesis has gained increasing consent in the last decade. The notion that a protein may act as the transmissible agent was originally proposed by Griffith[27] and Pattison and Jones[28] in 1967. Prusiner, Caughey and others provided most of the evidence that the central event in the pathogenesis of prion diseases is a change in conformation resulting in the conversion of PrP^C into a conformer (PrP^{res}) that has the same amino acid sequence and post-translational modifications of PrP^C but differs from PrP^C in the secondary structure, resistance to digestion with proteases, and pathogenicity (Fig. 1).[29–34]

According to the prion hypothesis,[35] the change in conformation of PrP^C into PrP^{res} would be: (i) induced by the exposure to exogenous PrP^{res} in the prion diseases transmitted by infection; (ii) an almost invariable consequence of the instability of PrP in the presence of a mutation in the familial or inherited form; and (iii) the result of a spontaneous, random event in the sporadic form.

Two major models have been proposed to account for the mechanism of PrP^{res}-induced PrP^C conversion.[35,36] According to one model,[35] (Fig. 2) a PrP^C and PrP^{res} molecules would combine to form a heterodimer which would be followed by the conversion of the PrP^C to the PrP^{res} form. Dissociation of the complex would release previously formed and newly formed PrP^{res} molecules, which would continue the conversion process in an autocatalytic chain-reaction.

The other model maintains that the conversion takes place following the interaction of PrP^C with an ordered aggregate of PrP^{res}, called 'nucleus' or 'seed' (Fig. 3).[36]

PrP^C–PrP^{res} dimerization and PrP^C conversion into PrP^{res} is thought to occur at the cell membrane and/or in the endosome shortly after internalization while storage of the newly formed PrP^{res} takes place in lysosomes.[37–40]

An increasing number of arguments are listed in favor of the prion hypothesis.

1. PrP^C knock out mice, genetically engineered not to express PrP^C, fail to develop a prion disease following inoculation with infected brain extracts.[41,42]
2. In experimental prion diseases, the transmissibility has been shown to be a function of the degree of amino acid sequence homology between the PrP^C of the donor and that of the recipient.[43] Moreover, evidence of the conversion of PrP^C into PrP^{res} primed by the presence of PrP^{res} has been obtained in a cell-free system.[44]
3. Brain extracts from subjects with inherited prion diseases in which the disease is linked to a *PRNP* mutation and is, therefore, unlikely to be the result of a virus infection, transmit the disease to recipient mice. Even more importantly, distinct sizes of the PrP^{res} fragment from the donor are reproduced in the recipient animals.[45] Since the generation of a PrP^{res} fragment of different size is thought to result from a PrP^{res} different conformation (see below), these findings imply that conformationally distinct donor's PrP^{res} acting as templates direct the single recipient's PrP^C to acquire their respective conformations, as predicted by the prion hypothesis.
4. Two proteins that share many of the characteristics of PrP^{res} have been identified in yeast.[46] According to their conformation, the yeast PrP induce alternative metabolic states that are transmissible by non-Mendelian

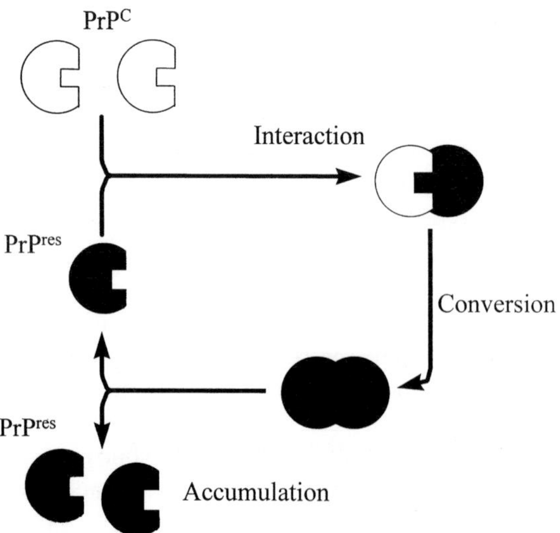

Fig. 2 PrP^C to PrP^{res} conversion according to the heterodimer formation model.

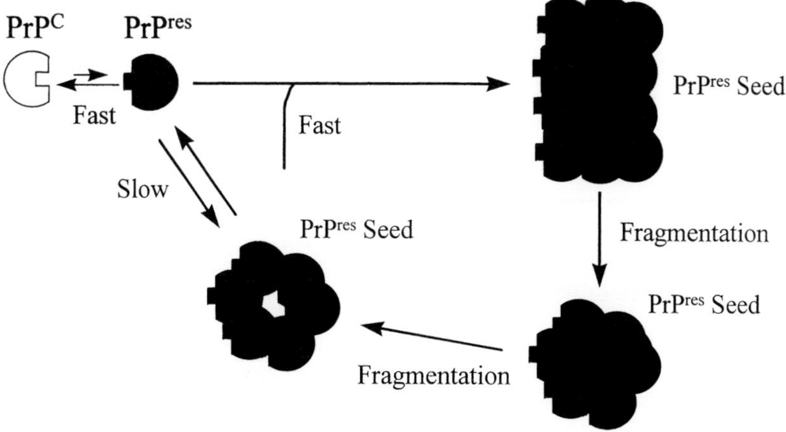

Fig. 3 PrP^C to PrP^{res} conversion according to the 'seed' or 'nucleus' model. The first spontaneous conversion between PrP^C and PrP^{res} is fast but the PrP^C conformation is thermodynamically favored. PrP^{res} accumulates only when it is captured by a pre-existing 'seed'. Fragmentation leads to multiformation of the PrP^{res} 'seeds' (adapted from Caughey and Chesebro[168]).

inheritance. Thus, the prion mechanism may not only be involved in the pathogenesis of prion diseases but may also provide a new mechanism of nucleic acid-independent inheritance.

5. Many attempts have failed to demonstrate significant amounts of nucleic acid associated with PrP^{res}

Combined, these lines of evidence strongly argue that: (i) PrP^C plays a central role in prion replication; and (ii) this process involves a PrP^C–PrP^{res} interaction. In addition, they support the hypothesis that PrP^{res} is the infectious agent and that the infectivity depends on conformation. However, objections are still raised.[47–50] Purified infectious brain fractions have been reported to contain small amounts of nucleic acid.[47] Occasionally, experimental prion diseases have been reported to occur and to be transmitted in the apparent absence of PrP^{res}.[48–50] Finally, all the findings supporting the prion hypothesis might also support the hypothesis that the infectious agent is an ubiquitous unconventional virus and that PrP^{res} acts as its receptor. Thus, the prion hypothesis awaits the proof that pure PrP^C can be converted in vitro into pure PrP^{res}, which in turn transmits the disease.

HUMAN PRION DISEASES

The cloning of the *PRNP* and the detection of the PrP^{res} in the brain of affected subjects have provided two powerful molecular tests for the diagnosis and characterization of prion diseases. This, in turn, has led not only to a better understanding of the prion diseases already known, but also to the identification of new variants, widening the spectrum of these disorders. The

Table 1 Classification of human prion diseases according to form and phenotype

Form	Phenotype
Inherited	Creutzfeldt-Jakob disease (fCJD) Fatal familial insomnia (FFI) Gerstmann-Sträussler-Scheinker (GSS) Mixed or undefined
Sporadic	CJD (sCJD) Sporadic form of FFI?
Acquired by an infectious mechanism	Iatrogenic CJD (iCJD) Kuru New variant of CJD (vCJD)?

three forms of human prion diseases, sporadic, inherited and acquired by infection, express three distinct, major phenotypes: CJD, FFI and GSS. A minority of cases of the inherited form, generally associated with insertional mutations, cannot be accommodated in any of these phenotypes and form an heterogeneous group. The classification of the human prion diseases, according to form and phenotype, is given in Table 1. The disease phenotype is determined by clinical, pathological and molecular features. Relevant clinical features are the duration of symptoms, the time of presentation of certain clinical signs, such as cognitive impairment or ataxia, and the presence or absence of pseudoperiodic sharp waves (PSW) on the electroencephalogram (EEG). The pathological phenotypes of prion diseases are defined by the individual relative amount and topography of five basic lesions: (i) spongiform degeneration; (ii) astrogliosis; (iii) loss of neurons; (iv) deposits of PrP^{res}; and (v) neurofibrillary tangles. The PrP deposits show distinct patterns and can be: (i) associated with structural lesions that are visible also following routine stains, like the punched out or kuru plaques, the multicentric plaques of GSS and the 'florid' plaques of the new variant CJD; or (ii) detectable only following immunostaining but not with routine histological stains.

SPORADIC CREUTZFELDT-JAKOB DISEASE

The history of CJD has been reported in detail.[51,52] Originally named spastic pseudosclerosis by Jakob, it subsequently received the current eponym from Spielmeyer. Only two of the five cases originally reported by Creutzfeldt and Jakob that have been re-examined appear to fulfil the current criteria for the diagnosis of this disease.[52] In 1924, the first case of familial CJD was reported.[51] It was later assessed that the inherited form accounts for approximately 15% of all cases of CJD.[53] With the observation of new cases, the phenotypic heterogeneity of the sporadic form became evident. The first variant was described by Heidenhain in 1929 and is characterized by a short disease duration and cortical blindness associated with a pathology that is more prominent in the occipital cortex.[51,52] Over the years, several other variants have been introduced which include the myoclonic, the cerebellar or ataxic, the thalamic and the

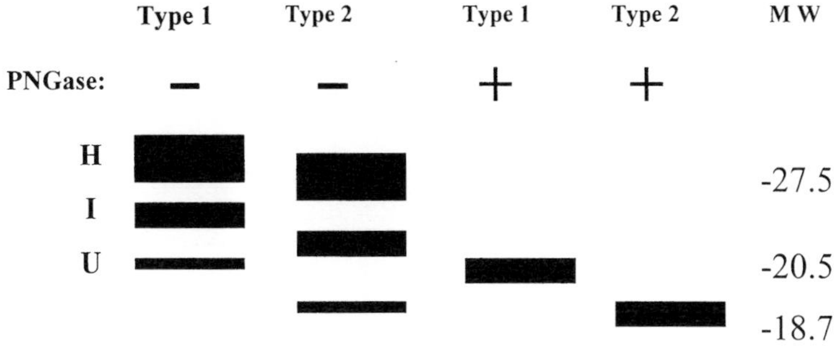

Fig. 4 Diagrammatic representation of PrP^{res} type 1 and type 2 patterns on Western blot. The three bands in the preparations not treated with protein glucosidase N (PNGase) represent the highly or fully glycosylated form (H), the intermediate glycosylated form (I) and the unglycosylated form (U). Following PNGase treatment, both PrP^{res} glycosylated forms co-migrate with the U form.

panencephalopathic.[52] Moreover, cases have been reported with an atypically long disease duration which made the diagnosis difficult.

Cloning of the gene coding for PrP and the characterization of the disease-related PrP allowed for the definitive separation of the sporadic from the inherited form. This also generated a complete re-examination of the clinical and pathological spectrum of sporadic CJD on the basis of molecular, rather than clinical and pathological features.[54]

MOLECULAR CLASSIFICATION OF SPORADIC CJD: PATHOLOGY

Four distinct groups or variants have been identified on the basis of the genotype at the *PRNP* codon 129 and of the characteristics of the PrP^{res} (Table 2, Fig. 4).[54]

Group 1

Group 1 includes subjects who are homozygous for methionine at codon 129 and have a PrP^{res} of type 1, i.e. PrP^{res} which has an electrophoretic mobility of approximately 20 kDa for the unglycosylated form and a distinctive ratio of the three glycoforms (Fig. 4). Group 1, which is by far the most common, is associated with the typical sporadic CJD phenotype but it also comprises the Heidenhain variant. Clinically, the subjects belonging to this group are characterized by a rapidly progressive myoclonic dementia of short duration (less than 1 year), often associated with visual cortical signs or ataxia. PSW are recorded at the EEG examination in about 90% of cases. The histopathology is characterized by a variable degree of spongiosis, gliosis and loss of neurons mainly affecting the cerebral cortex, neostriatum, thalamus and cerebellum. In the cerebral cortex, the vacuolization affects all layers and is often more prominent in the occipital lobe (Fig. 5A). The hippocampus, hypothalamus and brain stem are relatively spared. Immunohistochemistry demonstrates the fine punctate or 'synaptic' pattern of PrP staining[55] which colocalize with the distribution of spongiform degeneration (Fig. 5B). In a subgroup of patients, however, the 'coarse' or perivacuolar staining pattern is also seen (see below).

Table 2 Molecular and phenotypic features of the four sporadic Creutzfeldt-Jakob disease groups

	Codon 129	PrP^{res} Type	Symptom duration (months)	Symptoms at onset	EEG PSW	Neuropathology	PrP^{res} distribution	Immunostaining pattern
Group 1 (*n* = 14)	M/M	1	4 (1.5–7.0)	Dementia 12/14 Visual 3/14 Ataxia 3/14	13/14	Spongiosis[a] gliosis and neuronal loss of variable severity (according to duration) in all layers of the cerebral cortex, striatum, thalamus and cerebellum. Occipital cortex always affected	Highest amount in the cerebral cortex, striatum, thalamus and cerebellum	Punctate or coarse (more rarely and focally)
Group 2 (*n* = 2)	M/M	2	12, 36	Dementia	0/2	Spongiosis, gliosis and neuronal loss in all layers of the cerebral cortex, in the striatum and thalamus	Highest amount in the cerebral cortex, striatum and thalamus	Coarse
Group 3 (*n* = 4)	M/V	2	11 (5–18)	Ataxia/ dementia	0/4	Widespread spongiosis and gliosis in limbic lobe, striatum, diencephalus, brainstem and cerebellum with relative sparing of the neocortex in short duration (< 6–8 months) cases. Kuru[b] plaques in the cerebellum. Relative sparing of the occipital cortex	High amounts in all brain regions with the exception of the neocortex in short duration cases (< 6 months)	Plaque-like, coarse and punctate.[c] Laminar distribution in the deep layers of neocortex in short duration cases. Strong perineuronal staining
Group 4 (*n* = 5)	V/V	2	7 (4–20)	Ataxia	1/5 (after 10 months)	As in the M/V group but with more severe spongiosis, gliosis and granular cells loss in the cerebellum and no kuru plaques	As in M/V group but with highest amounts in the cerebellum	As in M/V group[c], but with no coarse pattern and less numerous plaque-like deposits

[a]The typical spongiosis, also called spongiform degeneration, is distinguished from the nonspecific status spongiosus by the type and cortical topography of the vacuoles which are fine and have variable topography, whereas the status spongiosus is coarse with large vacuoles and limited to layers 2 and 3. However, status spongiosus extended to the whole cortical thickness may be seen in Creutzfeldt-Jakob disease (especially Group 2)

[b]Kuru plaques refer to non-neuritic, punched-out plaques that are visible with hematoxylin-eosin stain and are Congo red positive

[c]PrP deposits are also present which react with PrP antibodies but are Congo red negative

Group 2

Group 2 includes subjects who also are homozygous for methionine at codon 129 but have PrP^{res} type 2, which is characterized by a PK-resistant unglycosylated fragment of approximately 19 kDa and a glycoform ratio slightly different from that of PrP^{res} type 1 (Fig. 4). Subjects of this group show a slower progression than those of group 1, having a duration of symptoms that varies between 1 and 4 years. Clinically, they present with cognitive impairment, while sustained myoclonus visual signs and the typical EEG with PSW are uncommon. In addition, cerebellar signs are usually mild or absent, even late in the course of the disease. Due to these clinical features, patients of this group sometimes receive the diagnosis of Alzheimer disease or of other non acute dementing illnesses.

The histopathological lesions have a similar distribution to that of the group 1, with the exception of the cerebellum which lacks significant spongiosis despite the long duration. Moreover, the spongiform degeneration is replaced by larger and coarser vacuoles similar to those associated with the so-called status spongiosus (Fig. 5C). The immunohistochemistry is characterized by a coarse pattern of immunoreactivity, also called perivacuolar, because of its prevalent localization at the rim of the large vacuoles (Fig. 5D). PrP^{res} accumulates in relatively large amounts in the cerebral cortex and basal ganglia, and to a lesser extent in the thalamus. In contrast, the protein is detected only in relatively low concentration in more caudal structures such as brain stem and cerebellum.

Groups 3 and 4

Groups 3 and 4 include subjects who are either heterozygous methionine/valine (group 3) or homozygous for valine at codon 129, and demonstrate PrP^{res} type 2 (Fig. 4). They have considerable similarities between them, but are quite different from groups 1 and 2. They include CJD cases that vary in duration between 4 and 20 months. Clinically, group 3 patients show cognitive impairment and ataxia from the onset, while ataxia is always the main presenting sign in group 4. Most patients in both groups lack PSW on the EEG. Pathologically, the cases of these groups show a moderate to severe spongiosis and gliosis with variable neuronal loss in the limbic cortex, striatum, thalamus, hypothalamus and brain stem. At variance with the cases of groups 1 and 2, the participation of the neocortex is a function of the disease duration and shows only mild spongiosis in cases of less than 8 month duration. Moreover, the spongiosis is often laminar and involves the deep cortical layers and the occipital cortex is less affected than the fronto-temporal cortex. The features that distinguish group 3 from 4 are the presence of kuru plaques in the molecular layer of the cerebellum and the paucity of other cerebellar lesions (Fig. 5E). These usually include only mild spongiosis and astrogliosis, while in group 4 the cerebellar lesions are much more severe. Following immunostaining both groups are characterized by the presence of plaque-like PrP positive deposits most of which are not visible with routine stainings and do not contain PrP amyloid, since they are Congo red negative and non-birefringent with the polarized light (Fig. 5F). The number of the PrP amyloid plaques, however, appears to increase with the duration of the disease. Another distinctive immunostaining feature, not seen in the other groups, is the strong reaction around some neuronal perikarya, while the

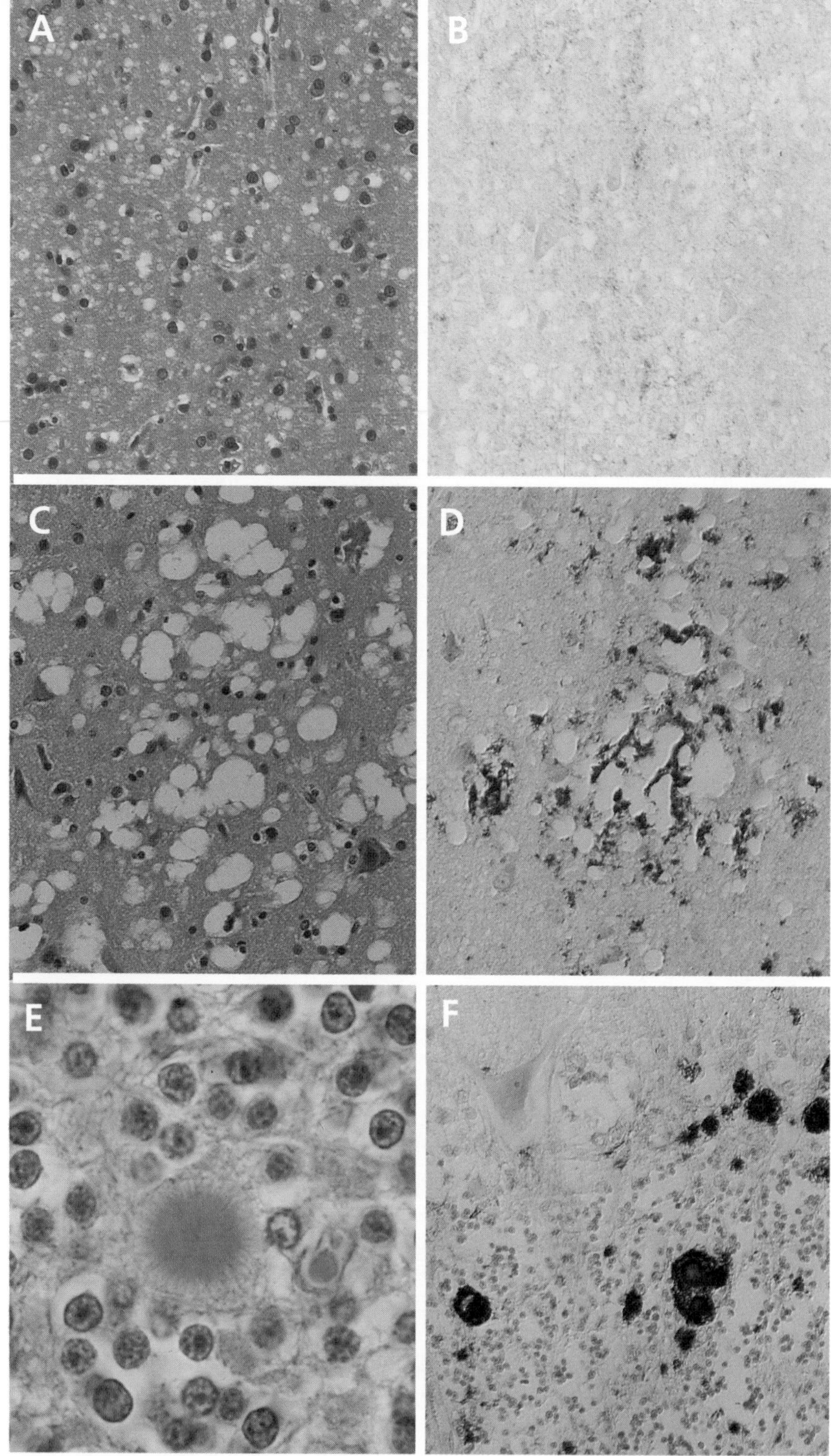

Fig. 5 (see page opposite for details)

Fig. 5 **A.** Classic spongiform degeneration in the cerebral cortex of a patient with typical sporadic CJD of group 1 (129M/M, PrP^{res} type 1). There are numerous vacuoles of relatively small size interspersed in the neuropil. H & E, × 375. **B.** Punctate or 'synaptic' PrP immunoreactivity in the cerebral cortex of a patient with typical sporadic CJD of group 1 (129M/M, PrP^{res} type 1). Immunolabeling with monoclonal antibody 3F4, × 375. **C.** Spongiform degeneration consisting of relatively large vacuoles, sometime with a 'grape-like' shape, in the cerebral cortex of a patient with sporadic CJD of group 2 (129 M/M, PrP^{res} type 2). H & E, × 375. **D.** Perivacuolar or coarse PrP immunoreactivity in the cerebral cortex of a patient with sporadic CJD of group 2 (129 M/M, PrP^{res} type 2). Immunolabeling with monoclonal antibody 3F4, × 375. **E.** A kuru plaque in the cerebellar granule cell layer of a patient with kuru. PAS staining, × 1428. **F.** Plaque-like PrP immunoreactivity in the cerebellum of a patient with sporadic CJD of group 3 (129/M/V, PrP^{res} type 2). Immunolabeling with monoclonal antibody 3F4, × 375

neuropil shows the punctate pattern. Moreover, cases with a less than 1 year duration are characterized by a laminar distribution of the immunostaining in the deep cortical layers corresponding to the spongiform degeneration. Overall, the distribution of the PrP^{res} is similar in groups 3 and 4 and, as observed in the distribution of the spongiform degeneration, is affected by the duration of the disease. In cases of less than a 5 month duration, PrP^{res} is present in relatively large and similar amounts throughout the brain except for the neocortex where it is barely detectable. This distribution is quite different from that of groups 1 and 2 in which the PrP^{res} is most abundant in the neocortex. In cases over 1 year duration, PrP^{res} also increases markedly in the neocortex so that it is present in comparable amounts virtually throughout the brain.

CURRENT VIEW ON THE ETIOLOGY OF SPORADIC CJD

The finding of two types of PrP^{res} associated with distinct clinico-pathological phenotypes in subjects with the same *PRNP* haplotype has provided strong evidence for the existence of prion strains in humans.[54] Distinct isolates or strains of the agent causing prion disease have been originally recognized in scrapie. When passaged in PrP syngenic mice, each strain shows highly preserved characteristics such as incubation times, neuropathological profile and distribution of PrP^{res}.[56,57] These observations imply the existence of an informational molecule which propagates the strain-specific properties. According to the prion hypothesis, the candidate molecule is the PrP^{res} itself and the agent strain differences are mediated by stable variations in its conformation. Although it is argued that the number of different PrP^{res} conformers required to account for the diversity of scrapie strains would be unreasonable, evidence for strain specific differences in PrP^{res} structure have, indeed, been recently described for scrapie,[58] transmissible mink encephalopathy,[59] and CJD.[45,54,60,61] The origin of prion strains in a naturally occurring disease such as sporadic CJD, however, remain difficult to explain. It has been proposed that sporadic CJD results from the random occurrence of an unfavorable event concerning *PRNP* and/or PrP^{C} such as a somatic mutation or an aberrant post-translational modification, which leads to the conversion of the aberrant PrP to PrP^{res}.[35] If this is the case, however, one would expect to observe a high phenotypic heterogeneity of the disease and no tendency to produce well-defined patterns with regard to type and distribution of lesions. In contrast, only two types of PrP^{res}, and a limited number of clinico-pathological phenotypes that are highly consistent among subjects are found, even following the examination of a large number of cases.[60] This indicates that the events leading to the formation of PrP^{res} in sporadic CJD are few, and stereotyped rather than stochastic.

Furthermore, the striking difference in the distribution of lesions and PrP^{res} accumulation in the early stages of the disease between sporadic CJD subjects of different variants (for example groups 1 and 4), even in subjects with the same *PRNP* haplotype, strongly suggest that distinct neuronal population are specifically targeted at onset. This implies a role for the putative informational molecule of the agent well before the occurrence of the first PrP^{C}–PrP^{res} conversion, the event that, according to the prion hypothesis, would make PrP^{res} the carrier of strain-specific information.

The epidemiology of sporadic CJD may also provide some clues with regard to the etiology of this disease. Increasing evidence indicates that codon 129 of *PRNP* modulates the susceptibility to the disease.[54,62–65] This notion is based on the findings that methionine and, possibly, valine homozygosity are, respectively, more prevalent among subjects with sporadic CJD than in the general population, and that methionine/valine heterozygosity is almost 3 times less prevalent.[62–65] Furthermore, the frequency distribution of age at onset in sporadic CJD is symmetrical around the mean of 60 years, and does not increase exponentially after a certain age.[66] Both these characteristics of sporadic CJD are difficult to explain by a stochastic event, and await clarification.

PRION DISEASES ACQUIRED BY INFECTIOUS MECHANISM

This important group of diseases includes kuru, the conditions acquired through medical or surgical treatments, called iatrogenic, and, possibly, the so-called new variant of CJD (vCJD), although the mode of acquisition of this variant has not yet been definitely established (Table 3). According to the prion hypothesis,[35] the prion diseases acquired by infection are caused by exogenous PrP^{res} that forms heterodimers with the endogenous PrP^{C} leading to the formation of endogenous PrP^{res}. The endogenous PrP^{res} would trigger an autocatalytic process resulting in the formation of sufficient PrP^{res} to cause the disease. The mechanism by which PrP^{res} reaches the brain when the port of entry of the exogenous PrP^{res} is in the GI tract, as in the case of kuru or, possibly, the vCJD, has not been determined. It is believed that the initial conversion occurs in the GI tract itself, where exogenous and endogenous PrP first meet. Then, in a step-wise or domino fashion, the PrP^{C}–PrP^{res} conversion continues through the lymphatic and/or the peripheral nervous system until it reaches the central nervous system. At this point, the high level of PrP^{C} expression and the stability of the neuronal cell population would facilitate the conversion and the accumulation of the abnormal protein.

KURU

First described[5] as an epidemic among the Fore people of New Guinea, kuru (which means shiver or shake) is believed to have been initiated and spread by

Table 3 Prion diseases acquired by an infectious mechanism.

Etiology	Codon 129 genotype	Clinical features	Pathology
IATROGENIC		**Central nervous system route of infection**	
Dura mater graft, corneal graft, stereotactic EEG electrodes	(*n* = 15) Met/Met 86% Met/Val 7% Val/Val 7%	Similar to sCJD of group 1 but with more frequent ataxia at onset and slower progression	Similar to sCJD of group 1, but (on average) with a more widespread and severe pathology
		Peripheral route of infection	
Growth hormone and gonadotrophin therapy	(*n* = 39) Met/Met 49% Met/Val 7% Val/Val 44%	Progressive cerebellar syndrome with late dementia and myoclonus. PSW on EEG usually absent	Like sCJD of groups 3 and 4. High frequency of kuru-like plaques, which are also present in M/M homozygotes
CONTAMINATED FOOD			
Kuru	(*n* = 39) Met/Met 30% (30%) Met/Val 50% (48%) Val/Val 20% (22%)	Ataxia, tremor, dysarthria with inconstant late dementia. PSW on EEG absent	Spongiosis, gliosis, neuronal loss and kuru plaques in cerebral cortex, basal ganglia, thalamus, and cerebellum. Plaques prominent in cerebellum
New variant?	(*n* = 11) Met/Met (100%)	Behavioral changes, dysesthesias followed by ataxia, myoclonus, and late dementia. No PSW on EEG	Spongiosis, gliosis, neuronal loss in cerebral cortex but more severe in basal ganglia and thalamus, less in cerebellum. Plaques 'kuru-like' but surrounded by spongiform vacuoles in cerebral cortex and cerebellar cortex, basal ganglia, thalamus and hypothalamus.

ritualistic endocannibalism when flesh from a CJD infected individual was consumed. Kuru has virtually disappeared following the end of this ritual. The original description of kuru pathology[67] was based on 12 cases of ages between 5 and 50 years and disease durations between 5 and 12 months. The histopathology and immunohistochemistry are similar to those of groups 3 and 4 of sporadic CJD. The 'punched out' or kuru plaques are present in about half of the cases, and occur more often in the granular cell layer of the cerebellum but are also in the cerebellar molecular layer, cerebral cortex and basal ganglia (Fig. 5E).[67] Other types of plaques such as diffuse and 'florid' are only occasionally present. The other consistent changes are neuronal loss, gliosis, and spongiosis, which, however, was only noted in subsequent examinations.[68,69] The lesions are present throughout the nervous system, but, as in sporadic CJD of group 3 and 4, they are often more severe in the basal ganglia, thalamus and brain stem. PrP immunostaining, recently performed in one case,[69] demonstrates a 'synaptic' pattern with strong perineuronal enhancement and a laminar distribution in the deep layers of the neocortex. In addition, it shows numerous immunoreactive PrP deposits and kuru plaques similar to group 3 and 4 of sporadic CJD. In agreement with these findings, PrP^{res} of type 2 has been observed in two examined cases.[60]

IATROGENIC CREUTZFELDT-JAKOB DISEASE

Since the first report of accidental human transmission of CJD following a corneal transplant in 1974,[10] at least 176 case of iatrogenic human transmission of CJD have been recorded.[70] Differences in incubation time, phenotypic expression of the disease, and genetic susceptibility have been observed among the affected individuals. The route of infection, which is either systemic or peripheral, as in hormone administration, or by direct contact with the central nervous system, as in transplants, is thought to play a major role in determining this variability. For example, methionine homozygosity at codon 129 increases over 2-fold the risk for the central type of iatrogenic CJD, while methionine/valine heterozygosity decreases the risk almost 7-fold. In contrast, valine homozygosity increases the risk of the peripheral type by over 3-fold, whereas methionine homozygosity increases it by only 0.2-fold.[70–72] Either PrP^{res} type 1 or 2 are associated with iatrogenic CJD.[60] Thus, the acquired forms of human prion diseases such as iatrogenic CJD and kuru reproduce the types of PrP^{res} seen in sporadic CJD, indicating that the PrP^{res} characteristics are reproduced after human-human transmission.[60] The PrP^{res} type appears to correlate better with the codon 129 rather than with the route of transmission, and PrP^{res} type 2 codistributes with the presence of the valine codon at position 129.[60]

The iatrogenic CJD acquired by the **central** route of infection has incubation times that vary between 16 and 28 months in subjects treated with neurosurgical procedures and intracerebral implanted electrodes, which directly expose the central nervous tissue to contamination. Incubation times are similar following corneal transplant, whereas they are much longer, 1.5–10 years, following dura mater implant.[73] In the cases associated with dura transplants, the most common clinical presentations appear to be a mixed cerebellar and cognitive syndrome, while an isolated cognitive impairment or cerebellar syndrome at the early stage is less common.[74–79] The typical EEG activity is present in the majority of the cases. The course is on average 14 months with a range of 3–27 months. The histopathology is characterized by the presence of spongiosis, gliosis and neuronal loss not only in the cerebral cortex and deep gray nuclei, but also in the cerebellum and brain stem. Kuru-like PrP plaques have been described in only one case.[79]

The iatrogenic CJD acquired by the **peripheral** route of infection has a mean incubation time that varies between 5 to 17 years, according to the country in which the infection occurred, having a mean of 17, 10 and 5 years in the USA, UK and France, respectively, with an overall range of 4–30 years. In 10 reported cases, the clinical presentation appears to be almost invariably a cerebellar syndrome while the typical EEG activity is lacking.[80-85] The mean duration is 15 months, with a range of 6–36 months. The histopathology is very similar to that of sporadic CJD of group 4, although the PrP amyloid plaques are more frequent in the iatrogenic form and are also present in subjects homozygous for methionine at codon 129.

NEW VARIANT OF CREUTZFELDT-JAKOB DISEASE

In 1996, Will et al reported 10 atypical cases of CJD in the UK recorded by the British National CJD Surveillance Unit.[86] These cases were remarkably homogeneous and differed from the typical CJD for both clinical and histopathological features. Shortly thereafter, a similar case was observed in France[87] and additional cases of the same variant were seen in the UK so that the current number of confirmed vCJD cases is 21. The clinical features that distinguish these cases from the typical sporadic CJD are the early age of onset, 16–48 years, the relatively long duration, 7.5–30 months, the presentation of behavioral changes requiring psychiatric consultation, dysesthesias and pain which are then followed by more common CJD signs such as ataxia, cognitive impairment and myoclonus. The typical EEG activity is lacking. The pathological hallmark of the vCJD is the presence of plaques encircled by a ring of spongiform vacuoles clearly visible with common histological stains (Fig. 6A). These plaques have a widespread distribution but are more prominent in the cerebral cortex, especially the occipital lobe, and the cerebellum.[88] These plaques, although seen in animal scrapie and named florid plaques, are only exceptionally seen in sporadic CJD, including CJD previously observed in young subjects. In addition, spongiform changes, astrogliosis and neuronal loss are present with a widespread distribution but more prominently in the basal ganglia and thalamus.[88] Immunostaining for PrP demonstrates, in addition to the florid plaques, the presence of a large number of nonamyloid PrP deposits throughout the cerebral and cerebellar cortices.[88]

Etiology of vCJD

The etiology of the vCJD is controversial. The evidence supporting the acquisition of this form from the bovine spongiform encephalopathy (BSE) is undeniable, but not definitive. The great majority of the cases of vCJD have

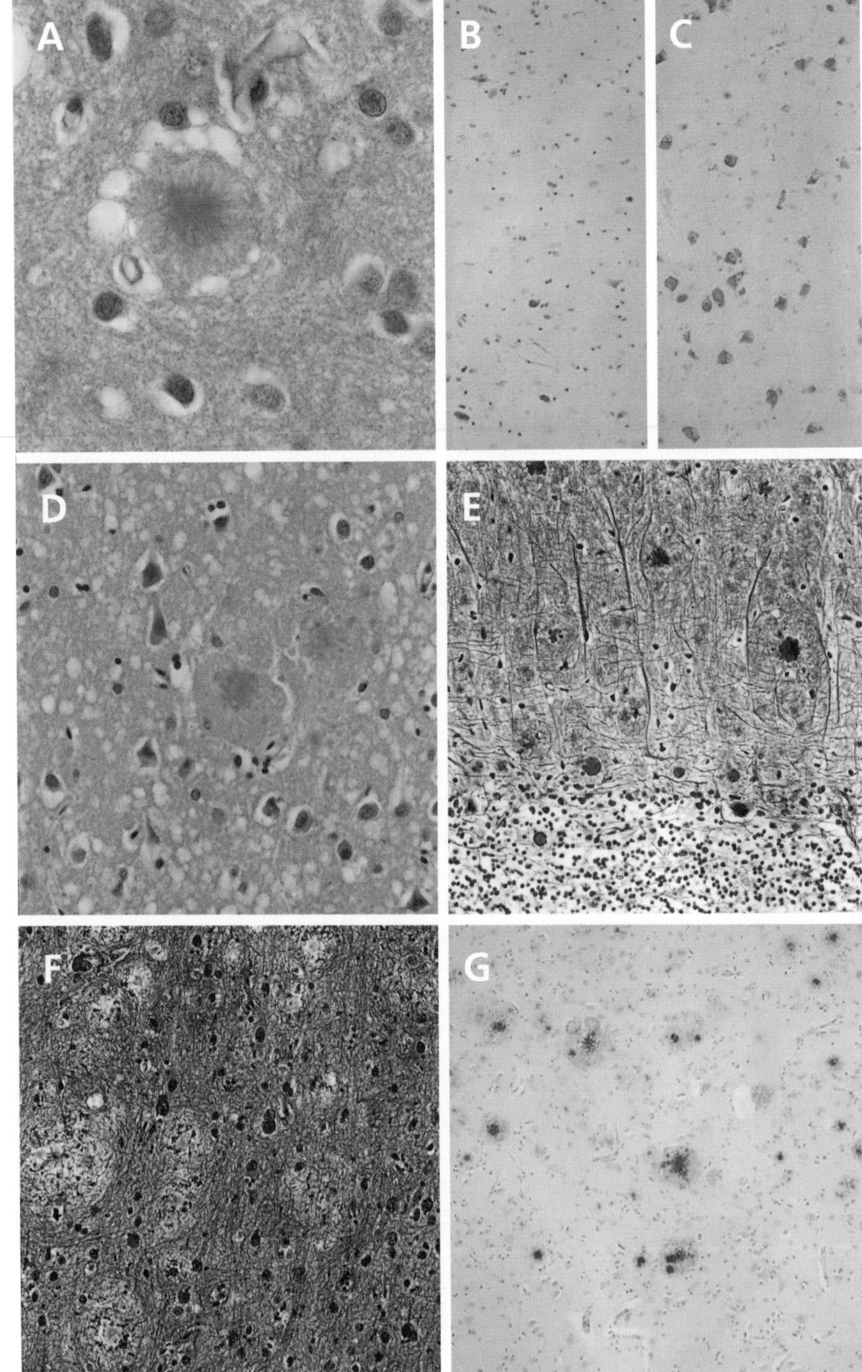

Fig. 6 **A**. A 'florid' plaque in the neocortex of a patient with vCJD. PAS staining, × 1492. **B**. Severe neuronal loss and gliosis in the antero-ventral thalamic nucleus of a patient with FFI. H&E staining, × 200. **C**. Antero-ventral thalamic nucleus of a control subject. H&E staining, × 200. **D**. A multicentric plaque in the cerebral cortex of a patient with GSS P102L–129M. H&E staining, × 608. (*continued on page opposite*)

Fig. 6 (continued) **E**. Cerebellar cortex of a patient with GSS F198S-129V. There are multiple plaques in the molecular and granule cell layers. Bodian staining, × 187. **F**. Cerebral cortex of a patient with GSS F198S-129V. There are multiple plaques with abundant neuritic component as well as numerous neurons undergoing neurofibrillary degeneration. Bodian stain, × 164. **G**. Cerebral cortex of a patient with GSS F198-129V. There are multiple multicentric PrP immunopositive plaques. Immunolabeling with a polyclonal antibody raised against synthetic peptide 90–102 (human PrP sequence), × 92

been observed in the UK where the human exposure to BSE is most likely to have occurred, since in the second half of 1980 there was an epidemic of this condition.[89] This would be consistent with an incubation time of 5–10 years, comparable to that of kuru and of the peripheral variant of iatrogenic CJD.[86] BSE can be transmitted to cynomologous macaque and the histopathology of the affected animals is similar to that described in humans but distinct from that of macaques inoculated with brain tissue from subjects with sporadic CJD.[90] There is a 94.4% homology between the human and cynomologous macaque and the macaque is homozygous for methionine at codon 129 as all subjects with vCJD reported to date.[86,87] Moreover, the PrP^{res} associated with the vCJD has a distinctive ratio of glycoforms, similar to that observed in wild-type mice inoculated with vCJD tissue and to that of the BSE PrP^{res} itself.[91] Finally, BSE PrP^{res} converts to PrP^{res} human PrP^{C} in a cell free system.[92] However, the efficiency of this conversion is not higher than that with which sheep scrapie PrP^{res} converts human PrP^{C}, although there is no evidence supporting the transmission of sheep scrapie to humans.[92] Therefore, the acquisition of vCJD from BSE, although likely, is still not proven.

INHERITED PRION DISEASES: GENERAL FEATURES

Modern techniques of molecular biology have brought about an explosion in the number and variety of the inherited prion diseases. At this time, there are 21 known *PRNP* mutations and three polymorphisms (Fig. 7 and Table 4). The mutations are of two types: (i) point mutations, which include 13 mutations distributed predominantly in the carboxyl two-thirds of the *PRNP* coding regions; and (ii) insertional mutations, made of 24 additional base pair (bp) repeats located between codon 51 and 91 (Fig. 7). The three polymorphisms include the methionine/valine at codon 129, the glutamic acid/lysine at codon 219 and the deletion of one 24 bp repeat. The polymorphism at codon 129 has a dual effect.

1. On the mutant allele, the polymorphic codons 129 and 219 affect basic aspects of the disease phenotype. Therefore, it is more appropriate to identify each *PRNP* genotype associated with inherited prion diseases not only by the mutation, but also by the codon 129 (or other polymorphic codons) present on the mutant allele, i.e. with the haplotype. Currently, 25 disease-associated *PRNP* haplotypes are known which result in CJD, FFI, GSS, mixed CJD and GSS, PrP-CAA and undefined phenotypes.

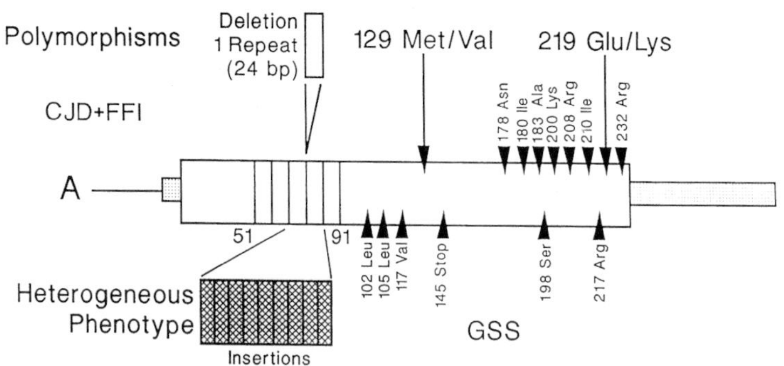

Fig. 7 Mutations and polymorphisms of the human prion protein gene. Polymorphisms are indicated with long arrows and open arrowhead. Mutations associated with the CJD or FFI phenotypes are displayed at the top. Mutations associated with the heterogeneous or GSS phenotypes are shown at the bottom. The insertion mutations include from 1 (24 base pairs) to 9 (216 base pairs) except for 3 (72 base pairs) insertion(s).

2. On the normal allele, the 129 polymorphism may influence some phenotypic features such as age at onset and duration of the disease. Genotypes and phenotypes of the *PRNP* pathogenic mutations known at this time are reported in Table 3.

INHERITED CJD

The histopathology of the inherited CJD is similar overall to that of the sporadic form. Therefore, only features that may help in differentiating the various haplotypes are reported (see also Table 4).

CJD E200K–129M and CJD D178N–129V

Clinically, the major phenotypic differences between these two haplotypes are the duration, the EEG, the occurrence of cerebellar and peripheral nerve signs, and seizures.[93–99] Although the duration may vary considerably, CJD E200K–129M has a shorter mean duration than the CJD D178N–129V. The typical EEG activity with PSW complexes, seizures, peripheral sensory and cranial nerve signs as well as presentation with cerebellar or visual signs are more common in the CJD E200K–129M.[93–99] Pathologically, the CJD E200K–129M subtype is very similar to the sporadic CJD group 1, while in the CJD D178N–129V phenotype the distribution of lesions is more similar to that of group 2. In the CJD E200K–129M the lesions mainly affect the cerebral cortex, striatum, thalamus and cerebellum. In the CJD D178N–129V, spongiosis, gliosis and neuronal loss are most marked in the cerebral cortex and striatum, and much less severe in the thalamus, while the cerebellum is generally uninvolved.[100] The histopathology of this subtype often shows intense cerebral cortical astrogliosis with large gemistocytic astrocytes and the loss of neurons resulting in the disorganization of the cerebral cortical layers.[100] The remaining neurons are occasionally ballooned and contain inclusions reminiscent of the cortical Lewy bodies. The immunostaining pattern is punctate and matches in severity the histopathology in both CJD haplotypes. In the CJD E200K–129M, immunostaining is consistently positive in the substantia gelatinosa of the spinal cord. No PrP-positive deposits, either in the form of amyloid or nonamyloid plaques, are present.

Other inherited CJD subtypes

Few cases are available with a detailed study of the phenotype. Overall, the clinical and pathological phenotype corresponds to that of groups 1 and 2 of the sporadic form. The CJD M232R–129M has been examined in three cases.[101,102] The age at onset and duration are variable. Clinically, cognitive impairment, myoclonus and mutism are common clinical signs along with typical EEG activity. The pathological features include gross cerebral cortical atrophy, spongiosis or status spongiosus, gliosis and neuronal loss that are often more prominent in the thalamus but are also present in the cerebral cortex, basal ganglia and brain stem. The cerebellum shows spongiosis in the molecular layer and atrophy of the granular layer. The cord also is mildly atrophic and shows demyelination. Immunostaining demonstrates the punctate pattern and the lack of PrP plaque-like deposits.[101,102] The CJD V210I–129M and the CJD H208R–129M phenotypes, which have been observed, respectively, in four cases and in one case, differ from the CJD M232R–129M by a consistently shorter duration, 3–5 months.[101,103–105] Other clinical signs and the histopathology including the PrP immunohistochemistry are very similar. CJD V180I–129M has been described in four subjects.[101] In one of them, the V180I mutation was heteroallelic with the M232R mutation. Clinically this subtype is characterized by a consistently longer duration of 1–2 years, and a lack of the typical EEG pattern. Pathologically, despite the long duration the CJD V180I–129M is similar to the group 1 of the sporadic form with typical spongiosis and some gliosis and neuronal loss in the cerebral cortex, basal ganglia and thalamus and a lack of status spongiosus. No plaque-like deposits are seen except for a case heterozygous at codon 129. CJD T183A–129M has been described in nine members of one kindred.[106] The hallmark of this subtype is the long duration, an average of over 4 years, with a relatively early onset, similar to that of CJD D178N–129V. Personality changes are the presenting sign, followed by behavioral abnormalities and often Parkinsonian signs. The EEG changes are not typical. The histopathology is characterized by spongiosis, which is severe in the frontal and temporal cortexes and decreases in severity in parietal and occipital cortices, and basal ganglia but is not present in the hippocampal region, thalamus, brain stem, or cerebellum.

GERSTMANN-STRÄUSSLER-SCHEINKER DISEASE

GSS is a chronic hereditary autosomal dominant cerebellar syndrome accompanied by pyramidal signs and a cognitive decline, which may evolve into severe dementia.[107] Amyotrophy and Parkinsonian signs may be present either early or late in the course of the disease. The characteristic pathological

Table 4 Genotype and phenotype of inherited prion diseases

Genotype	Onset (yr)	Duration	*Clinical and **pathological features
Creutzfeldt-Jakob disease (CJD) phenotype			
D178N-129V	26–56	9–51 months	*Dementia, ataxia, myoclonus, extrapyramidal and pyramidal signs **Spongiosis, neuronal loss and astrogliosis in the cerebral cortex (most severe), striatum and thalamus (least severe), while the cerebellum is spared
V180I-129M	66–85	1–2 years	*Similar to group 1 sCJD but with slower progression. **Like group 1 sCJD
T183A-129M	45	4 years	*Personality changes followed by dementia and Parkinsonism **Atrophy with spongiform degeneration in the cerebral cortex and, to a lesser extent, in the basal ganglia
E200K-129M	35–66	2–41 months	*Similar to group 1 sCJD. Atypical signs such as supranuclear palsy and peripheral neuropathy in some cases **Like group 1 sCJD.
H208R-129M	60	7 months	*Like group 1 sCJD. **Like group 1 sCJD.
V210I-129M	49–70	3–5 months	*Like group 1 sCJD. **Like group 1 sCJD.
M232R-129M	55–70	4–24 months	*Like group 1 sCJD. **Like group 1 sCJD.
Fatal familial insomnia (FFI) phenotype			
D178N-129M	20–71	6–33 months	*Reduction of total sleep time, enacted dreams, sympathetic hyperactivity, myoclonus, ataxia; late dementia, pyramidal and extrapyramidal signs in the cases with a relatively long duration (> 1 year). **Preferential thalamic and olivary atrophy. Spongiform changes in the cerebral cortex in the subjects with a duration of symptoms longer than 1 yr
Gerstmann-Sträussler-Scheinker syndrome (GSS) phenotype			
P102L-129M	30–62	1–10 years	*Slowly progressive cerebellar syndrome with late dementia, extrapyramidal and pyramidal signs. Rare cases (shorter duration) overlap with CJD **PrP amyloid deposits in the cerebellum and, to a lesser extent, in the cerebrum. Variable degree of spongiosis, neuronal loss and astrogliosis. No NFT
P102L-129M -219L	31–34	4 years	*Differ from the above P102L form for the less prominent cerebellar signs **Few PrP plaques in the cerebral and cerebellar cortices. No spongiosis
P102L-129V	33	12 years	*Seizures, numbness, gait difficulties, dysarthria, long tract signs. No dementia **Widespread PrP plaques. No spongiosis
P105L-129V	40–50	6–12 years	*Spastic paraparesis progressing to quadriparesis; late dementia; no myoclonus and only mild cerebellar signs **PrP amyloid deposits, neuronal loss and gliosis in the cerebral cortex and, to a lesser extent, in the striatum and thalamus. No spongiform changes.

Genotype	Onset (yr)	Duration	*Clinical and **pathological features
A117V-129V	20–64	1–11 years	*Dementia, Parkinsonism, pyramidal signs. Occasional cerebellar signs **Widespread PrP amyloid deposits in the cerebrum and, more rarely, in the cerebellum associated with variable degree of spongiform changes, neuronal loss and astrogliosis.
Y145STOP-129M	38	21 years	*Slowly progressive dementia **PrP amyloid angiopathy in most gray matter structuresassociated with NFT in the neocortex, hippocampus and subcortical nuclei. No spongiosis
F198S-129V	34–71	3–12 years	*Like 102 GSS subtype, but with a more chronic course (no overlap with CJD) **Like 102 GSS subtype but with more extensive PrP amyloid deposits, NFT in the cerebral cortex and subcortical nuclei and inconspicuous spongiosis
Q217R-129V	62–66	5–6 years	*Slowly progressive dementia, cerebellar and extrapyramidal signs **Like 198 GSS subtype but with the most severe lesions in the cerebral cortex, thalamus and amygdala
Heterogeneous phenotype: the insertional mutations			
ins 24 bp-129M	73	4 months	*Like group 1 sCJD. **NA
ins 48 bp-129M	58	3 months	*Like group 1 sCJD. **Like group 1 sCJD.
ins 96 bp-129M	56	2 months	*Like group 1 sCJD. **Like group 1 sCJD, but with PrP patches in cerebellum (IHC)
ins 96 bp-129V	82	4 months	*Examined at terminal stage showed akinetic mutism, diffuse myoclonus and pyramidal signs. **NA
ins 120 bp-129M	31,45	5,15 years	*Progressive dementia, myoclonus, cerebellar and extrapyramidal signs **Spongiosis, gliosis and neuronal loss (no information on topography, severity and presence of PrP deposits). CJD phenotype
ins 144 bp-129M	22–53	3 months –18 years	*Similar to 120 bp insertion subtype **Most cases show a CJD phenotype with spongiosis, gliosis and neuronal loss. One case had kuru-like plaques in the cerebellum. Some cases show only mild aspecific gliosis and neuronal loss. PrP patches in the cerebellum
ins 168 bp-129M	23–35	7–13 years	*Similar to 120 bp insertion subtype. **Mild gliosis and neuronal loss, and no spongiosis in 1 case, CJD phenotype in another
ins 192 bp-129V	21–54	5 months –6 years	*Similar to 120 bp insertion subtype **Spongiosis, gliosis and neuronal loss, PrP multicentric amyloid plaques with widespread distribution. GSS-like phenotype
ins 216 bp-129M	32–55	2.5–4 years	*Similar to 120 bp insertion subtype **PrP amyloid plaques in the cerebellum, cerebral cortex and striatum. No obvious neuronal loss, gliosis or spongiosis. GSS-like phenotype

NA = not available; PrP = prion protein; NFT = neurofibrillary tangles.

phenotype is the presence of PrP-amyloid plaques in the cerebellar cortex in association with pyramidal tract degeneration. Specific features such as spongiform changes, neurofibrillary tangles (NFT) and Lewy bodies may be differentiating the various GSS haplotypes. The *PRNP* mutations associated with GSS disease are shown in Table 4 and Figure 5. In view of the consistent presence of PrP amyloid deposits, the term hereditary prion protein amyloidosis has also been introduced. This nomenclature would allow us to also include in this group the recently recognized phenotype characterized clinically by severe dementia and pathologically by the presence of a prion protein cerebral amyloid angiopathy (CAA) and NFT. This entity, which is rare, is referred to as PrP-CAA.[108] Although classified among prion diseases, transmissibility is not a consistent feature of PrP amyloidosis.

In GSS, the symptomatology occurs in the third to seventh decades; the mean duration of illness is 5 years. Although the incidence of GSS is believed to be less than 2 per 10^8, it is probably underestimated, since GSS may present as a syndrome mimicking spinocerebellar degeneration, olivopontocerebellar atrophy, spastic paraparesis, Parkinsonism, or dementia.[107]

The neuropathologic diagnosis of GSS is based on the presence of PrP-amyloid deposits, the distribution and extent of which differ widely between families. Amyloid is accompanied by glial proliferation and by the loss of neuronal processes and perikarya, leading to variable degrees of atrophy of the affected regions. The clinical phenotypes are associated with mutations of *PRNP*, allelic polymorphisms, and, possibly, with environmental and tissue-specific factors.

GENOTYPES AND CLINICOPATHOLOGICAL PHENOTYPES

Mutation of PrP residue 102 in coupling with methionine at residue 129 (P102L–129M)

A proline (CCG) to leucine (CTG) substitution on a methionine 129 allele has been found in at least 32 families from the US, Canada, UK, Germany, France, Austria, Italy, Israel, Japan and Mexico and is the most common cause of GSS.[109–114]

A progressive cerebellar syndrome with ataxia, dysarthria, incoordination of saccadic movements, and pyramidal signs are associated with mental and behavioral deterioration. Dementia or akinetic mutism occur in the late stages of the disease. The age at the onset of clinical signs is in the fourth to sixth decades of life and the duration of the disease ranges from 5 months to 6 years. Considerable intrafamilial phenotypic variability is visible.[109,112,113] Myoclonus and PSW on EEG, a finding of diagnostic relevance in CJD, occur in some P102L patients; some of them present a rapid course of 5–9 months with a clinical picture indistinguishable from that of CJD.[109,112,113] Neuropathologically, deposits of fibrillar and non-fibrillar PrP in the cerebral and cerebellar parenchyma are consistently found (Fig. 6D).[109,112,114,115] Spongiform changes, neuronal loss and astrocytosis vary in severity even among patients of the same kindred, and are most severe when the course of the illness is rapid.[109,112,113]

Mutation of PrP residue 102 in coupling with methionine at residue 129 and lysine at residue 219 (P102L–129M–219K)

This mutation has been associated with either dementia or cerebellar signs in a Japanese family. Neuropathologically, mild PrP deposits are detected in the cerebral and cerebellar cortex and basal ganglia, with no visible amyloid or spongiform changes.[116]

Mutation of PrP residue 102 in coupling with valine 129 (P102L–129V)

This has been seen in two patients. In one patient, studied clinically and pathologically,[117] seizures, numbness of the extremities, spastic paraparesis, weakness, dysarthria, swallowing difficulty and no dementia were observed. Degeneration of the corticospinal, spinal cerebellar and gracile tracts were seen. A moderate amount of PrP deposits in the cerebellar cortex and mild amounts in the cerebral cortex were also present. Spongiform changes were absent. The duration of the disease was 12 years.

Mutation of PrP residue 105 (P105L)

A proline (CCA) to leucine (CTA) substitution at codon 105 on a valine 129 allele has been found in patients with hereditary spastic paraparesis in four Japanese families.[118–122]

Clinically, pyramidal signs are prominant in the initial stages.[120,121] Extrapyramidal signs such as fine finger tremor and rigidity of limbs may be seen. Paraparesis progresses to tetraparesis and is accompanied by emotional incontinence and dementia. Myoclonus and PSW on EEG, or severe cerebellar signs, have not been reported. The age at the onset of the clinical signs is in the fourth and fifth decades of life, and the duration of the disease ranges from 6–12 years.

Neuropathologically, PrP deposits are found in the neocortex, especially the motor area, striatum and thalamus. Multicentric PrP-amyloid plaques and diffuse deposits are respectively detected in superficial and deep layers of the neocortex, in association with neuronal loss and astrocytosis. NFT are occasionally seen, but not spongiform changes. Amyloid plaques are rare in the cerebellum, while axonal losses occur in the pyramidal tracts.[118–122]

Mutation of PrP residue 117 (A117V)

An alanine (GCA or GCG) to valine (GTG) substitution on a valine 129 allele has been described in a French (Alsatian) family and in two US kindreds, one being of German origin.[123–125]

The clinical phenotypes are presenile dementia in the Alsatian family,[125–128] presenile dementia, pyramidal signs, and Parkinsonism in the US-German kindred.[123,129] Severe ataxia, dysarthria, mild Parkinsonism and dementia are present in a patient from a third family.[123] In the Alsatian and in the US-German families, the age at the onset of the clinical signs is between the second and sixth decades.[127,129] The duration of the disease ranges from 1–11 and 2–6 years, respectively. The clinical phenotype in the Alsatian family is variable.[125] Three patients studied in the first and second generations of the published pedigree exhibited dementia as the main clinical symptom, while affected subjects from subsequent generations showed the association of dementia, pyramidal and pseudobulbar signs with ataxia, extrapyramidal symptoms, amyotrophy, myoclonus and tonic-clonic seizures. The EEG did not show PSW.

Neuropathologically, PrP-amyloid deposits and PrP deposits without the tinctorial properties of amyloid are widespread throughout the cerebrum, and are rare in the cerebellum of subjects with dementia alone.[124–129] Numerous PrP-amyloid deposits in the cerebral cortex, basal ganglia and thalamus, as well as in the cerebellum, were found in three patients from the Alsatian family,[125] who had died at 24, 39 and 73 years of age. In the lattermost, who survived 9 years after the onset of the clinical signs, NFT were numerous in the cerebral cortex, in contrast with the rare deposits of Aβ. Spongiform changes were absent. In patients of the US-German family, PrP-amyloid deposits were prominent in the cerebral cortex and striatum, but not in the cerebellum; NFT were occasionally found. In the recently reported third family, there is a conspicuous deposition of PrP amyloid in the cerebellum.[125]

Mutation at PrP residue 198 (F198S): the Indiana kindred

A phenylalanine (TTC) to serine (TCC) substitution at codon 198 on a valine 129 allele has been described in patients from an Indiana kindred.[131]

The clinical phenotype is characterized by a gradual loss of short-term memory and progressive clumsiness in walking, bradykinesia, rigidity, dysarthria, and dementia. Signs of cognitive impairment and eye-movement abnormalities may be detected by specific tests before the clinical onset of symptoms. Psychotic depression has been seen in several patients, and tremor is mild or absent. Symptoms may progress slowly over 5 years or rapidly over as little as 1 year. The age at onset of clinical signs is 40–71 years. Patients homozygous for valine at codon 129 have, on average, clinical signs 10 years earlier than heterozygous patients.[132] The duration of the disease ranges from 2–12 years.[107,133] On immunoblot patients with the F198S mutation have a distinct pattern of PrP^{res} isoforms comprising three major peptides of approximately 27–29, 18–19 and 8 kDa.

The neuropathologic phenotype is characterized by the presence of severe PrP deposition and amyloid formation in the cerebral and cerebellar parenchyma as well as neurofibrillary lesions in the cerebral gray matter (Fig. 6E–G).[107,134–136] Unicentric and multicentric PrP-amyloid deposits are distributed throughout the gray structures of the cerebrum, cerebellum, and midbrain. Amyloid deposition is severe in the lower layers of frontal, insular, temporal and parietal cortex, and is moderate in the hippocampus, where plaques occur predominantly within the stratum lacunosum-moleculare of the CA1 sector and subiculum. PrP deposits are numerous in the claustrum, the caudate nucleus, putamen, the anterior, dorsomedial, ventrolateral and lateral dorsal nuclei of the thalamus, the cerebellar molecular layer, the mesencephalic tegmentum, the substantia nigra, and periaqueductal grey matter; however, the degree of amyloid formation in these areas varies. Amyloid deposits are surrounded by astrocytes, astrocytic processes and microglial cells. In the neocortex, amyloid cores associated with abnormal neurites have morphological similarity to neuritic plaques of Alzheimer disease (Fig. 6F).[134] The neurites immunoreact with antibodies to tau, ubiquitin, and to N- and C-terminal domains of the β-amyloid precursor protein.[107]

NFT and neuropil threads are found in large number in the neocortex and in most of the subcortical nuclei.

Moderate to severe cerebral and cerebellar atrophy, nerve cell loss and gliosis are found in the neocortex, striatum, red nucleus, substantia nigra, cerebellum, locus coeruleus, and inferior olivary nucleus. Spongiform changes are inconspicuous. On immunoblot, patients with the F1985 mutation have a distinct pattern of PrP^{res} isoforms comprising three major peptides of approximately 27–29, 18–19, and 8 kDa.

Mutation at PrP residue 217 (Q217R)

A glutamine (CAG) to arginine (CGG) substitution[131] on a Val129 allele has been described in two patients from an American family of Swedish origin. Clinically, gradual memory loss, progressive ataxia, Parkinsonism and dementia are seen in the seventh decade of life. The duration of the disease is 5–6 years.[107]

Neuropathologically, PrP-amyloid deposits in the cerebrum and cerebellum and abundant NFT in the cerebral cortex and several subcortical nuclei are seen.

Mutation at PrP residue 145 (Y145STOP)

A tyrosine (TAT) to stop codon (TAG) substitution on a methionine 129 allele[108] has been found through studies of a Japanese patient with a clinical diagnosis of Alzheimer disease.[137] Clinically, memory disturbance, disorientation, and a progressively severe dementia were observed in the fourth decade of life; the EEG did not show PSW. The duration of the disease was 21 years.

Neuropathologically, there are PrP-amyloid deposits in the walls of the small and the medium-sized parenchymal and leptomeningeal blood vessels and in the perivascular neuropil as well as neurofibrillary lesions in the cerebral gray matter. The neurofibrillary tangles are composed of paired helical filaments with a periodicity of 70–80 nm and were decorated with monoclonal antibodies recognizing abnormally phosphorylated tau. Diffuse atrophy of the cerebrum, dilation of the lateral ventricles, neuronal loss and gliosis are severe; there are no spongiform changes.

AMYLOID IN GSS DISEASE AND PRP-CAA

The biochemical composition of PrP amyloid has been determined in brain tissue samples obtained from patients with mutations F198S and Q217R.[138,139] The amyloid preparations from amyloid cores contain two major peptides of ~11 and ~7 kDa spanning residues 58–150 and 81–150 of PrP, respectively.[138,139] The finding that the amyloid protein was an N- and C-terminal truncated fragment of PrP was verified by immunostaining brain sections with antisera raised against synthetic peptides homologous to residues 23–40, 90–102, 127–147 and 220–231 of human PrP.

In GSS F198S and Q217R, the amyloid protein does not include the region containing the amino acid substitution. Analyzing patients who are heterozygous methionine/valine at codon 129 and using 129 valine as a marker for the mutant allele it has been possible to establish that only mutant PrP was involved in amyloid formation.[139]

Limited data are available on the amyloid of GSS P102L. Western blot analysis of amyloid-enriched fractions, using antibodies to PrP, showed two broad bands of 25–30 and 15–20 kDa and an amino acid sequence analysis of HPLC purified peptides generated by enzymatic digestion of the 25–30 and 15–20 kDa bands revealed that mutant leucine at position 102 is contained in the amyloid fractions.[140,141] Recent immunohistochemical data have shown that the amyloid deposits are best recognized by antibodies directed to epitopes in PrP region 90–165. These results indicate that GSS P102L differs from the other GSS variants in that the amyloid peptide is more extended toward the C-terminus of PrP.[115]

In PrP-CAA, amyloid deposits in tissue sections are immunoreactive with antibodies to PrP spanning the region 90–147 and not with antibodies to Aβ. Immunoblot analysis of proteins extracted from amyloid fibrils showed that the smallest amyloid subunit is a 7.5 kDa peptide immunoreactive with antibodies to epitopes located within residues 90–147 of PrP, and unreactive to antisera to N- and C-termini. In addition, immunohistochemistry shows that a substantial amount of PrP deposits is labeled by an antiserum to the C-terminus. These findings suggest that C-terminal fragments of PrP encoded by the normal allele contribute to PrP deposits, since the genetic defect in PrP-CAA is a stop codon, resulting in a C-terminal truncated protein. In PrP-CAA, regions of the cerebrum are characterized by severe PrP vascular deposition regardless of amyloid formation; neurofibrillary changes are present in a large quantity.

GSS AND NEUROFIBRILLARY TANGLES

NFT in cell bodies and in neurites are a major feature of the neuropathologic phenotype in the GSS variants F198S and Q217R as well as PrP-CAA (Y145STOP).[108,134,136,142] By electron microscopy, paired helical filaments appear as the main constituents of the NFT. Each member of the pair is a filament about 10 nm in diameter. The pair of filaments measure about 22–24 nm at its maximum width, and the helical twist has a period of about 70–80 nm. NFT have also been observed in some GSS patients with P105L and A117V variants.

Immunohistochemical studies of NFT in F198S, Q217R and PrP-CAA using phosphorylation-dependent and independent anti-tau antibodies do not reveal differences between NFT of Alzheimer disease and those of PrP amyloidosis. Paired helical filament-enriched fractions obtained from the neocortex of F198S patients contained SDS-soluble tau isoforms with electrophoretic mobility and an immunochemical profile corresponding to those of A68 extracted from the brain of patients with Alzheimer disease.

GSS AND ANIMAL TRANSMISSION

Tissue homogenates from the brain of patients from families with GSS P102L and eight repeat insertion, inoculated into non-human primates, marmosets and mice may induce a spongiform encephalopathy in the recipient animals.[143] No transmission has occurred following inoculation of tissue from patients carrying other GSS mutations.

HETEROGENOUS PHENOTYPE: INSERTIONAL MUTATIONS

To date, insertional mutations have been found in 10 kindreds and 9 affected individuals from uninformative families (Table 4). The phenotype associated with the insertional mutations is highly variable, particularly regarding the duration of the disease, ranging between 2 months and 18 years and the clinical and pathological features, including the typical CJD phenotype, a phenotype more consistent with GSS and conditions of several years' duration lacking specific histopathology.[144,145] Despite this remarkable heterogeneity, this group appears to follow some general rules. Clinically, approximately two-thirds of the subjects with four or fewer octapeptide insertions, or 24 to 96 bp, have a phenotype indistinguishable from the sporadic CJD group 1 phenotype, i.e. rapidly progressive dementia of less than 1 year duration, often associated with ataxia and visual disturbances, myoclonus and PSW on the EEG.[144] The penetrance is low in these subjects so that the familial incidence of the disease may be undetectable. In contrast, less than 10% of the subjects with 5 or more octapeptide inserts, 120–216 bp, present the typical CJD clinical phenotype. The pathological phenotype shows a similar distribution between affected subjects with a low and high number of octapeptide repeats. Almost 90% (13 out of 15) of the subjects with 6 or fewer octapeptide inserts that have undergone autopsy examination show histopathological changes consistent with those of CJD, even though the majority of these cases have a disease duration of more than 1 year. These changes include spongiform degeneration or status spongiosus, astrogliosis and neuronal loss in different combinations with no PrP amyloid plaques outside the granular cell layer of the cerebellum. In contrast, the great majority (6 out of 7) of autopsied subjects with 7 or more octapeptide inserts show a different histopathological phenotype. Five of these cases, along with one

Table 5 FFI kindreds with D178N mutation

	Nationality		Number
Kindreds			
	Italian[148,152,a,b]		3
	French[153]		2
	American[152,159]		4
	Australian[169,c]		2
	German[d]		2
	Austrian[e]		1
	British[f]		2
	Canadian[g]		1
		Total	**17**
Isolated cases			
	Italian[152]		2
	Japanese[170]		1
		Total	**3**

Personal communication from: [a]Tagliavini F & Bugiani O; [b]Vignolo LA & Padovani A; [c]Masters CL & Brown P; [d]Kretzschmar HA; [e]Budka H; [f]Will RG; [g]Green G.

carrying six octapeptide insertions, have a histopathology consistent with that of GSS. In addition to various degrees of spongiosis, gliosis and neuronal loss, there are PrP amyloid plaques often multicentric in the molecular layer of the cerebellum and often in the cerebral gray matter, a distribution not seen in CJD. Rarely (1 subject from this group and one with 6 octapeptide repeat insertions out of a total of 22 autopsied cases) are there minimal or not distinctive histological changes such as astrogliosis and neuronal loss without spongiosis, and PrP amyloid plaques. In conclusion, the CJD-like histopathological phenotype is very common in association with up to 6 octapeptide insertional mutations. The GSS-like phenotype is common in association with 8 and 9 octapeptide insertional mutations. Although a less than 1 year disease duration is more often associated with the CJD than with the GSS pathological phenotype, overall, such a duration is relatively rare and was reported in only 5 of the 22 autopsied cases. Significant amyloid formation occurs only in association with 6 or more octapeptide repeats and does not require a long course since PrP amyloid plaques were present in a subject with a 3 month course.

FATAL FAMILIAL INSOMNIA

EPIDEMIOLOGY

Currently, we are aware of 17 families and 3 isolated individuals that carry the FFI mutation (Table 5). To date, the FFI haplotype appears to be the third most common after the E200K–129M and P102L–129M haplotypes.

CLINICAL PHENOTYPE

The disease begins between 20 and 71 years of age (mean = 49 years) and may have either a relatively short (6–13 months) or long (24–48 months) duration. This variability in the symptom duration is, at least in part, genetically determined (see below). The cardinal clinical features are: insomnia (better defined as an increasing incapacity to generate sleep), dysautonomia and motor signs. The sleep disturbance when searched with polysomnography, is usually present at the onset of the disease, and progressively worsens.[146]

Impairment of autonomic function is also an early sign. It is characterized by increased sweating and salivation, constipation, impotence, hypertension, tachycardia, tachypnea, and mild fever.[146,147] Motor manifestations include dysarthria and ataxia and may predominate as presenting signs.[146,148–150] The cognitive functions show impairment of vigilance and attention associated to a selective impairment of memory with a relative preservation of global intelligence.[150]

HISTOPATHOLOGY

The hallmark is loss of neurons and astrogliosis in the thalamus, which is present in all subjects, independent of the disease duration (Fig. 6B,C).[151–153] The medio-dorsal and anterior ventral thalamic nuclei are invariably and severely affected, while the involvement of other thalamic nuclei varies. The

Table 6 Two FFI phenotypes

	Codon 129	
	Met/Met	Met/Val
Clinical course (range)*	7–18 months	11-33 months
Periodic EEG activity*	0/6	2/3
Presentation*	Insomnia, dysautonomia	Ataxia, dysarthria
PET study** (hypometabolic regions)	Thalamus	Thalamus + cortex
Pathology*		
Thalamic atrophy	+++	+++
Neocortical spongiosis	±	++

*Based on nine subjects, six homozygous, and three heterozygous at codon 129[153]
**Based on seven subjects, 4 homozygous and three heterozygous.[171]

inferior olives also show neuronal loss and gliosis in most cases. In contrast, the pathology of the cerebral cortex varies in proportion to the disease duration and is more severe in the limbic lobe than in the neocortex.[151,152] The entorhinal cortex and, to a lesser extent, the pyriform and paraolfactory cortices, show spongiosis and astrogliosis in most subjects. Instead, the neocortex is virtually spared in the subjects with a disease duration of less than 1 year, but focally affected by spongiosis and gliosis in those with a course between 12 and 20 months, and diffusely involved only in subjects with a disease of more than 20 months duration. In addition, the frontal, temporal, and parietal lobes are affected more severely than the occipital lobe. The other structures are virtually normal or show mild focal pathology. Overall, the thalamus is more severely and consistently involved than any other brain region. Therefore, on the basis of the pathology, FFI can be defined as a preferential thalamic degeneration.

GENOTYPE-PHENOTYPE CORRELATION

FFI share the same mutation of the CJD D178N–129V subtype (CJD178), but have a significantly different phenotype, which is determined by the genotype at codon 129 on the mutated allele.[154] The methionine codon is linked to FFI, while the valine codon is linked to CJD178.[154]

Some heterogeneity in the clinical and histopathological features has been noted even within the FFI affected subjects (Table 6).[152] The differences observed are consistent with the existence of two slightly different phenotypes which are determined by the genotype at codon 129 of the normal allele. FFI patients homozygous for methionine at codon 129 manifest, on average, a more rapid course and prominent sleep and autonomic disturbances, while signs of motor and cognitive dysfunction are mild. In contrast, the methionine/valine heterozygotes have a more chronic course and manifest motor signs as a prominent clinical feature at onset while sleep disturbances and autonomic signs are less severe. Additionally, signs of cortical involvement also appear in these subjects, although late in the course of the disease. As noted above, the histopathology varies as a function of the disease duration which, in turn is a function of the 129 methionine/valine polymorphism. Overall, the thalamus is similarly affected in all subjects, but the cerebral cortex is generally more severely affected in the heterozygotes at codon 129.

PRION PROTEIN IN FFI AND CJD178

The PrP^{res} fragments associated with FFI and CJD178 differ both in the size of the core protein and in the percent ratio of the three PrP^{res} glycoforms.[155] The size of the PrP^{res} fragments generated by exogenous PK in CJD178 and FFI matches the PrP^{res} type 1 and 2, respectively, observed in sporadic CJD (Fig. 4). The distinctive glycoform ratio of FFI and CJD178 PrP^{res} which is characterized by the under-representation of the unglycosylated form, is the result of the under-representation of this mutant glycoform prior to the conversion to the PrP^{res} isoform, probably because of the more pronounced instability of this D178N mutant glycoform.[21] These findings are consistent with the conclusion that the PrP^{res} associated with FFI and CJD178 have different protein conformations and/or distinct ligand binding interactions. Therefore, the FFI and CJD178 phenotypes are likely to be determined by the codon 129 of the mutant allele which, coupled with the D178N mutation, results in the expression of PrP^{res} with distinct biophysical characteristics.

TRANSMISSIBILITY OF FFI

Transgenic mice expressing a chimeric human-mouse PrP^{C} develop a prion disease 200 days after the intracerebral inoculation with a homogenate from FFI brains.[45] The pathology as well as the presence of PrP^{res} are predominant in the thalamus. This transmission experiment, along with others,[156,157] not only demonstrates that FFI shares transmissibility with other prion diseases but may also provide important clues about the mechanisms of PrP^{C}–PrP^{res} conversion. This was demonstrated by the finding that the size of the PrP^{res} fragment expressed by the inoculated transgenic mice is identical in electrophoretic mobility to the PrP^{res} fragment present in the inoculum from subjects with FFI. Replication of the PrP^{res} fragment size was also observed in the transmission of sporadic and inherited CJD associated with PrP^{res} type 1.[45] Since the recipient mice did not carry any of the donor's *PRNP* mutations, this remarkable finding indicates that the distinct conformations associated with PrP^{res} type 1 and 2 can be reproduced independently of the genetic information, probably on the basis of information contained in the conformation of the donor's PrP^{res}. This mechanism explains the old dilemma of prion strain diversity in a way that does not require the participation of nucleic acids.

FFI AND ITS RELATIONSHIP WITH THALAMIC DEMENTIA: DOES THE SPORADIC FORM OF FFI EXIST?

The concept of thalamic dementia or thalamic degeneration was introduced by Stern in 1939 when he described a subject with severe cognitive impairment of approximately 6 months duration that, at autopsy, showed only severe atrophy of ventral anterior and medial dorsal thalamic nuclei and a variable degree of astrogliosis in the cerebral cortex.[158] Thalamic degeneration has been subsequently classified by Martin into three groups:[159] (i) the thalamic degeneration associated with multisystem atrophies; (ii) the so-called preferential thalamic degeneration; and (iii) the thalamic form of CJD. Groups 1 and 2 included familial and sporadic forms, whereas thalamic CJD was described only in sporadic cases. The nosologic position of preferential thalamic degeneration and, in particular, its delineation from thalamic CJD, however, remained unclear. After the description of FFI, it has been shown that previously reported familial cases of preferential thalamic degeneration or dementia have the same PRNP D178N–129M haplotype as FFI. Therefore, the condition previously identified as familial thalamic dementia and FFI are one and the same disease.[159,160] In contrast, no mutations in *PRNP* are found in the multiple system atrophy with thalamic degeneration;[159] it, therefore, does not belong to the group of prion diseases.

However, in contrast to the familial forms, only one incidence of the sporadic cases of preferential thalamic degeneration has been analyzed for the presence of PrP^{res}.[160] Clinically and histopathologically this case is similar to that of Stern; however, insomnia was reported by clinical observation. Immunoblotting demonstrated the presence of PrP^{res} type 2 as in FFI in the cerebral cortex (unpublished results), while sequencing ruled out the presence of the D178N mutation. The presence of PrP^{res}, insomnia, dysautonomia, and endocrine disturbances must be proven in more cases in order to definitely clarify the nosology of the sporadic form of preferential thalamic degeneration and to decide whether these cases should now be classified as a thalamic form of sporadic CJD or as a sporadic form of fatal insomnia.

MECHANISMS OF PHENOTYPIC HETEROGENEITY

Phenotypic variability is one of the challenging features of prion diseases. As mentioned above, the phenotype appears the result of the concerted action of different variables. The two main determinants appear to be the *PRNP* genotype, specified either by mutations or polymorphisms in the gene, and the type of PrP^{res} fragment that form in the brain. As exemplified in sporadic CJD, the two variables are relatively independent, although the *PRNP* haplotype clearly favors the formation of a certain PrP^{res} type. Since distinct PrP^{res} types may represent the molecular basis of prion strains, or at least their molecular signature, it might be argued that the *PRNP* haplotype acts as a modulator of the host susceptibility to distinct strains of prion.

Another mechanism likely to play a role in phenotypic heterogeneity of prion diseases is the allelic origin of PrP^{res}. Inherited prion diseases are overwhelmingly heterozygous for the pathogenic mutation. Therefore, not only the ease with which the mutant PrP (PrP^{M}) converts into the PrP^{res}, but also the potential conversion of the PrP expressed by the normal or wild type allele (PrP^{Wt}) is important. These two variables influence the rate of production and, therefore, the amount and distribution of the PrP^{res} formed, which, in turn, have been shown to be related to the severity and topography of the lesions in human and in animal prion diseases.[54,152,161,162] Recent studies have documented a variable, mutation specific, contribution of the PrP^{Wt} to the pathogenesis of inherited prion diseases. In the CJD subtype associated with the V210I mutation, PrP^{res} is formed by both PrP^{Wt} and PrP^{M}.[163] A similar observation has been made for the inherited forms carrying insertional mutations.[164] In the CJD subtype linked to the E200K mutation,[165] only PrP^{M} is resistant to proteases, but both PrP^{M} and PrP^{Wt} are insoluble in nonionic detergents indicating that wild type PrP, although not converted to PrP^{res}, is aggregated and, therefore, abnormal. PrP^{Wt} is different in FFI and CJD178. In both of these diseases, PrP^{res} derives exclusively from PrP^{M}. Similarly, in the GSS subtypes associated with the A117V and the F198S mutations, only PrP^{M} is present in the PrP amyloid deposits that characterize these diseases.[139,166] It appears, therefore, that, in inherited prion diseases, the amount of PrP^{res} that accumulates in the brain not only depends on the conversion of PrP^{M} to PrP^{res} but also on the variable, mutation specific, conversion of PrP^{Wt}.

In order to fully understand phenotypic heterogeneity in prion diseases the role of each of the above mechanisms, and possibly other mechanisms, needs to be clarified. The challenge is to understand the role that these variables, and probably other variables that will undoubtedly be uncovered, play individually as well as jointly in the pathogenesis of human prion diseases.

The first step in this research endeavor is the detailed and accurate characterization of the clinical, laboratory, and histopathological features of each subject affected by a prion disease.

ADDENDUM

Bruce ME et al. recently provided strong evidence that the same agent strain is involved in both BSE and vCJD.[172]

ACKNOWLEDGMENTS

We thank Prof. Peter Lantos for providing tissue of kuru and new variant CJD. This work was supported in part by NIH grants AG08012, AG08155, AG08992, AG10133, SN29822 and the Britton Fund.

REFERENCES

1. Creutzfeldt HG. Über eine eigenartige herdförmige Erkrankung des Zentralnervensystems. *Z Neurol Psychiat* 1920; **57**: 1–18
2. Jakob A. Über eine eigenartige Erkrankungen des Zentralnervensystems mit bemerkenswertem anatomichen Befunde (Spastische Pseudosklerose-Encephalomyelopathie mit anatomishen disseminierten Degenerationsherden). *Z Gesamte Neurol Psychiat* 1921; **64**: 147–228
3. Gerstmann J. Über ein noch nicht beschriebenes Reflexphanomen bei einer Erkrankung des zerebellaren Systems. *Wiener Med Wochenschr* 1928; **78**: 906–908
4. Gerstmann J, Sträussler E, Scheinker I. Über eine eigenartige hereditär-familiäre Erkrankung des Zentralnervensystems. Zugleich ein Beitrag zur Frage des vorzeitigen lokalen Alterns. *Z Neurol Psychiat* 1936; **154**: 736–762
5. Gajdusek DC, Zigas V. Degenerative disease of the central nervous system in New Guinea. The endemic occurrence of 'Kuru' in the native population. *N Engl J Med* 1957; **257**: 974–978
6. Hadlow WJ. Scrapie and kuru. *Lancet* 1959; **2**: 289–290
7. Gajdusek DC, Gibbs Jr CJ, Alpers M. Experimental transmission of a Kuru-like syndrome to chimpanzees. *Nature* 1966; **209**: 794–796

8. Gibbs Jr CJ, Gajdusek DC, Asher DM et al. Creutzfeldt-Jakob disease (spongiform encephalopathy): transmission to the chimpanzee. *Science* 1968; **161**: 388–389
9. Masters CL, Gajdusek DC, Gibbs Jr CJ. Creutzfeldt-Jakob disease virus isolations from the Gerstmann-Sträussler syndrome. *Brain* 1981; **104**: 559–588
10. Duffy P, Wolf J, Collins G, De Voe AG, Streeten B, Cowen D. Possible person to person transmission of Creutzfeldt-Jakob disease. *N Engl J Med* 1974; **290**: 692–693
11. Merz PA, Somerville RA, Wisniewski HM, Iqbal K. Abnormal fibrils from scrapie-infected brain. *Acta Neuropathol* 1981; **54**: 63–74
12. Bolton DC, McKinley MP, Prusiner SB. Identification of a protein that purifies with the scrapie prion. *Science* 1982; **218**: 1309–1311
13. Prusiner SB. Novel proteinaceous infectious particles cause scrapie. *Science* 1982; **216**: 136–144
14. Chesebro B, Race R, Wehrly K et al. Identification of scrapie prion protein-specific mRNA in scrapie-infected and uninfected brain. *Nature* 1985; **315**: 331–333
15. Oesch B, Westaway D, Wälchli M et al. A cellular gene encodes scrapie PrP 27–30 protein. *Cell* 1985; **40**: 735–746
16. Sparkes RS, Simon M, Cohn VH et al. Assignment of the human and mouse prion protein genes to homologous chromosomes. *Proc Natl Acad Sci USA* 1986; **83**: 7358–7362
17. Stahl N, Borchelt DR, Hsiao K, Prusiner SB. Scrapie prion protein contains a phosphatidylinositol glycolipid. *Cell* 1987; **51**: 229–240
18. Caughey B, Race RE, Ernst D, Buchmeier MJ, Chesebro B. Prion protein biosynthesis in scrapie-infected and uninfected neuroblastoma cells. *J Virol* 1989; **63**: 175–181
19. Endo T, Groth D, Prusiner SB, Kobata A. Diversity of oligosaccharide structures linked to asparagines of the scrapie prion protein. *Biochemistry* 1989; **28**: 8380–8388
20. Chen SG, Teplow DB, Parchi P, Teller JK, Gambetti P, Autilio-Gambetti L. Truncated forms of the human prion protein in normal brain and in prion diseases. *J Biol Chem* 1995; **270**: 19173–19180
21. Petersen RB, Parchi P, Richardson SL, Urig CB, Gambetti P. Effect of the D178N mutation and the codon 129 polymorphism on the metabolism of the prion protein. *J Biol Chem* 1996; **271**: 12661–12668
22. Shyng SL, Huber MT, Harris DA. A prion protein cycles between the cell surface and an endocytic compartment in cultured neuroblastoma cells. *J Biol Chem* 1993; **268**: 15922–15928
23. Borchelt DR, Koliatsos VE, Guarnieri M, Pardo CA, Sisodia SS, Price DL. Rapid anterograde axonal transport of the cellular prion glycoprotein in the peripheral and central nervous systems. *J Biol Chem* 1994; **269**: 14711–14714
24. Collinge J, Whittington MA, Sidle KC et al. Prion protein is necessary for normal synaptic function. *Nature* 1994; **370**: 295–297
25. Whittington MA, Sidle KCL, Gowland I et al. Rescue of neurophysiological phenotype seen in PrP-null mice by transgene encoding human prion protein. *Nat Genet* 1995; **9**: 197–201
26. Tobler I, Gaus SE, Deboer T et al. Altered circadian activity rhythms and sleep in mice devoid of prion protein. *Nature* 1996; **380**: 639–642
27. Griffith JS. Self-replication and scrapie. *Nature* 1967; **215**: 1043–1044
28. Pattison IH, Jones KM. The possible nature of the transmissible agent of scrapie. *Vet Rec* 1967; **80**: 2–4
29. Hope J, Morton LJD, Farquhar CF, Multhaup G, Beyreuther K, Kimberlin RH. The major polypeptide of scrapie-associated fibrils (SAF) has the same size, charge distribution and N-terminal protein sequence as predicted for the normal brain protein (PrP). *EMBO J* 1986; **5**: 2591–2597
30. Turk E, Teplow DB, Hood LE, Prusiner SB. Purification and properties of the cellular and scrapie hamster prion proteins. *Eur J Biochem* 1988; **176**: 21–30
31. Caughey BW, Dong A, Bhat KS, Ernst D, Hayes SF, Caughey WS. Secondary structure analysis of the scrapie-associated protein PrP 27–30 in water by infrared spectroscopy. *Biochemistry* 1991; **30**: 7672–7680
32. Gasset M, Baldwin MA, Fletterick RJ, Prusiner SB. Perturbation of the secondary structure of the scrapie prion protein under conditions that alter infectivity. *Proc Natl Acad Sci USA* 1993; **90**: 1–5
33. Pan KM, Baldwin M, Nguyen J et al. Conversion of α-helices into β-sheets features in the formation of the scrapie prion proteins. *Proc Natl Acad Sci USA* 1993; **90**: 10962–10966

34. Safar J, Roller PP, Gajdusek DC, Gibbs CJ Jr. Conformational transitions, dissociation, and unfolding of scrapie amyloid (prion) protein. *J Biol Chem* 1993; **268**: 20276–20284
35. Prusiner SB. Molecular biology of prion diseases. *Science* 1991; **252**: 1515–1522
36. Jarrett JT, Lansbury PT Jr. Seeding 'one-dimensional crystallization' of amyloid: a pathogenic mechanism in Alzheimer's disease and scrapie? *Cell* 1993; **73**: 1055–1058
37. Borchelt DR, Taraboulos A, Prusiner SB. Evidence for synthesis of scrapie prion proteins in the endocytic pathway. *J Biol Chem* 1992; **267**: 16188–16199
38. Caughey B, Raymond GJ, Ernst D, Race RE. N-terminal truncation of the scrapie-associated form of PrP by lysosomal protease(s): implications regarding the site of conversion of PrP to the protease-resistant state. *J Virol* 1991; **65**: 6597–6603
39. Taraboulos A, Raeber AJ, Borchelt DR, Serban D, Prusiner SB. Synthesis and trafficking of prion proteins in cultured cells. *Mol Biol Cell* 1992; **3**: 851–863
40. McKinley MP, Taraboulos A, Kenaga L et al. Ultrastructural localization of scrapie prion proteins in cytoplasmic vesicles of infected cultured cells. *Lab Invest* 1991; **65**: 622–630
41. Büeler H, Aguzzi A, Sailer A et al. Mice devoid of PrP are resistant to scrapie. *Cell* 1993; **73**: 1339–1347
42. Sailer A, Büeler H, Fischer M, Aguzzi A, Weissmann C. No propagation of prions in mice devoid of PrP. *Cell* 1994; **77**: 967–968
43. Prusiner SB, Scott M, Foster D et al. Transgenic studies implicate interactions between homologous PrP isoforms in scrapie prion replication. *Cell* 1990; **63**: 673–686
44. Kocisko DA, Come JH, Priola SA et al. Cell-free formation of protease-resistant prion protein. *Nature* 1994; **370**: 471–474
45. Telling GC, Parchi P, DeArmond SJ et al. Evidence for the conformation of the pathologic isoform of the prion protein enciphering and propagating prion diversity. *Science* 1996; **274**: 2079–2082
46. Wickner RB, Masison DC, Edskes HK. [PSI] and [URE3] as yeast prions. *Yeast* 1995; **11**: 1671–1685
47. Akowitz A, Sklaviadis T, Manuelidis L. Endogenous viral complexes with long RNA cosediment with the agent of Creutzfeldt-Jakob disease. *Nucleic Acids Res* 1994; **22**: 1101–1107
48. Xi YGL, Ingrosso L, Ladogana A, Masullo C, Pocchiari M. Amphotericin B treatment dissociates in vivo replication of the scrapie agent from PrP accumulation. *Nature* 1992; **356**: 598–601
49. Lasmezas CI, Deslys JP, Robain O et al. Transmission of the BSE agent to mice in the absence of detectable abnormal prion protein. *Science* 1997; **275**: 402–405
50. Manuelidis L, Fritch W, Xi YG. Evolution of a strain of CJD that induces BSE-like plaques. *Science* 1997; **277**: 94–98
51. Kirschbaum WR. *Jakob-Creutzfeldt Disease*. Amsterdam: Elsevier, 1968; 1–25
52. Richardson EP Jr, Masters CL. The nosology of Creutzfeldt-Jakob disease and conditions related to the accumulation of PrPCJD in the nervous system. *Brain Pathol* 1995; **5**: 33–41
53. Masters CL, Gajdusek DC, Gibbs CJ Jr. The familial occurrence of Creutzfeldt-Jakob disease and Alzheimer's disease. *Brain* 1981; **104**: 535–558
54. Parchi P, Castellani R, Capellari S et al. Molecular basis of phenotypic variability in sporadic Creutzfeldt-Jakob disease. *Ann Neurol* 1996; **39**: 767–778
55. Kitamoto T, Shin RW, Doh-ura K et al. Abnormal isoform of prion proteins accumulates in the synaptic structures of the central nervous system in patients with Creutzfeldt-Jakob disease. *Am J Pathol* 1992; **140**: 1285–1294
56. Fraser H, Dickinson AG. Scrapie in mice. Agent-strain differences in the distribution and intensity of grey matter vacuolation. *J Comp Pathol* 1973; **83**: 29–40
57. Bruce ME, McConnell I, Fraser H, Dickinson AG. The disease characteristics of different strains of scrapie in Sinc congenic mouse lines: implications for the nature of the agent and host control of pathogenesis. *J Gen Virol* 1991; **72**: 595–603
58. Kascsak RJ, Rubenstein R, Merz PA et al. Immunological comparison of scrapie-associated fibrils isolated from animals infected with four different scrapie strains. *J Virol* 1986; **59**: 676–683
59. Bessen RA, Marsh RF. Distinct PrP properties suggest the molecular basis of strain variation in transmissible mink encephalopathy. *J Virol* 1994; **68**: 7859–7868
60. Parchi P, Capellari S, Chen SG et al. Typing prion isoforms. *Nature* 1997; **386**: 232–233
61. Parchi P, Capellari S, Chen SG et al. Similar posttranslational modifications of the prion protein in familial, sporadic, and iatrogenic Creutzfeldt-Jakob disease. *Soc Neurosci Abstr* 1996; 711
62. Palmer MS, Dryden AJ, Hughes JT, Collinge J. Homozygous prion protein genotype predisposes to sporadic Creutzfeldt-Jakob disease. *Nature* 1991; **352**: 340–342

63. Laplanche JL, Delasnerie-Laupretre N, Brandel JP et al. Molecular genetics of prion diseases in France. *Neurology* 1994; **44**: 2347–2351
64. Salvatore M, Genuardi M, Petraroli R, Masullo C, D'Alessandro M, Pocchiari M. Polymorphisms of the prion protein gene in Italian patients with Creutzfeldt-Jakob disease. *Hum Genet* 1994; **94**: 375–379
65. Windl O, Dempster M, Estibeiro JP et al. Genetic basis of Creutzfeldt-Jakob disease in the United Kingdom: a systematic analysis of predisposing mutations and allelic variation in the PRNP gene. *Hum Genet* 1996; **98**: 259–264
66. Brown P, Gibbs CJ Jr, Rodgers-Johnson P et al. Human spongiform encephalopathy: the National Institutes of Health series of 300 cases of experimentally transmitted disease. *Ann Neurol* 1994; **35**: 513–529
67. Klatzo I, Gajdusek DC, Zigas V. Pathology of kuru. *Lab Invest* 1959; **8**: 799–847
68. Scrimgeour EM, Masters CL, Alpers MP, Kaven J, Gajdusek DC. A clinico-pathological study of a case of kuru. *J Neurol Sci* 1983; **59**: 265–275
69. Hainfellner JA, Liberski PP, Guiroy DC et al. Pathology and immunocytochemistry of a kuru brain. *Brain Pathol* 1997; **7**: 547–553
70. Brown P, Cervenakova L, Goldfarb LG et al. Iatrogenic Creutzfeldt-Jakob disease: an example of the interplay between ancient genes and modern medicine. *Neurology* 1994; **44**: 291–293
71. Collinge J, Palmer MS, Dryden AJ. Genetic predisposition to iatrogenic Creutzfeldt-Jakob diseae. *Lancet* 1991; **337**: 1441–1442
72. Deslys JP, Marce D, Dormont D. Similar genetic susceptibility in iatrogenic and sporadic Creutzfeldt-Jakob disease. *J Gen Virol* 1994; **75**: 23–27
73. Brown P, Preece MA, Will RG. 'Friendly fire' in medicine: hormones, homografts, and Creutzfeldt-Jakob disease. *Lancet* 1992; **340**: 24–27
74. Martinez-Lage JF, Poza M, Sola J et al. Accidental transmission of Creutzfeldt-Jakob disease by dural cadaveric grafts. *J Neurol Neurosurg Psychiatry* 1994; **57**: 1091–1094
75. Miyashita K, Inuzuka T, Kondo H et al. Creutzfeldt-Jakob disease in a patient with a cadaveric dural graft. *Neurology* 1991; **41**: 940–941
76. Esmonde T, Lueck CJ, Symon L, Duchen LW, Will RG. Creutzfeldt-Jakob disease and lyophilised dura mater grafts: report of two cases. *J Neurol Neurosurg Psychiatry* 1993; **56**: 999–1000
77. Willison HJ, Gale AN, McLaughlin JE. Creutzfeldt-Jakob disease following cadaveric dura mater graft. *J Neurol Neurosurg Psychiatry* 1991; **59**: 940
78. Lane KL, Brown P, Howell DN et al. Creutzfeldt-Jakob disease in a pregnant woman with an implanted dura mater graft. *Neurosurgery* 1994; **34**: 737–740
79. Yamada S, Aiba T, Endo Y, Hara M, Kitamoto T, Tateishi J. Creutzfeldt-Jakob disease transmitted by a cadaveric dura mater graft. *Neurosurgery* 1994; **34**: 740–743
80. Billette de Villemeur T, Gelot A, Deslys JP et al. Iatrogenic Creutzfeldt-Jakob disease in three growth hormone recipients: a neuropathological study. *Neuropathol Appl Neurobiol* 1994; **20**: 111–117
81. Weller RO, Steart PV, Powell-Jackson JD. Pathology of Creutzfeldt-Jakob disease associated with pituitary-derived human growth hormone administration. *Neuropath Appl Neurobiol* 1986; **12**: 117–129
82. Holmes SJ, Ironside JW, Shalet SM. Neurosurgery in a patient with Creutzfeldt-Jakob disease after pituitary derived growth hormone therapy in childhood. *J Neurol Neurosurg Psychiatry* 1996; **60**: 333–335
83. Ellis CJ, Katifi H, Weller RO. A further British case of growth hormone induced Creutzfeldt-Jakob disease. *J Neurol Neurosurg Psychiatry* 1992; **55**: 1200–1202
84. Masson C, Delalande I, Deslys JP et al. Creutzfeldt-Jakob disease after pituitary-derived human growth hormone therapy: two cases with valine 129 homozygous genotype. *Neurology* 1994; **44**: 179–180
85. Cochius JI, Hyman N, Esiri MM. Creutzfeldt-Jakob disease in a recipient of human pituitary-derived gonadotrophin: a second case. *J Neurol Neurosurg Psychiatry* 1992; **55**: 1094–1095
86. Will RG, Ironside JW, Zeidler M et al. A new variant of Creutzfeldt-Jakob disease in the UK. *Lancet* 1996; **347**: 921–925
87. Chazot G, Broussolle E, Lapras C, Blättler T, Aguzzi A, Kopp N. New variant of Creutzfeldt-Jakob disease in a 26-year-old French man. *Lancet* 1996; **347**: 1181
88. Ironside JW. Review: Creutzfeldt-Jakob disease. *Brain Pathol* 1996; **6**: 379–388
89. Wells GAH, Wilesmith JW. The neuropathology and epidemiology of bovine spongiform encephalopathy. *Brain Pathol* 1995; **5**: 91–103

90. Lasmezas CI, Deslys JP, Demalmay R et al. BSE transmission to macaques. *Nature* 1996; **381**: 743–744
91. Collinge J, Sidle KCL, Meads J, Ironside J, Hill AF. Molecular analysis of prion strain variation and the aetiology of 'new variant' CJD. *Nature* 1996; **383**: 685–690
92. Raymond GJ, Hope J, Kocisko DA et al. Molecular assessment of the potential transmissibilities of BSE and scrapie to humans. *Nature* 1997; **388**: 285–288
93. Hsiao K, Meiner Z, Kahana E et al. Mutation of the prion protein in Libyan Jews with Creutzfeldt-Jakob disease. *N Engl J Med* 1991; **324**: 1091–1097
94. Chapman J, Brown P, Goldfarb LG, Arlazoroff A, Gajdusek DC, Korczyn AD. Clinical heterogeneity and unusual presentations of Creutzfeldt-Jakob disease in Jewish patients with the PRNP codon 200 mutation. *J Neurol Neurosurg Psychiatry* 1993; **56**: 1109–1112
95. Collinge J, Palmer MS, Campbell T, Sidle KCL, Carrol D, Harding A. Inherited prion disease (PrP lysine 200) in Britain: two case reports. *BMJ* 1993; **306**: 301–302
96. Bertoni JM, Brown P, Goldfarb LG, Rubenstein R, Gajdusek DC. Familial Creutzfeldt-Jakob disease (codon 200 mutation) with supranuclear palsy. *JAMA* 1992; **268**: 2413–2415
97. Antoine JC, Laplanche JL, Mosnier JF, Beavdry P, Chatelain J, Michel D. Demyelinating peripheral neuropathy with Creutzfeldt-Jakob disease and mutation at codon 200 of the prion protein gene. *Neurology* 1996; **46**: 1123–1127
98. Inoue I, Kitamoto T, Doh-ura K, Shii H, Goto I, Tateishi J. Japanese family with Creutzfeldt-Jakob disease with codon 200 point mutation of the prion protein gene. *Neurology* 1994; **44**: 299–301
99. Brown P, Goldfarb LG, Kovanen J et al. Phenotypic characteristics of familial Creutzfeldt-Jakob disease associated with the codon 178Asn PRNP mutation. *Ann Neurol* 1992; **31**: 282–285
100. Parchi P, Capellari S, Sima AAF et al. Creutzfeldt-Jakob disease associated with the 178Asn mutation in the prion protein gene: neuropathological and molecular features. *J Neuropath Exp Neurol* 1996; 55: **635**
101. Kitamoto T, Tateishi J. Human prion diseases with variant prion protein. *Phil Trans R Soc Lond [Biol]* 1994; **343**: 391–398
102. Hoque MZ, Kitamoto T, Furukawa H, Muramoto T, Tateishi J. Mutation in the prion protein gene at codon 232 in Japanese patients with Creutzfeldt-Jakob disease: a clinicopathological, immunohistochemical and transmission study. *Acta Neuropathol* 1996; **92**: 441–446
103. Ripoll L, Laplanche JL, Salzmann M et al. A new point mutation in the prion protein gene at codon 210 in Creutzfeldt-Jakob disease. *Neurology* 1993; **43**: 1934–1938
104. Pocchiari M, Salvatore M, Cutruzzola F et al. A new point mutation of the prion protein gene in Creutzfeldt-Jakob disease. *Ann Neurol* 1993; **34**: 802–807
105. Mastrianni JA, Iannicola C, Myers RM, DeArmond S, Prusiner SB. Mutation of the prion protein gene at codon 208 in familial Creutzfeldt-Jakob disease. *Neurology* 1996; **47**: 1305–1312
106. Nitrini R, Rosemberg S, Passos-Bueno MR et al. Familial spongiform encephalopathy associated with a novel prion gene mutation. *Ann Neurol* 1997; **42**: 138–146
107. Ghetti B, Dlouhy SR, Giaccone G et al. Gerstmann-Sträussler-Scheinker disease and the Indiana kindred. *Brain Pathol* 1995; **5**: 61–75
108. Ghetti B, Piccardo P, Spillantini MG et al. Vascular variant of prion protein cerebral amyloidosis with tau-positive neurofibrillary tangles: The phenotype of the stop codon 145 mutation in PRNP. *Proc Natl Acad Sci USA* 1996; **93**: 744–748
109. Hainfellner JA, Brantner-Inthaler S, Cervenáková L et al. The original Gerstmann-Sträussler-Scheinker family of Austria: divergent clinicopathological phenotypes but constant PrP genotype. *Brain Pathol* 1995; **5**: 201–211
110. Hsiao K, Baker HF, Crow TJ et al. Linkage of a prion protein missense variant to Gerstmann-Sträussler syndrome. *Nature* 1989; **338**: 342–345
111. Kretzschmar HA, Honold G, Seitelberger F et al. Prion protein mutation in family first reported by Gerstmann, Sträussler, and Scheinker. *Lancet* 1991; **337**: 1160
112. Adam J, Crow TJ, Duchen LW, Scaravilli F, Spokes E. Familial cerebral amyloidosis and spongiform encephalopathy. *J Neurol Neurosurg Psychiatry* 1982; **45**: 37–45
113. Barbanti P, Fabbrini G, Salvatore M et al. Polymorphism at codon 129 or codon 219 of PRNP and clinical heterogeneity in a previously unreported family with Gerstmann-Sträussler-Scheinker disease (PrP–P102L mutation). *Neurology* 1996; **47**: 734–741
114. Young K, Jones CK, Piccardo P et al. Gerstmann-Sträussler-Scheinker disease with mutation at codon 102 and methionine at codon 129 of PRNP in previously unreported patients. *Neurology* 1995; **45**: 1127–1134

115. Piccardo P, Ghetti B, Dickson DW et al. Gerstmann-Sträussler-Scheinker disease (PRNP P102L): amyloid deposits are best recognized by antibodies directed to epitopes in PrP region 90–165. *J Neuropathol Exp Neurol* 1995; **54**: 790–801
116. Furukawa H, Kitamoto T, Tanaka Y, Tateishi J. New variant prion protein in a Japanese family with Gerstmann-Sträussler syndrome. *Mol Brain Res* 1995; **30**: 385–388
117. Young K, Clark HB, Piccardo P, Dlouhy SR, Ghetti B. Gerstmann-Sträussler-Scheinker disease with the PRNP P102L mutation and valine at codon 129. *Mol Brain Res* 1997; **44**: 147–150
118. Tateishi J, Kitamoto T, Doh-ura K et al. Immunochemical, molecular genetic, and transmission studies on a case of Gerstmann-Sträussler-Scheinker syndrome. *Neurology* 1990; **40**: 1578–1581
119. Nakazato Y, Ohno R, Negishi T, Hamaguchi K, Arai E. An autopsy case of Gerstmann-Sträussler-Scheinker's disease with spastic paraplegia as its principal feature. *Clin Neurol* 1991; **31**: 987–992
120. Amano N, Yagishita S, Yokoi S et al. Gerstmann-Sträussler-Scheinker syndrome – a variant type: amyloid plaques and Alzheimer's neurofibrillary tangles in cerebral cortex. *Acta Neuropathol* 1992; **84**: 15–23
121. Kitamoto T, Amano N, Terao Y et al. A new inherited prion disease (PrP–P105L mutation) showing spastic paraparesis. *Ann Neurol* 1993; **34**: 808–813
122. Yamada M, Itoh Y, Fujigasaki H et al. A missense mutation at codon 105 with codon 129 polymorphism of the prion protein gene in a new variant of Gerstmann-Sträussler-Scheinker disease. *Neurology* 1993; **43**: 2723–2724.
123. Doh-ura K, Tateishi J, Sasaki H, Kitamoto T, Sakaki Y. Pro–Leu change at position 102 of prion protein is the most common but not the sole mutation related to Gerstmann-Sträussler syndrome. *Biochem Biophys Res Commun* 1989; **163**: 974–979
124. Hsiao KK, Cass C, Schellenberg GD et al. A prion protein variant in a family with the telencephalic form of Gerstmann-Sträussler-Scheinker syndrome. *Neurology* 1991; **41**: 681–684
125. Mastrianni JA, Curtis MT, Oberholtzer JC et al. Prion disease (PrP–A117V) presenting with ataxia instead of dementia. *Neurology* 1995; **45**: 2042–2050
126. Mohr M, Tranchant C, Heldt N, Warter JM. Alsatian variant of codon 117 form of Gerstmann-Sträussler-Scheinker syndrome: autopsic study of 3 cases. *Brain Pathol* 1994; **4**: 524
127. Tranchant C, Doh-ura K, Steinmetz G et al. Mutation du codon 117 du géne du prion dans une maladie de Gerstmann-Sträussler-Scheinker. *Rev Neurol (Paris)* 1991; **147**: 274–278
128. Tranchant C, Doh-ura K, Warter JM et al. Gerstmann-Sträussler-Scheinker disease in an Alsatian family – clinical and genetic studies. *J Neurol Neurosurg Psychiatry* 1992; **55**: 185–187
129. Warter JM, Steinmetz G, Heldt N et al. Demence pre-senile familiale: syndrome de Gerstmann-Sträussler-Scheinker. *Rev Neurol (Paris)* 1982; **138**: 107–121
130. Nochlin D, Sumi SM, Bird TD et al. Familial dementia with PrP-positive amyloid plaques: a variant of Gerstmann-Sträussler syndrome. *Neurology* 1989; **39**: 910–918
131. Hsiao K, Dlouhy SR, Farlow MR et al. Mutant prion proteins in Gerstmann-Sträussler-Scheinker disease with neurofibrillary tangles. *Nat Genet* 1992; **1**: 68–71
132. Dlouhy SR, Hsiao K, Farlow MR et al. Linkage of the Indiana kindred of Gerstmann-Sträussler-Scheinker disease to the prion protein gene. *Nat Genet* 1992; **1**: 64–67
133. Farlow MR, Yee RD, Dlouhy SR, Conneally PM, Azzarelli B, Ghetti B. Gerstmann-Sträussler-Scheinker disease. I. Extending the clinical spectrum. *Neurology* 1989; **39**: 1446–1452
134. Ghetti B, Tagliavini F, Masters CL et al. Gerstmann-Sträussler-Scheinker disease. II. Neurofibrillary tangles and plaques with PrP-amyloid coexist in an affected family. *Neurology* 1989; **39**: 1453–1461
135. Giaccone G, Verga L, Bugiani O et al. Prion protein preamyloid and amyloid deposits in Gerstmann-Sträussler-Scheinker disease, Indiana kindred. *Proc Natl Acad Sci USA* 1992; **89**: 9349–9353
136. Tagliavini F, Giaccone G, Prelli F et al. A68 is a component of paired helical filaments of Gerstmann-Sträussler-Scheinker disease, Indiana kindred. *Brain Res* 1993; **616**: 325–329
137. Kitamoto T, Iizuda R, Tateishi J. An amber mutation of prion protein in Gerstmann-Sträussler-Scheinker syndrome with mutant PrP plaques. *Biochem Biophys Res Commun* 1993; **192**: 525–531
138. Tagliavini F, Prelli F, Ghiso J et al. Amyloid protein of Gerstmann-Sträussler-Scheinker disease (Indiana kindred) is an 11 kD fragment of prion protein with an N-terminal glycine at codon 58. *EMBO J* 1991; **10**: 513–519

139. Tagliavini F, Prelli F, Porro M et al. Amyloid fibrils in Gerstmann-Sträussler-Scheinker disease (Indiana and Swedish kindreds) express only PrP peptides encoded by the mutant allele. *Cell* 1994; **79**: 695–703
140. Kitamoto T, Muramoto T, Hilbich C, Beyreuther K, Tateishi J. N-terminal sequence of prion protein is also integrated into kuru plaques in patients with Gerstmann-Sträussler syndrome. *Brain Res* 1991; **545**: 319–321
141. Kitamoto T, Yamaguchi K, Doh-ura K, Tateishi J. A prion protein missense variant is integrated in kuru plaque cores in patients with Gerstmann-Sträussler syndrome. *Neurology* 1991; **41**: 306–310
142. Giaccone G, Tagliavini F, Verga L et al. Neurofibrillary tangles of the Indiana kindred of Gerstmann-Sträussler-Scheinker disease share antigenic determinants with those of Alzheimer disease. *Brain Res* 1990; **530**: 325–329
143. Baker HF, Duchen LW, Jacobs JM, Ridley RM. Spongiform encephalopathy transmitted experimentally from Creutzfeldt-Jakob and familial Gerstmann-Sträussler-Scheinker diseases. *Brain* 1990; **113**: 1891–1909
144. Capellari S, Vital C, Parchi P et al. Familial prion disease with a 144 bp insertion in the prion protein gene in a Basque family. *Neurology* 1997; 49: 133–141
145. Cochran EJ, Bennett DA, Cervenakova L et al. Familial Creutzfeldt-Jakob disease with a five-repeat octapeptide insert mutation. *Neurology* 1996; **47**: 727–733
146. Lugaresi E, Medori R, Montagna P et al. Fatal familial insomnia and dysautonomia with selective degeneration of thalamic nuclei. *N Engl J Med* 1986; **315**: 997–1003
147. Cortelli P, Parchi P, Contin M et al. Cardiovascular dysautonomia in fatal familial insomnia. *Clin Autonom Res* 1991; **1**: 15–21
148. Medori R, Tritschler HJ, LeBlanc A et al. Fatal familial insomnia is a prion disease with a mutation at codon 178 of the prion protein gene. *N Engl J Med* 1992; **326**: 444–449
149. Medori R, Montagna P, Tritschler HJ et al. Fatal familial insomnia: a second kindred with mutation of prion protein gene at codon 178. *Neurology* 1992; **42**: 669–670
150. Gallassi R, Morreale A, Montagna P et al. Fatal familial insomnia: behavioral and cognitive features. *Neurology* 1996; **46**: 935–939
151. Manetto V, Medori R, Cortelli P et al. Fatal familial insomnia: Clinical and pathological study of five new cases. *Neurology* 1992; **42**: 312–319
152. Parchi P, Castellani R, Cortelli P et al. Regional distribution of protease-resistant prion protein in fatal familial insomnia. *Ann Neurol* 1995; **38**: 21–29
153. Gambetti P, Parchi P, Petersen RB, Chen SG, Lugaresi E. Fatal familial insomnia and familial Creutzfeldt-Jakob disease: clinical, pathological and molecular features. *Brain Pathol* 1995; **5**: 43–51
154. Goldfarb LG, Petersen RB, Tabaton M et al. Fatal familial insomnia and familial Creutzfeldt-Jakob disease: disease phenotype determined by a DNA polymorphism. *Science* 1992; **258**: 806–808
155. Monari L, Chen SG, Brown P et al. Fatal familial insomnia and familial Creutzfeldt-Jakob disease: different prion proteins determined by a DNA polymorphism. *Proc Natl Acad Sci USA* 1994; **91**: 2839–2842
156. Tateishi J, Brown P, Kitamoto T et al. First experimental transmission of fatal familial insomnia. *Nature* 1995; **376**: 434–435
157. Collinge J, Palmer MS, Sidle KC et al. Transmission of fatal familial insomnia to laboratory animals. *Lancet* 1995; **346**: 569–570
158. Stern K. Severe dementia associated with bilateral symmetrical degeneration of the thalamus. *Brain* 1939; **62**: 157–171
159. Petersen RB, Tabaton M, Berg L et al. Analysis of the prion protein gene in thalamic dementia. *Neurology* 1992; **42**: 1859–1863
160. Mizusawa H, Ohkoshi N, Sasaki H, Kanazawa I, Nakanishi T. Degeneration of the thalamus and inferior olives associated with spongiform encephalopathy of the cerebral cortex. *Clin Neuropathol* 1988; **7**: 81–86
161. Jendroska K, Heinzel FP, Torchia M et al. Proteinase-resistant prion protein accumulation in Syrian hamster brain correlates with regional pathology and scrapie infectivity. *Neurology* 1991; **41**: 1482–1490
162. Castellani R, Parchi P, Stahl J, Capellari S, Cohen M, Gambetti P. Early pathologic and biochemical changes in Creutzfeldt-Jakob disease: study of brain biopsies. *Neurology* 1996; **46**: 1690–1693
163. Silvestrini MC, Cardone F, Maras B et al. Identification of the prion protein allotypes which accumulate in the brain of sporadic and familial Creutzfeldt-Jakob disease patients. *Nat Med* 1997; **3**: 521–525

164. Chen SG, Parchi P, Brown P et al. Allelic origin of the abnormal prion protein in familial prion diseases. *Nat Med* 1997; **3**: 1009–1015
165. Gabizon R, Telling G, Meiner Z, Halimi M, Kahana I, Prusiner SB. Insoluble wild-type and protease-resistant mutant prion protein in brains of patients with inherited prion disease. *Nat Med* 1996; **2**: 59–64
166. Tagliavini F, Prelli F, Porro M et al. Only mutant PrP participates in amyloid formation in Gerstmann-Sträussler-Scheinker disease with Ala–Val substitution at codon 117. *J Neuropathol Exp Neurol* 1995; **54**: 416
167. Riek R, Hornemann S, Wider G, Billeter M, Glockshuber R, Wüthrich K. NMR structure of the mouse prion protein domain PrP (121–231). *Nature* 1997; **382**: 180–182
168. Caughey B, Chesebro B. Prion protein and the transmissible spongiform encephalopathies. *Trends Cell Biol* 1997; **7**: 56–62
169. Silburn P, Cervenakova L, Varghese P, Tannenberg A, Brown P, Boyle R. Fatal familial insomnia: a seventh family. *Neurology* 1996; **47**: 1326–1328
170. Nagayama M, Shinohara Y, Furukawa H, Kitamoto T. Fatal familial insomnia with a muatation at codon 178 of the prion protein gene: first report from Japan. *Neurology* 1996; **47**: 1313–1316
171. Cortelli P, Perani D, Parchi P et al. Cerebral metabolism in fatal familial insomnia: Relation to duration, neuropathology, and distribution of protease-resistent prion protein. *Neurology* 1997; **49**: 126–133
172. Bruce ME, Will RG, Ironside JW et al. Transmissions to mice indicate that 'new variantæ CJD is caused by the BSE agent. *Nature* 1997; **389**: 498–501

4

Telomeres, tumour-suppressors and lifespan checkpoints: implications for tumour pathology

David Wynford-Thomas

BIOLOGY OF CELLULAR AGING

THEORIES OF AGING

It is now 30 years since Hayflick first quantified the finite proliferative lifespan of normal human fibroblasts and defined the essential features of cellular senescence.[1] It has, of course, since become well-established that such limited proliferative capacity is a fundamental characteristic of all normal mammalian somatic cells, albeit varying in magnitude with species and cell type. Even stem cells should probably not be considered an exception since, although sustained, their proliferation is asymmetric, always yielding one mortal daughter cell.

Two theories of cellular (and by inference organismal) senescence have competed over these last three decades. The 'random error' hypothesis[2] views senescence as the passive consequence of accumulated damage to cellular macro-molecules and is essentially a 'wear and tear' concept of aging which has been difficult to either prove or refute. While it is clear that 'damage', particularly that due to reactive oxygen species, can reduce proliferative lifespan,[3,4] as a fundamental **cause** of aging this has been increasingly overshadowed during the last 5 years by the concept of 'programmed' senescence. This regards aging as an active, predetermined, process based on some form of cell division counter, and owes its recent popularity to the emergence of a highly plausible candidate for such a biological clock: the erosion of chromosomal telomeres.[5]

Prof. David Wynford-Thomas, Department of Pathology, University of Wales College of Medicine, Heath Park, Cardiff CF4 4XN, UK

THE TELOMERE CLOCK

Telomeres form the specialised ends of chromosomes in all species and in vertebrates are composed of a tandem array of thousands of copies of a single repeat sequence (TTAGGG), together with associated telomere binding proteins.[6] Although probably evolved to serve a number of functions concerned with protection of chromosomal integrity (see below), their significance as a timer stems from the so-called 'end-replication' problem[7] which is the intrinsic inability of DNA polymerases to complete replication of the 3′ end of a DNA duplex due to the obligate requirement for an upstream RNA primer. This means that, in every round of replication, the newly synthesised lagging strand is missing the extreme 5′-terminus, which sets up a progressive erosion of telomere sequence, amounting in mammalian cells to 50–200 bp per generation. Germ cells (and perhaps stem cells[8,9]) escape this problem by expressing an enzyme – telomerase – which opposes the effect of erosion by synthesising new terminal repeat elements using an RNA template containing the telomere array sequence. The activity of this enzyme is normally repressed at a specific point in embryonic development,[10] whereafter the telomere clock begins to tick.

Published measurements of telomere lengths have been notoriously variable due to true biological variation in telomere repeat number between chromosomes plus the fact that Southern blot measurements rely upon measuring a terminal restriction fragment (TRF) which also includes a sub-telomeric region which itself varies between chromosomes. Nevertheless, the prediction has held true that telomere length does shorten as a function of proliferative age[11,12] and, therefore, represents a plausible basis on which to construct a clock. Human diploid fibroblasts, for example, have a mean TRF length of 7–9 kbp in the adult, which falls to around 5–7 kbp by the time the cells reach the senescence limit described by Hayflick.[11–13]

TWO-STAGE MORTALITY: SENESCENCE AND CRISIS

The classic state of 'senescence' in normal fibroblasts represents a phenotype in which, although proliferatively arrested, cells remain biochemically active and viable for long periods.[14] This is programmed aging *par excellence*, as evidenced for example by the induction of specific genes known to inhibit cell proliferation, notably ($p21^{WAF1}$)[15] and ($p16^{INK4a}$).[16] Also consistent with this idea of an active process of growth arrest is its abrogation by many DNA tumour virus gene products which target specific cellular regulatory proteins, in particular the tumour suppressor gene products p53 and p105Rb.[17]

At least in the human, however, such escape from senescence is only temporary, cells eventually entering a second state of growth arrest originally termed 'crisis',[18,19] in the case of fibroblasts reached after a further 20–30 population doublings. Unlike senescence, this is characterised not so much by a fall in birth rate as by an increase in death rate, accompanied by nuclear pleomorphism and abnormal mitoses. At a cytogenetic level, there is also gross disruption of chromosomal structure and number. Although the stochastic nature of much of this 'damage' is reminiscent of the 'error theory' of aging, it is in fact the predictable consequence of the further running of the telomere clock, in this case resulting from loss of telomere function rather than from activation of a growth arrest switch. Indeed, crisis can be thought of as an interesting convergence of the 'programmed' and 'error' theories. Escape from crisis, which is much rarer in human than rodent cells, appears to depend on restoration of telomere stability by reactivation of telomerase or an equivalent mechanism.[19,20]

These two hurdles, senescence and crisis, which the normal cell must overcome to escape mortality, correspond to mortality stage 1 (M1) and stage 2 (M2) in the now much cited model of Shay and Wright (Fig. 1).[5,18]

THE TELOMERE CLOCK AND M2 CRISIS

Telomeres and their associated proteins may preserve chromosome integrity by preventing exonuclease attack, by permitting nuclear matrix attachment, and perhaps most importantly by preventing end-to-end fusion. These functions appear to be critically diminished when **mean** telomere length falls to around 1–2 kb, although this probably reflects the near-total loss of telomeres from a sub-set of chromosomes. (Proof of this should soon be available with the development of more sensitive methods for *in situ* detection and measurement of telomere length.[21]) Most of the cytogenetic features of cells in crisis are readily explicable on the basis of loss of end-protecting function, for example, telomeric associations, dicentrics, and the broken chromosomes and aneuploidy which follow from the resulting fusion-bridge-breakage cycles.[22]

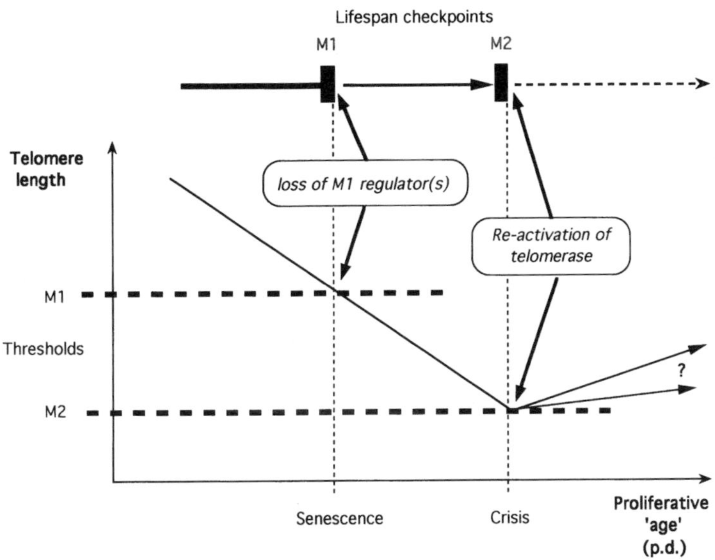

Fig. 1 Proliferative aging programmed by telomere erosion. Schematic illustrating the basic mortality control model (adapted from Wynford-Thomas et al[83] and Holt et al.[89]) To become immortal a cell needs to overcome two check-points: escape from M1 (senescence) is achieved by abrogation of growth-arrest signals; escape from M2 requires stabilisation of telomere length, by telomerase activation or an equivalent mechanism.

Measurement of proliferative lifespan in cells induced to escape M1, e.g. by tumour virus oncogenes in tissue culture, suggest that crisis does not supervene until cells have completed as many as 50 or more population doublings beyond their normal adult state (although, of course, only a limited range of cell types have been studied, notably fibroblasts,[18] breast[23,24] and squamous[25] epithelium). This is consistent with observed normal telomere lengths of > 8 kbp in most adult cells and an erosion rate of 50–200 bp per population doublings.

At first sight, therefore, given that 50 population doublings corresponds to a clonal expansion of 2^{50}, i.e. 10^{15} cells, one might imagine that crisis could never represent a biologically significant barrier to normal (or tumour) cell proliferation! Why this is not so for tumour growth is explained below; for normal tissues, it is a misleading calculation since it is, of course, based on pure exponential growth. In reality, it should impose a very real potential hurdle for the life-long proliferation of stem cells in renewing tissues such as surface epithelia, since even assuming the longest estimates of cell cycle time, many stem cells (e.g. those of intestinal epithelium) would need to complete many hundreds if not thousands of population doublings in a normal human lifespan.[26] This has led some to believe that stem cells must be spared from telomere erosion by constitutive expression of telomerase. Although telomerase activity can be detected in some renewing tissues, notably bone marrow,[27–29] its significance remains uncertain,[30] not least because of the difficulty in defining the stem cell population quite apart from measuring its telomere length, and the confounding influence of cell growth state on telomerase activity.[31] (Clarification may be forthcoming when *in situ* assays of telomere length and telomerase activity are developed.)

The alternative possibility is that the process of telomere erosion, although occurring in stem cells, does not affect the length of telomeres in the retained daughter cell because the eroded newly-synthesised DNA strand is always preferentially segregated to the differentiating daughter cell. Such asymmetric retention of ‘immortal DNA strands’ was suggested many years ago in a different context to account for unexpectedly low rates of mutation in stem cell populations.[32,33] Viewed in this way, the low level telomerase activity detected in bone marrow may simply be required to repair random damage to the immortal-strand telomeres, rather than to prevent replication-related erosion.

On either basis, the notion that stem cells are preferentially protected from telomere erosion provides an interesting prediction in relation to the pathology of epithelial dysplasia. The fundamental proliferative abnormality in this process is usually assumed to be the retention of proliferating post-stem cells which have escaped the normally inevitable fate of differentiation and cell death, such that, although there may be still an overall balance between birth and death rate in the epithelium, the normal asymmetry of stem cell division has been disrupted. If such neoplastic cells, although escaping differentiation, have nevertheless lost the telomere-preserving mechanism postulated above for true stem cells, then, with time, they should eventually approach the M2 barrier. It is interesting, therefore, that many of the cytological and cytogenetic features of dysplasia closely resemble those seen in tissue culture cells in crisis. Further progression of such early dysplastic lesions is presumably dependent on the random reactivation of telomerase which although rare (probably less than 1 per million cell divisions in human fibroblasts, for example[34,35]) will, nevertheless, be expected given the total target cell population size involved.

THE TELOMERE CLOCK AND M1 SENESCENCE

THE COUNTER

While it can be seen from the above that telomere erosion is almost certainly the underlying cause for the breakdown of normal chromosome function at crisis, how good is the evidence that it also represents the biological clock driving the **programmed** arrest at M1 senescence? The basic observation, that telomere length shortens both in vitro and in vivo as a function of the number of cell doublings, rather than simply elapsed time, has so far held true.[11,12,19,25] It has also been shown that in isolates from donors of differing age, the remaining proliferative capacity of cells varies predictably with the initial telomere length.[36] Finally, although somewhat less convincing, there is also evidence that telomere length tends, as predicted, to reach a constant lower limit at senescence.[13]

Many of these observations have been hampered by the technical difficulty of obtaining accurate measurements of telomere repeat length, most relying on the rather imprecise measurement of the mean TRF length by Southern blotting which, as noted above, contains a variable component contributed by the sub-telomeric region.[13] There is also a considerable true variation in the length of telomere repeats and it is still not clear whether the senescence signal is generated in response to the mean or to the shortest telomeres in any given cell. Overall, though, there is a powerful, if still correlative, body of evidence to support the view that telomere shortening is the fundamental signal for M1. What is needed now is a critical interventional experiment, for example the demonstration that introduction of a normal chromosome with senescent telomere length will induce senescence in a young fibroblast, thereby reproducing the result already obtained by somatic cell hybridisation between senescent and young cells. Some progress towards this aim was provided by the demonstration that experimentally-induced **elongation** of telomeres resulted in extension of lifespan,[37] although since this experiment was done in SV40-expressing cells it probably addresses the role of telomere erosion in signalling M2 rather than M1.

THE SENSOR

Two (not necessarily exclusive) hypotheses have been put forward to explain how telomere attrition might trigger growth arrest in senescent cells (reviewed in Wright & Shay[5]). The 'chromatin conformation' mechanism postulates that telomere erosion exerts a *cis*-acting influence on sub-telomeric heterochromatin resulting in altered expression (presumably on just one or a few chromosomes) of genes signalling growth arrest. Similar mechanisms can be envisaged, based on altered association of telomere binding proteins on eroded telomeres.

The second, conceptually-different proposal is that the essential trigger results not from the change in the average telomere length, but from a greater degree of erosion occurring in a random sub-set of chromosomes. It is known that there is an increasing spread of telomere length as cells approach senescence and there is long-standing cytogenetic data to suggest that in the last few divisions there is failure of the end-protecting function of at least a few telomeres per cell, as evidenced by the onset of telomere association events.[38] This suggests that some telomeres may have been eroded to the point where, either directly, or indirectly through the consequences of end-to-end fusion, a DNA 'damage' signal is generated which is of course a well-established stimulus for cell cycle arrest.[39,40] This also provides a highly plausible basis for the role of p53 in mediating M1 growth arrest (as discussed at length below).

THE EFFECTORS

Since DNA tumour viruses have evolved efficient ways of preventing senescence in their host cells, it is not surprising that they have provided important clues to the key cellular effectors of senescence. Two major common targets are the products of the tumour suppressor genes p53[41,42] and the retinoblastoma-susceptibility gene RB,[43] which play a key role in two growth-inhibitory signal pathways which appear to function either alternatively or co-operatively, depending upon cell type (see below and Fig. 2). Here we will describe their role in the most well-characterised model – the human fibroblast – before, in a later section, discussing potentially more relevant epithelial cell types.

p53: 'guardian of cellular senescence'

Initial experiments suggested that in fibroblasts both pRb and p53 needed to be inactivated before cells could begin to escape M1.[23] This work relied, however, on transfection of young fibroblasts, which exhibit a wide range of variability in remaining lifespan, sufficient to potentially blur the effect of any genetic manipulation. We re-analysed this question,[44] exploiting the ability of amphotropic retroviral vectors to target a near-senescent cell population, in which most of this lifespan variablity had been removed by the synchronising effect of growth to within a few population doublings of M1. In this way, it could be shown conclusively that expression of a dominant-negative p53 mutant was able to extend the normal lifespan of human fibroblasts by an average of 17, and in some cases over 25 population doublings.[44] The conclusion, that wild-type p53 function is essential for normal entry into M1 senescence, is now also supported by complementary findings in fibroblasts from Li-Fraumeni syndrome (LFS) patients, which again indicate that loss of wild-type p53 delays entry into senescence by at least 20–30 population doublings.[45]

An extension of this sort of magnitude may not seem great in comparison with the normal lifespan of the cell, and indeed further escape to generate an immortal line is exceedingly rare in LFS (and was never observed in our experiments). Nevertheless, 20–30 population doublings is more than sufficient to represent a strong selective pressure for loss of p53 in a tumour clone which is reaching senescence and is, of course, enough to allow a high probability for additional mutations leading to yet further extension of proliferative lifespan.

Given that wild-type p53 function is necessary (if not sufficient) for the normal operation of the M1 lifespan checkpoint, it is important to determine whether it is acting as a direct switch in this process or is simply needed at a constant permissive level to allow the operation of some other inducer. Strong support for an active role has recently been obtained by studying one of the major biochemical functions of p53, its ability to act as a transcription factor.[41,46] Using a clone of normal human fibroblasts stably expressing a p53-driven reporter construct (expressing the histochemically-detectable enzyme β-galactosidase), we have shown that as cells approach senescence, in the last few population doublings there is a dramatic increase in expression of the reporter, in almost perfect inverse correlation to the rate of cell proliferation.[47] This, together with complementary data from Atadja et al,[48] provides strong, albeit correlative, evidence that activation of the *trans*-activating function of p53 plays an essential role in normal entry to senescence (although of course it does not formally exclude an additional requirement for one of the other less well-characterised biochemical functions of p53,[41] such as transcriptional repression, transcription-independent signalling, or direct inhibition of DNA replication).

An obvious downstream target for transcriptional activation by p53 is the major cell cycle inhibitor p21$^{sdi1/WAF1}$, which was originally cloned on the basis of its marked induction in senescent cells.[15] This protein inhibits several of the key cyclin-dependent kinases which are essential for normal passage through the G1 phase of the cell cycle.[49] In our hands at least, however, we have found that the induction of p21 in senescent fibroblasts is not abolished by mutant p53,[50] leaving open, therefore, the identity of the downstream targets of p53 in these cells (Z in Fig. 2). Possibilities could include any of a wide range of growth inhibitory target genes, including GADD45[51] and IGF BP3.[52]

pRb: the 'back-up' pathway?

Although abrogation of p53 function clearly leads to a failure to enter M1 after the normal number of divisions, the extension of lifespan is always finite and indeed is significantly less than that produced by a dual knockout of both pRb and p53 (Bond et al, unpublished observations).[23] Similarly, single knockout of pRb (as obtained, for example, with the human papilloma virus HPVE7 oncogene) produces a sub-maximal extension of lifespan, similar to that produced by loss of p53 alone. This leads to a model (Fig. 2) in which two parallel pathways, one dependent on p53, the other on pRb, co-operate to bring about normal M1 in an additive manner. If either is eliminated, however, it can be envisaged that the other undergoes hyper-induction as cells proliferate past M1, until its activity eventually reaches a point where it can bring about growth arrest on its own, albeit at a later than normal proliferative age.

The pRb protein is a very plausible candidate mediator for such a second pathway, since it stands at a key 'gateway' in cell cycle progression. Normal G1 to S phase cell-cycle transition is dependent on inactivation of its growth-repressor activity through phosphorylation,[43] and a well-established

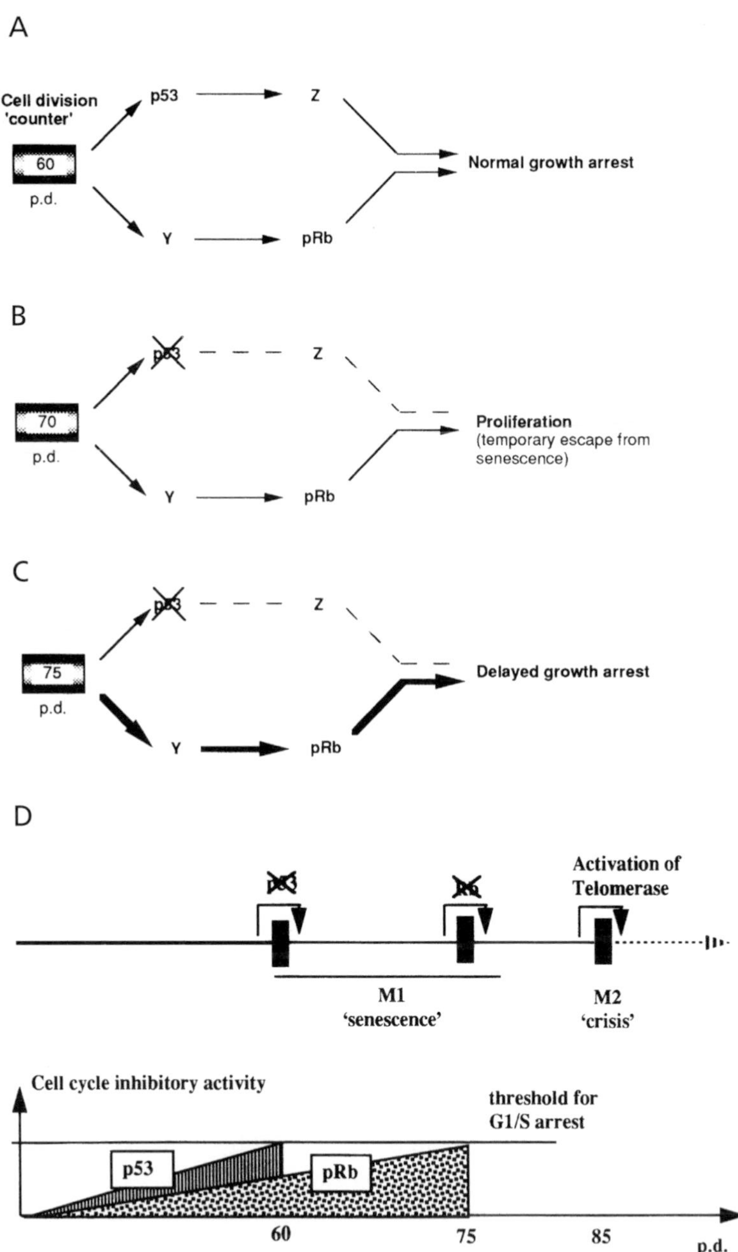

Fig. 2 'Dual circuit braking' in the human fibroblast. Highly simplified signal diagrams (A–C) illustrating how the interaction between p53 and pRb-dependent pathways provides a 'back-up' against escape from senescence. **(A)** Normal growth arrest at senescence (~60 population doublings) requires the concerted action of both p53 and pRb dependent pathways; **(B)** if one pathway is lost (p53 in this example), the overall growth inhibitory signal becomes insufficient, and proliferation continues past the normal M1; **(C)** ultimately, however, a delayed growth arrest is achieved by further up-regulation the remaining pathway (in this case Rb), to the point where it substitutes for the missing pathway. This allows M1 to be effectively divided into two successive lifespan checkpoints **(D)**. Only if both are eliminated can the cell proceed to M2. (See text for further discussion.)

biochemical feature of senescent fibroblasts is their failure to phosphorylate pRb, despite the presence of adequate extra-cellular growth signals.[53] The most likely explanation for this is the overactivity in senescent cells of inhibitors of Rb kinases of which one, p21$^{sdi1/WAF1}$, has already been mentioned.[15] Another major candidate is the cyclin kinase inhibitor (p16^{INK4a}),[54] which is also markedly induced in senescence[16] and is now known to be a frequent target for mutational loss in tumours and immortal cell lines.[54] What is currently not so clear is the nature of the detector (Y in Fig. 2) which could link the telomere clock to expression of such genes, independently of p53. Perhaps this pathway is activated, not by a 'DNA damage' related mechanism as postulated for p53, but by the alternative telomere-related signal based on altered expression of sub-telomeric genes.[5] More provocatively, of course, a non-telomere-dependent clock for this pathway can still not be formally excluded! Indeed, this would explain the worrying anomaly that fibroblasts from the laboratory mouse (*Mus musculus*) senesce more rapidly than human cells, despite having enormously long telomeres.[55]

Finally, for completeness, it should be mentioned that somatic cell hybridisation experiments point to the existence of at least one more independent pathway capable of inducing senescence, since some lines which have lost both p53 and Rb can be shown to cross-complement each other.[56]

HOW TUMOURS EVADE THE TELOMERE CLOCK

EVASION OF M2 CRISIS: ROLE OF TELOMERASE

The first evidence that reactivation of telomerase may allow tumour cells to escape the otherwise lethal consequence of loss of functional telomeres came from in vitro immortalisation models. In an elegant study of human embryo kidney cell transformation by SV40T or adenovirus 5, Counter and colleagues[19] demonstrated that mean telomere (TTAGGG repeat) length declined progressively at a rate of around 65 bp per generation until at a lower limit of around 1.5 kbp, the culture entered crisis. Those rare sub-clones which escaped to give rise to immortal lines all showed stabilised telomere length at or slightly above this value, and were shown to express telomerase activity as measured on an in vitro substrate. Similar results were soon obtained in other cell types, for example, EBV-expressing lymphocytes[57] and cervical epithelial cells and keratinocytes expressing HPVE6/E7.[25] In all cases, escape from crisis was tightly correlated to telomerase reactivation, although the subsequent behaviour of telomere length varied, in some cases remaining just above the crisis level, in others growing to reach significantly higher levels.[25]

Extension of this work to real human tumours was thwarted for some time by the onerous nature of the biochemical assay for telomerase activity, which required preparing extract from around 10^8 cells. Nevertheless, Counter and colleagues[58] succeeded in demonstrating the existence of such activity in metastatic ovarian cancer by making use of ascitic fluid as a convenient source of cells.

The development[59,60] of a PCR-based telomerase assay (TRAP) allowing analysis of very small cell numbers and tiny biopsies opened the way to a flood of investigations on clinical samples.[59,61] In general, these have confirmed the initial expectation, i.e. that the vast majority of cancers have reactivated telomerase, presumably as a requirement for escape from crisis. The broadly 'late' timing of reactivation observed so far in most experimental[62] and human[59,63] tumours is also consistent with this view. Of course, the exact relationship with clinico-pathological 'stage' is expected to be complex, since it is difficult from current knowledge to predict the point at which critical telomere erosion will occur during the development of any given tumour type. This will depend on the initial telomere length of the cell of origin, the rate of telomere erosion and the number of prior population doublings which have been undergone by the tumour cell population. The latter is not simply related to tumour size, since it will vary depending on the number of successive clonal selection steps undergone, and on the prevailing rates of cell death during the tumour's history.[61] Where these parameters are favourable, a tumour population may achieve malignant transformation and reach a clinically significant size without the need to activate telomerase – good examples being some neuroblastomas[64] and retinoblastoma,[61] and many low-grade hematological malignancies.[29] In most tissues, however, telomerase activation becomes necessary at some point in this progression, corresponding to the benign-malignant transition in the multi-step models analysed to date,[59,63], and making telomerase a potentially useful marker of malignancy.

The mechanism for reactivation of telomerase remains one of the key unanswered questions at present and will require a much greater understanding of its normal control. In human tissues, activity does not correlate well with expression of the RNA component of the enzyme,[65] suggesting that the critical level of control may be at the expression of the protein component. The prevailing assumption, of course, is that the underlying mechanism for reactivation is somatic mutation resulting in loss of expression or function of a repressor of telomerase expression, which is assumed to be constitutively present in normal somatic cells. Fusions between mortal and immortal cells[37] support this, and suggest that chromosome transfer experiments may provide a starting point for cloning of such repressors.[66]

Some current puzzles

There are now a significant number of observations which would not have been predicted from the original telomerase theory. Perhaps most surprising is the finding that some immortal, transformed human cell lines have stable, and indeed often exceptionally long, telomeres with no evidence of telomerase activity, even using the highly sensitive TRAP assay.[20] So far, this has been restricted to cell lines transformed by DNA tumour viral oncogenes suggesting[20] that it may not be relevant to real human cancers. Nevertheless, it points to the existence of a telomerase-independent mechanism for maintaining long stable telomeres, which by analogy with lower organisms, could be achieved by recombination.

The opposite paradox has also now been described, i.e. tumour cells which are telomerase-positive but, nevertheless, show progressive telomere erosion. This appears to be a characteristic feature of haematological malignancies, particularly chronic leukemias.[29] In this case, the explanation appears to be that the normal cell of origin is itself telomerase-positive (at least when assessed by the TRAP assay). As discussed above, this appears to be a feature of many bone marrow derived cells (including mature stages) the biological role of which is not clear, particularly given the evidence for continuing shortening of telomeres in these cells with age in vivo.[30] It may reflect a requirement for low levels of telomerase activity to repair spontaneous telomere damage. Alternatively, it may simply be a pitfall of the in vitro TRAP assay's insensitivity to additional levels of control operating only in the intact cell. For example, modulatory proteins which normally limit access of the telomerase to its substrate[67] may not function in the test-tube assay.

We have recently observed a similar phenomenon in lines derived from differentiated thyroid cancers which display substantial levels of telomerase activity by TRAP assay in culture but, nevertheless, show progressive telomere decline (Jones et al, manuscript in preparation). Interestingly, long-term culture shows that telomere length eventually stabilises at a lower limit rather longer than that observed in most post-crisis cells and without there being any corresponding increase in telomerase activity. Furthermore, the dynamics of telomere length correlated very poorly with the actual level of telomerase activity in different sub-clones. Again, these data support the idea that additional levels of control operate in the intact cell which are not reflected in the TRAP assay. As suggested by de Lange,[67] telomere binding proteins are an obvious candidate and indeed may play an essential homeostatic role in determining the length at which telomeres stabilise for any given level of telomerase activity.

In thyroid, in contrast to bone marrow, telomerase activity was not detectable in normal cells (even with TRAP) so, unlike in the case of hematological malignancies, the activity seen in thyroid cancer cells must be due to its re-activation at some point in clonal evolution. Our observation that this activity appears to be ineffective, however, in preventing telomere erosion, calls into question what selective advantage it could have for the tumour cell! Currently, the most likely explanation is that there is none and that this represents an example of telomerase activation as a **secondary** consequence of some other genetic event (e.g. tumour suppressor gene, TSG, inactivation) for which there **is** selective pressure. This idea is supported by the finding that DNA virus oncogenes known to target TSG's (e.g. HPVE6) have been shown to induce telomerase re-activation in some cases.[68]

Similarly, in a model of murine breast carcinogenesis induced by the wnt-1 oncogene,[55] a marked increase in telomerase activity occurs apparently before any significant telomere erosion has taken place. Indeed, it is now clear that in telomerase-competent cells (most cancers), wide variations in the level of telomerase activity can occur merely as a secondary accompaniment of changes in the rate of cell proliferation.[31] Clearly, such observations are a major source of potential misinterpretation when analysing clinical samples, for which information on the dynamic behaviour of telomere length will of course be lacking.

EVASION OF M1 SENESCENCE: CELL-SPECIFIC LIFESPAN CHECKPOINTS

Whereas escape from M2 would appear to involve a very limited set of mechanisms, the same is not true of M1, where it is now becoming clear that a range of 'options' exist, reflecting the diversity of the normal control pathways maintaining senescence in different cell types. Indeed, the 'choice' of cell lifespan checkpoint control in a normal cell may well have a profound influence on the subsequent behaviour of its tumours. In the case of fibroblasts, for example, escape from M1 should require loss of function of both the p53 and Rb pathways, either directly, or indirectly – through expression of inhibitors such as mdm2[69] or loss of mediators such as ($p16^{INK4a}$)[16] – and this accords broadly with molecular analysis of human sarcomas.[70, 71] The same dual-knockout applies to epithelial populations in which both pathways are involved, a good example being carcinomas of the head and neck derived from squamous epithelium in which again p53 mutation often coincides with loss of ($p16^{INK4a}$).[72] This is also consistent with in vitro experiments demonstrating the need to lose both pathways for efficient immortalisation of squamous epithelium.[25,73] In some other cell types, however, the picture appears to be surprisingly simpler, with only one of the two major pathways apparently playing a role. Although, unfortunately, only a few cell types have been analysed in sufficient detail, examples of each of these 'extreme' cases can now be cited.

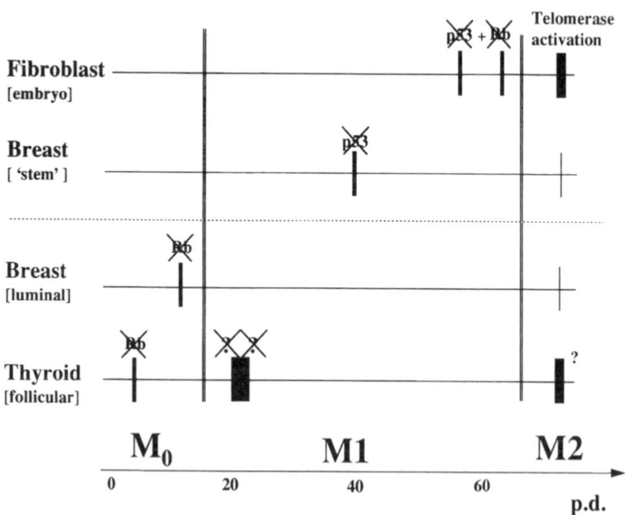

Fig. 3 Cell-type diversity in the nature and timing of lifespan check-points. For each cell type, the vertical bars indicate the approximate timing of checkpoints (based on population doublings observed in tissue culture). For M_0/M1, the cell cycle regulator(s) whose loss is sufficient to allow escape are shown (where known). For M2 escape, it is assumed that telomerase activation will be common to all. The width of the bars indicates the probability that escape will occur (thickest = least likely). The four human cell types appear to fall into two groups: (i) fibroblasts and 'stem-type' (poorly differentiated) breast epithelium show a classic 'late' M1 block regulated minimally by p53 (plus pRb in the fibroblast); a,d (ii) well-differentiated breast (luminal) and thyroid (follicular) epithelial cells have a much earlier (M_0), p53-independent, checkpoint regulated by pRb (in the case of thyroid there is also a later block mediated by an, as yet, undefined mechanism).

Control by a p53-dependent pathway only

Band and colleagues[74] first made the observation that primary cultures derived from normal (mammoplasty) breast tissue contained an epithelial population which could surprisingly be immortalised efficiently by introduction of just a single DNA tumour virus oncogene (HPV E6) which was known to target p53 without affecting the function of pRb. Subsequently, Shay confirmed and extended this result by showing[23] that, in sharp contrast to fibroblasts, in these breast epithelial cells expression of E6 not only extends lifespan but also confers immortalisation competence (and with a surprisingly high frequency). This result has now also been reproduced with vectors expressing mutant p53 (as opposed to viral genes), albeit with only one of a series of mutants.[75] Additional expression of HPV E7 (thereby abrogating pRb) in breast cells expressing E6 conferred no extra proliferative capacity at any stage, and when expressed alone E7 has no effect on their lifespan, both results contrasting sharply with fibroblast data.

Taken together, these data strongly suggest, therefore, that in this population of breast cells, loss of p53 function is sufficient to fully escape M1 and argues that the putative Rb-dependent pathway (Y in Fig. 2) is either absent or incapable of generating a significant inhibitory signal even in post-M1 cultures. It also emphasises the importance of the Rb-independent signal pathway (Z in Fig. 2) in mediating the action of p53.

It can readily be imagined that the apparent dependence of these cells on just a single control mechanism should make them more vulnerable than fibroblasts to spontaneous escape from senescence.[76] This, together with their apparently higher intrinsic ability to escape M2,[34] may well contribute to their greater tumorigenic potential in vivo. At the very least it would predict a major selective advantage for loss of p53 function in an emerging tumour clone.

Control by a p53-independent pathway only

It is now becoming clear that the cells analysed in the above studies are not representative of the major component of breast epithelium in vivo, but represent instead a small sub-population which has been highly selected for by the in vitro conditions used. These cells show features intermediate between that of myo-epithelial and luminal cells,[77] characterised by expression of 'basal' markers vimentin and cytokeratin 14, together with luminal markers 8 and 18 (but not 19), and lack expression of estrogen receptor (ER). They are likely to correspond to the 'basal' phenotype postulated by Papadimitriou and colleagues[78] to represent a stem cell population, which importantly appears to give rise to a more aggressive sub-set of breast cancers (see below).

The major in vivo population, which displays the classic luminal phenotype (positive for cytokeratin 8, 18 and 19 and ER; negative for vimentin) has been less adequately investigated, due to greater technical difficulties in cell culture. Recent studies, however,[24,79] are now pointing to a remarkable difference in the control of senescence between these and the 'basal/ stem-cell' population.

Luminal cells, isolated from early passage mammoplasty samples, undergo growth arrest which resembles M1 senescence but occurs after a much smaller number of population doublings than in fibroblasts or 'basal' breast cells, leading some workers to distinguish it as an M_0 state.[79] Abrogation of p53 function, e.g. by expression of HPVE6, is strikingly without effect on the timing of this arrest in these cells. In contrast, abrogation of pRb is apparently sufficient, alone, to produce full escape from senescence and confers the same degree of immortalisation competence as expression of both E7 and E6. Escape from senescence by abrogation of pRb function clearly occurs despite the presence of wild-type p53 and, indeed, levels of the protein are increased in such cells,[79] suggesting that the p53 pathway is being partially activated but is in some way prevented from achieving growth arrest. Control of senescence in luminal cells, therefore, appears to be the inverse of that in 'basal' cells, i.e. p53-independent but pRb-dependent.

A closely similar situation has been observed by our laboratory in thyroid follicular epithelial cells (Bond et al, unpublished observations).[80] These also show a limited proliferative potential in culture entering a state of viable quiescence from which they can be rescued by expression of HPVE7 alone, but not by HPVE6 or mutant p53,[81] to which they are totally indifferent. Again, thyroid epithelial cells growing in response to HPVE7, express high levels of wild-type p53, to which they apparently fail to respond. Since in these primary culture experiments there is insufficient 'opportunity' for additional spontaneous genetic events to have occurred, one is forced to conclude that wild-type p53, although clearly modified sufficiently to be stabilised, is either not fully activated or else its activity is blocked by an endogenous inhibitor, such as mdm2.[69]

One fascinating implication of these observations is the existence of physiological cell-type-specific differences in sensitivity to p53-mediated growth arrest. If some cell types are indeed intrinsically resistant to p53 activation, this may have critical implications for the design of new p53-based therapies[82] which rely on the assumption that only tumour cells have lost functional p53!

SOME NOVEL IMPLICATIONS FOR TUMOUR PATHOLOGY

AN EXPLANATION FOR THE SELECTION OF P53 MUTATION IN HUMAN CANCERS

Current dogma views p53 as a mediator of growth arrest in response to generalised DNA damage incurred through exposure to exogenous (e.g. UV) or endogenous (e.g. free radical) agents thereby limiting the propagation of mutations. While this 'guardian of the genome' role[40] readily explains why tumour cells bearing loss-of-function p53 mutations should show increased genomic instability, it does not provide an obvious explanation for the **selection** of these mutations in the first place. In contrast, the direct role in senescence discussed here provides a clear selective advantage,[83] and one which will be expected to act not just on a random sub-set of tumour cells at any one time but on the entire tumour clone as it approaches M1. Indeed, such a dual function for p53 as a final common pathway for growth arrest in response to both senescence and generalised DNA damage could contribute to its being such a unique weak point in the cellular defence against malignancy,[84] since p53 mutations acquired primarily in order to escape senescence will secondarily entail a loss of genomic stability hence predisposing the cell to yet more mutational events. (Hypoxia has recently been proposed as an alternative p53-activating selection pressure in expanding tumours,[85] but it is difficult to reconcile this with the frequent occurrence of p53 mutation in some neoplasms while still at a thin *in situ* stage.)

P53 MUTATION AND BREAST CANCER BIOLOGY

On the above reasoning, it would be predicted that the minority of human cancer types which do **not** show high frequencies of p53 mutation might be those derived from cells which do not have a p53-dependent M1 lifespan checkpoint. The limited studies of this point to date are indeed tantalisingly suggestive of this, as seen in the analysis of breast and thyroid cells,[24,74,75,79,80] discussed at length above, and especially for breast are perhaps of even greater significance than has been appreciated.

It is widely accepted that a minority (around one-third) of invasive ductal breast cancers fall into a more aggressive sub-group which can be defined on the basis of a range of clinico-pathological parameters including poor differentiation (high grade), high proliferative rate, ER-negativity (with hormone-independence), and high expression of EGF-R.[86] These features, together with their intermediate filament profile (expression of some luminal markers together with basal markers CK14 and vimentin), has led to the suggestion[78] that this sub-group in contrast to the majority, arises not from the luminal cell but from a less-differentiated breast epithelial cell with features intermediate between classical luminal and basal (myo-epithelial), perhaps representing a stem-cell.

Clearly, this distinction in vivo corresponds strikingly with the two populations of normal breast epithelium identified in vitro in mammoplasty cultures by Band[24] and Galloway,[79] the highly proliferative 'stem' type being regulated by a p53-dependent life-span checkpoint only, contrasting with the more restricted proliferative capacity of the luminal cell, regulated by a p53-independent pathway.

Analysis of p53 status of breast cancers has consistently indicated a very strong correlation between the occurrence of p53 mutation and the ER-negative, EGFR-positive, poorly differentiated phenotype.[87,88] Of course, such correlations can never be expected to be absolute, since for example p53 function may be lost in indirect ways, and some ER-negative tumours may be derived from luminal cells which have lost ER expression (p53 status has not as far as we are aware been directly correlated with cytokeratin profile). Nevertheless, if these clinical data are put together with the cell biology then a novel explanation emerges for the two different phenotypes, namely that the majority well-differentiated 'luminal' tumour type retains wild-type p53 because it arises form a cell having only a p53-**independent** lifespan control, in which there is, therefore, no selection for p53 mutation, whereas the converse accounts for the need to mutate p53 in the 'stem-cell type' tumours.

Viewed in this way, the significance of the association of p53 mutation with the more aggressive phenotype is quite different from the conventional view, i.e. it is not that the tumour is aggressive and less differentiated **because** it has a mutant p53, but that the p53 mutation is merely an inevitable reflection of the controls operating in the cell of origin. This is, of course, a specific example of the general principle (frequently ignored in molecular oncology) that the phenotype of a tumour is determined as much by the properties of its cell of origin as by the nature of its somatic mutations.

TUMOUR PROGRESSION

The above argument is particularly pertinent to studies attempting to define the molecular basis of progression to hormone insensitivity in breast cancer. The assumption in such work is nearly always that tumours become unresponsive through some further mutational event. The line of reasoning above, however, suggests that the switch in behaviour may instead reflect the partial or complete *trans*-differentiation of the tumour cell from luminal to stem type, selected for by therapy-induced hormone-deprivation. It will be of interest to test the prediction that such tumours should have acquired the need to inactivate p53.

Our laboratory has recently obtained strong evidence that it is exactly this co-operation between an epigenetic and a genetic mechanism which is responsible for another major switch in human cancer behaviour, the transition from differentiated to anaplastic carcinoma of the thyroid.[80]

ACKNOWLEDGEMENTS

Work in the author's laboratory is supported by the Cancer Research Campaign and the Medical Research Council.

REFERENCES

1. Hayflick L. The limited in vitro lifetime of human diploid cell strains. Exp Cell Res 1965; 37: 614–636
2. Holliday R. Minireview: the limited proliferation of cultured human diploid cells: regulation or senescence? Gerontology 1990; 36: 1–6
3. Chen Q, Fischer A, Reagan JD, Yan L-J, Ames BN. Oxidative DNA damage and senescence of human diploid fibroblast cells. Proc Natl Scad Sci USA 1995; 92: 4337–4341
4. Sohal RS, Weindruch R. Oxidative stress, caloric restriction and aging. Science 1996; 273: 59–63
5. Wright WE, Shay JW. Time, telomeres and tumours: is cellular senescence more than an anticancer mechanism? Trends Cell Biol 1995; 5: 293–297
6. Blackburn EH. Telomeres: no end in sight. Cell 1994; 77: 621–623
7. Cech TR. Chromosome end games. Science 1994; 266: 387–388
8. Greaves M. Is telomerase activity in cancer due to selection of stem cells and differentiation arrest? Trends Genet 1996; 12: 127–128
9. Shay JW, Wright WE. The reactivation of telomerase activity in cancer progression. Trends Genet 1996; 12: 129–131
10. Wright WE, Piatyszek MA, Rainey WE, Byrd W, Shay JW. Telomerase activity in human germline and embryonic tissues and cells. Dev Genet 1996; 18: 173–179
11. Harley CB, Futcher AB, Greider CW. Telomeres shorten during aging of human fibroblasts. Nature 1990; 345: 458–460
12. Allsopp RC, Chang E, Kashefi-Aazam M et al. Telomere shortening is associated with cell division in vitro and in vivo. Exp Cell Res 1995; 220: 194–200
13. Allsopp RC, Harley CB. Evidence for a critical telomere length in senescent human fibroblasts. Exp Cell Res 1995; 219: 130–136

14. Goldstein S. Replicative senescence: the human fibroblast comes of age. Science 1990; 249: 1129–1132
15. Noda A, Ning Y, Venable SF, Pereira-Smith OM, Smith JR. Cloning of senescent cell-derived inhibitors of DNA synthesis using an expression screen. Exp Cell Res 1994; 211: 90–98
16. Hara E, Smith R, Parry D, Tahara H, Stone S, Peters G. Regulation of p16^{CDKN2} expression and its implications for cell immortalization and senescence. Mol Cell Biol 1996; 16: 859–867
17. Bryan TM, Reddel RR. SV40-induced immortalization of human cells. Crit Rev Oncong 1994; 5: 331–357
18. Wright WE, Pereira-Smith OM, Shay JW. Reversible cellular senescence: implications for immortalisation of normal human diploid fibroblasts. Mol Cell Biol 1989; 9: 3088–3092
19. Counter CM, Avillion AA, Le Feuvre CE et al. Telomere shortening associated with chromosome instability is arrested in immortal cells which express telomerase activity. EMBO J 1992; 11: 1921–1929
20. Bryan TM, Englezou A, Gupta J, Bacchetti S, Reddel RR. Telomere elongation in immortal human cells without detectable telomerase activity. EMBO J 1995; 14: 4240–4248
21. Lansdorp PM, Verwoerd NP, van de Rijke FM et al. Heterogeneity in telomere length of human chromosomes. Hum Mol Genet 1996; 5: 685–691
22. Hastie ND, Dempster M, Dunlop MG, Thompson AM, Green DK, Allshire RC. Telomere reduction in human colorectal carcinoma and with aging. Nature 1990; 346: 866–868
23. Shay JW, Wright WE, Brasiskyte D, Van der Hagen BA. E6 of human papillomavirus type 16 can overcome the M1 stage of immortalisation in human mammary epithelial cells but not human fibroblasts. Oncogene 1993; 8: 1407–1413
24. Wazer DE, Liu X-L, Chu Q, Gao Q, Band V. Immortalization of distinct human mammary epithelial cell types by human papilloma virus 16 E6 or E7. Proc Natl Acad Sci USA 1995; 92: 3687–3691
25. Klingelhutz AJ, Barber SA, Smith PP, Dyer K, McDougall JK. Restoration of telomeres in human papillomavirus-immortalized human anogenital epithelial cells. Mol Cell Biol 1994; 14: 961–969
26. Potten CS, Loeffler M. Stem-cells – attributes, cycles, spirals, pitfalls and uncertainties – lessons for and from the crypt. Development 1990; 110: 1001–1020
27. Broccoli D, Young JW, De Lange T. Telomerase activity in normal and malignant hematopoietic cells. Proc Natl Acad Sci USA 1995; 92: 9082–9086
28. Hiyama K, Hirai Y, Kyoizumi S et al. Activation of telomerase in human lymphocytes and hematopoietic progenitor cells. J Immunol 1995; 3711–3715
29. Counter CM, Gupta J, Harley CB, Leber B, Bacchetti S. Telomerase activity in normal leukocytes and in hematologic malignancies. Blood 1995; 85: 2315–2320.
30. Vaziri H, Dragowska W, Allsopp RC et al. Evidence for a mitotic clock in human hematopoietic stem cells: loss of telomeric DNA with age. Proc Natl Acad Sci USA 1994; 91: 9857–9860
31. Holt SE, Wright WE, Shay JW. Regulation of telomerase activity in immortal cell lines. Mol Cell Biol 1996; 16: 2932–2936
32. Cairns J. Mutation selection and the natural history of cancer. Nature 1975: 255: 197–200
33. Potten CS, Hume WJ, Reid P, Cairns J. The segregation of DNA in epithelial stem cells. Cell 1978; 15: 899–906
34. Shay JW, Van der Haegen BA, Ying Y, Wright WE. The frequency of immortalization of human fibroblasts and mammary epithelial cells transfected with SV40 large T-antigen. Exp Cell Res 1993; 209: 45-52
35. Shay JW, Wright WE. Quantitation of the frequency of immortalisation of normal human diploid fibroblasts by SV40 large T-antigen. Exp Cell Res 1989; 184: 109–118
36. Allsopp RC, Vaziri H, Patterson C et al. Telomere length predicts replicative capacity of human fibroblasts. Proc Natl Acad Sci USA 1992; 89: 10114–10118
37. Wright WE, Brasiskyte D, Piatyszek MA, Shay JW. Experimental elongation of telomeres extends the lifespan of immortal x normal cell hybrids. EMBO J 1996; 15: 1734–1741
38. Benn PA. Specific chromosome aberrations in senescent fibroblast cell lines derived from human embryos. Am J Hum Genet 1976; 28: 465–473
39. Kastan MB, Onyekwere O, Sidransky D, Vogelstein B, Craig RW. Participation of p53 protein in the cellular response to DNA damage. Cancer Res 1991; 51: 6304-6311

40. Lane DP. p53, guardian of the genome. Nature 1992; 358: 15–16
41. Cox LS, Lane DP. Tumour suppressors, kinases and clamps: how p53 regulates the cell cycle in response to DNA damage. BioEssays 1995; 17: 501–508
42. Wynford-Thomas D, Jones CJ, Wyllie FS. The tumour suppressor gene p53 as a regulator of proliferative life-span and tumour progression. Biol Signals 1997; In press
43. Weinberg RA. The retinoblastoma protein and cell cycle control. Cell 1995; 81: 323–330
44. Bond JA, Wyllie FS, Wynford-Thomas D. Escape from senescence in human diploid fibroblasts induced directly by mutant p53. Oncogene 1994; 9: 1885–1889
45. Rogan EM, Bryan TM, Hukku B et al. Alterations in p53 and p16^{ink4} expression and telomere length during spontaneous immortalization of Li-fraumeni syndrome fibroblasts. Mol Cell Biol 1995; 15: 4745–4753
46. Thut CJ, Chen J-L, Klemm R, Tjian R. p53 transcriptional activation mediated by coactivators TAFII40 and TAFII60. Science 1995; 267: 100–105
47. Bond JA, Haughton M, Blaydes JP, Gire V, Wynford-Thomas D, Wyllie FS. Evidence that transcriptional activation by p53 plays a direct role in the induction of cellular senescence. Oncogene 1997; In press
48. Atadja P, Wong H, Garkavtsev I, Geillette C, Riabowol K. Increased activity of p53 in senescing fibroblasts. Proc Natl Acad Sci USA 1995; 92: 8348–8352
49. Sherr CJ, Roberts JM. Inhibitors of mammalian G_1 cyclin-dependent kinases. Genes Dev 1995; 9: 1149–1163
50. Bond JA, Blaydes JP, Rowson J, Haughton MF, Smith JR, Wynford-Thomas D. Mutant p53 rescues human diploid cells from senescence without inhibiting the induction of SD11/WAF1. Cancer Res 1995; 55: 2404–2409
51. Kearsey JM, Coates PJ, Prescott AR, Warbrick E, Hall PA. Gadd45 is a nuclear cell cycle regulated protein which interacts with p21^{Cip1}. Oncogene 1995; 11: 1675–1683
52. Buckbinder L, Talbott R, Velasco-Miguel S et al. Induction of the growth inhibitor IGF-binding protein 3 by p53. Nature 1995; 377: 646–649
53. Stein GH, Beeson M, Gordon L. Failure to phosphorylate the retinoblastoma gene product in senescent human fibroblasts. Science 1990; 249: 666–669
54. Kamb A. Cell-cycle regulators and cancer. Trends Genet 1995; 11: 136–140
55. Broccoli D, Godley LA, Donehower LA, Varmus HE, De Lange T. Telomerase activation in mouse mammary tumors: lack of detectable telomere shortening and evidence for regulation of telomerase RNA with cell proliferation. Mol Cell Biol 1996; 16: 3765–3772
56. Whitaker NJ, Bryan TM, Bonnefin P et al. Involvement of RB-1, p53 p16^{INK4} and telomerase in immortalisation of human cells. Oncogene 1995; 11: 971–976
57. Counter CM, Botelho FM, Wang P, Harley CB, Bacchetti S. Stabilisation of short telomeres and telomerase activity accompany immortalisation of Epstein-Barr virus-transformed human B lymphocytes. J Virol 1994; 68: 3410–3414
58. Counter CM, Hirte HW, Bacchetti S, Harley CB. Telomerase activity in human ovarian carcinoma. Proc Natl Acad Sci USA 1994; 91: 2900–2904
59. Kim NW, Piatyszek MA, Prowse KR et al. Specific association of human telomerase activity with immortal cells and cancer. Science 1994; 266: 2011–2015
60. Piatyszek MA, Kim NW, Weinrich SL et al. Detection of telomerase activity in human cells and tumors by a telomeric repeat amplification protocol (TRAP). Methods Cell Sci 1995; 17: 1–15
61. Bacchetti S, Counter CM. Telomeres and telomerase in human cancer. Int J Oncol 1995; 7: 423–432
62. Blasco MA, Rizen M, Greider CW, Hanahan D. Differential regulation of telomerase activity and telomerase RNA during multi-stage tumorigenesis. Nature Genet 1996; 12: 200–204
63. Chadeneau C, Hay K, Hirte HW, Gallinger S, Bacchetti S. Telomerase activity associated with acquisition of malignancy in human colorectal cancer. Cancer Res 1995; 55: 2533–2536
64. Hiyama E, Hiyama K, Yokoyama T, Matsuura Y, Piatyszek MA, Shay JW. Correlating telomerase activity levels with human neuroblastoma outcomes. Nature Med 1995; 1: 249–255
65. Feng J, Funk WD, Wang S-S et al. The RNA components of human telomerase. Science 1995; 269: 1236–1241
66. Vojta PJ, Carl Barrett J. Genetic analysis of cellular senescence. Biochim Biophys Acta 1995; 1242: 29–41

67. De Lange T. In search of vertebrate telomeric proteins. Semin Cell Dev Biol 1996; 7: 23–29
68. Klingelhutz AJ, Foster SA, McDougall JK. Telomerase activation by the E6 gene product of human papillomavirus type 16. Naure 1996; 380: 79–82
69. Momand J, Zambetti GP, Olson DC, George D, Levine AJ. The mdm-2 oncogene product forms a complex with the p53 protein and inhibits p53-mediated transactivation. Cell 1992; 69: 1237–1245
70. Knight JC, Fletcher CDM. Soft tissue tumours. In: Lemoine N, Neoptolemos J, Cooke T (eds). Cancer. Oxford: Blackwell, 1994: 262–275
71. Stratton MR, Moss SD, Warren W et al. Mutations of the p53 gene in human soft tissue sarcomas: association with abnormalities of the RB1 gene. Oncogene 1990; 5: 1297–1301
72. Loughran O, Malliri A, Owens D et al. Association of CDKN2A/p16^{INK4a} with human head and neck keratinocyte replicative senescence: relationship of dysfunction to immortality and neoplasia. Oncogene 1996; 13: 561–568
73. Halbert CL, Demers GW, Galloway DA. The E7 gene of human papillomavirus type 16 is sufficient for immortalization of human epithelial cells. J Virol 1991; 65: 473–478
74. Band V, De Caprio JA, Delmolino L, Kulesa V, Sager R. Loss of p53 protein in human papillomavirus type 16 E6-immortalised human mammary epithelial cells. J Virol 1991; 65: 6671–6676
75. Gollahon LS, Shay JW. Immortalization of human mammary epithelial cells transfected with mutant p53 (273^{his}). Oncogene 1996; 12: 715–725
76. Shay JW, Tomlinson G, Piatyszek MA, Gollahon LS. Spontaneous in vitro immortalisation of breast epithelial cells from a patient with Li-fraumeni syndrome. Mol Cell Biol 1995; 15: 425–432
77. Van der Haegen BA, Shay JW. Immortalization of human mammary epithelial cells by SV40 large T-antigen involves a two step mechanism. In Vitro Cell Dev Biol 1993; 29A: 180–182
78. Taylor-Papadimitriou J, Berdichevsky F, D'Souza B, Burchell J. Human models of breast cancer. In: Lemoine NR and Wright NA (eds). The Molecular Pathology of Cancer, Cancer Surveys 16. Cold Spring Harbor: Cold Spring Harbor Laboratory, 1993; 59–78
79. Foster SC, Galloway DA. Human papillomavirus type 16 E7 alleviates a proliferation block in early passage human mammary epithelial cells. Oncogene 1996; 12: 1773-1779
80. Bond JA, Ness GO, Rowson J, Ivan M, White D, Wynford-Thomas D. Spontaneous de-differentiation correlates with extended lifespan in transformed thyroid epithelial cells: An epigenetic mechanism of tumour progression. Int J Cancer 1996; 67:563–572
81. Wyllie FS, Lemoine NR, Barton CM, Dawson T, Bond D, Wynford-Thomas D. Direct growth stimulation of normal human epithelial cells by mutant p53. Mol Carcinogen 1993; 7: 83–88
82. Bischoff Jr, Fattaey A, Kirn D. An adenovirus mutant that replicates selectively in p53-deficient human tumor cells. Science 1996; 274: 373–376
83. Wynford-Thomas D, Bond JA, Wyllie FS, Jones CJ. Does telomere shortening drive selection for p53 mutation in human cancer? Mol Carcinogen 1995; 12: 119–123
84. Wynford-Thomas D. p53: guardian of cellular senescence. J Pathol 1997; 180: 118–121
85. Graeber TG, Osmanian C, Jacks T et al. Hypoxia-mediated selection of cells with diminished apoptotic potential in solid tumours. Nature 1996; 379: 88–91
86. Nicholson RI, Gee JMW. Growth factors and modulation of endocrine response in breast cancer. In: Vedeckis WV (ed). Hormones and Cancer. Boston: Birkhauser, 1996; 227–264
87. Thor AD, Moore II DH, Edgerton SM et al. Accumulation of p53 tumor supressor gene protein: an independent marker of prognosis in breast cancers. J Natl Cancer Inst 1992; 84: 845–855
88. Mazars R, Spinardi L, BenCheikh M et al. p53 mutations occur in aggressive breast cancer. Cancer Res 1992; 52: 3918–3923
89. Holt SE, Shay JW, Wright WE. Refining the telomere-telomerase hypothesis of aging and cancer. Nature Biotechnol 1996; 14: 836–839

5

Hodgkin's disease and immunoglobulin genetics

Freda K. Stevenson Dennis H. Wright

PATHOLOGY OF HODGKIN'S DISEASE

The original description of what has come to be known as Hodgkin's disease (HD) was based on the clinical features and gross pathology of six patients reported by Hodgkin in 1832. One hundred years later, a histological review of tissue from these patients concluded that only three were likely to have been true HD. In fact, the diagnostically important Reed-Sternberg (RS) cells were only clearly recognized at the turn of the century. It is the identification of the RS cells, in a background appropriate for one of the four subtypes of the Rye classification of HD, which is now central to the histological definition of this disease. In spite of its importance, the nature of the RS cell remains the subject of conjecture and debate, and intensive immunohistological study in recent years has not resolved this issue. It has, however, delineated the immunophenotype of classical and variant RS cells, and influenced our understanding of the nature and classification of HD. This is reflected in the REAL classification[1] which, for the first time, incorporates HD into an overall category of lymphomas.

Lymphocyte-predominant HD

The atypical cells seen in lymphocyte predominant HD (LPHD) do not usually resemble classical RS cells. They have the nuclear structure of centroblasts, but they are often multilobated and have been given the name of 'pop-corn' cells (Fig. 1A). They have an immunophenotype distinct from that of classic RS cells in that they express B cell antigens, including immunoglobulin J chain, but do

Prof. Freda K. Stevenson DPhil FRCPath, Consultant Immunologist and Professor of Immunology, Molecular Immunology Group, Tenovus Laboratory, Southampton University Hospitals, Tremona Road, Southampton SO16 6YD, UK

Prof. Dennis H. Wright MD FRCPath, Emeritus Professor of Pathology, Department of Pathology, Southampton University Hospitals, Tremona Road, Southampton SO16 6YD, UK

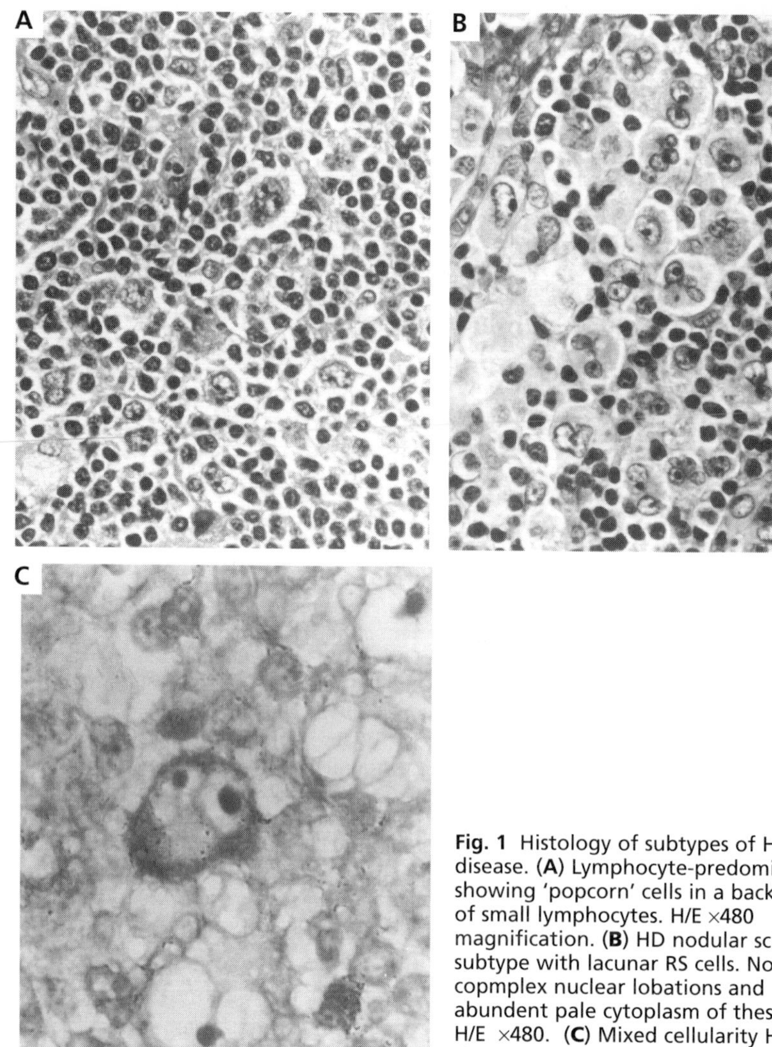

Fig. 1 Histology of subtypes of Hodgkin's disease. (**A**) Lymphocyte-predominant HD showing 'popcorn' cells in a background of small lymphocytes. H/E ×480 magnification. (**B**) HD nodular sclerosing subtype with lacunar RS cells. Note copmplex nuclear lobations and abundent pale cytoplasm of these cells. H/E ×480. (**C**) Mixed cellularity HD showing classical binucleate RS cells. Giemsa ×1200 magnification.

not express either CD30 or CD15.[2] Reports on the clonality of the pop-corn cells as determined by light chain restriction are conflicting. In many cases it is difficult to establish light chain restriction either by immunohistochemistry or by *in situ* hybridisation for mRNA. The apparent polyclonal nature of many cases of LPHD raises the question of whether these are neoplasms or abnormal (pre-neoplastic) follicle centre cell reactions.[3] The long natural history of nodular LPHD lends support to the latter possibility.

The number of pop-corn cells within the nodules of LPHD varies. Large numbers of such cells raises the question of neoplastic progression, although, if the proliferation remains confined within the follicles, it is usually regarded as part of the spectrum of nodular LPHD. A small proportion of cases, however, do progress to a diffuse, high grade B cell lymphoma. In such cases, the disease often remains localised and appears to have a better prognosis than other high grade B-cell lymphomas.

The number of T cells in the nodules of LPHD varies widely, although, even in nodules with a B cell predominance, the pop-corn cells themselves are tightly rosetted by T cells. These T cells are CD2, CD3, CD4 and CD57-positive, a phenotype characteristic of T cells found in the germinal centres of secondary follicles. T cells with a similar phenotype are found in increased numbers in progressive transformation of germinal centres, a condition that may precede or follow the development of LPHD. The T cells that rosette the atypical cells in LPHD are CD57 positive, whereas those that rosette classical RS cells are not. CD57-positive T cells, isolated from the tonsil, regularly express mRNA for IL-4, whereas CD57-negative T cells do not. It appears likely that the CD57-positive subset of CD4 T cells is involved in control of B cell maturation in the light zone of germinal centres.[5]

The relationship between nodular LPHD and diffuse proliferations with a similar cytomorphology has been the subject of debate. Some nodular LPHD cases show diffuse areas and it appears likely that forms of this disease with diffuse growth pattern can occur. Such cases should, however, be approached with diagnostic caution. If the atypical cells have the morphology and phenotype of classic RS cells, the case probably falls into the most recently defined category of lymphocyte-rich classical HD.[1] If the atypical cells have a B cell phenotype, the possibility of T cell rich B cell lymphoma should be entertained. In this disease, the neoplastic cells more closely resemble other large B cell lymphoma cells and do not have the morphology of pop-corn cells. The presence of CD57-positive T cells may be helpful in identifying diffuse LPHD.

Nodular sclerosing HD

The defining characteristic of nodular sclerosing (NS) HD is the presence of banded sclerosis. This subtype of HD is also characterised by lacunar RS cells (Fig. 1B). These cells have complex multilobated nuclei and lack the prominent eosinophilic nucleoli of classical RS cells. The cytoplasm of these cells is pale staining and abundant. Retraction of the cytoplasm in formalin fixed tissues gives the lacunar appearance. Although this appearance is artefactual in that it is not seen in frozen section, it reflects the abundant, relatively organelle-free, cytoplasm of these cells. Dogma states that classic RS cells should be identified before a diagnosis of NSHD is made, and such cells are occasionally encountered. The reality of the situation, however, is that lacunar RS cell variants in an appropriate cellular setting are usually accepted as being diagnostic of NSHD.[6] Variant RS cells may form apparent syncytial sheets often with areas of necrosis giving rise to so-called syncytial HD (NSHD Grade 2). The importance of this feature is that it may raise problems of differential diagnosis from metastatic carcinoma or melanoma, or of anaplastic large cell lymphoma.

Biopsies that show lacunar type RS cells but do not have banded fibrosis may be categorized as NSHD cellular phase. The justification for this designation is that biopsies at other sites or subsequent biopsies from such cases often show typical NSHD.[7] In many HD trials, however, cases without banded sclerosis are placed in the mixed cellularity category on the grounds that lacunar cells can be found in biopsies that otherwise look like MCHD, blurring the distinction between this category and cellular phase NS.

Mixed cellularity HD

Mixed cellularity HD typically has obvious classical RS cells (Fig. 1C) and mononuclear Hodgkin's cells in a background of small lymphocytes and histiocytes often, but not always, accompanied by eosinophils and neutrophils. Interfollicular HD in which paracortical infiltrates of HD are seen between reactive secondary follicles is usually categorized as MCHD.

Lymphocyte-depleted HD

The category of lymphocyte-depleted HD underwent rapid attrition following the introduction of immunohistochemistry.[6] Several publications reported that a high proportion of cases previously given this designation were, in fact, anaplastic carcinomas or high grade non-Hodgkin's lymphomas, including anaplastic large cell lymphoma. The diagnosis of lymphocyte-depleted HD of either the reticular or the diffuse fibrosis subtypes should be made with caution and be based on the presence of morphologically and immunophenotypically characteristic RS cells.

CELL OF ORIGIN

It is now generally accepted that the atypical cell seen in LPHD is a B cell, and that it is probably of follicle centre origin.[2,3] The histogenesis of classic and lacunar type RS cells is less certain. The majority of RS cells express CD30 and CD15 and, although these are widely used as markers for HD, they are not specific, and give no clue to histogenesis. RS cells do not express the lymphocyte common antigen and the reported expression of T and B cell lineage markers is variable. The tight rosetting of RS cells by T cells makes the detection of T lineage markers in paraffin sections difficult, although expression of CD1, CD2, CD3, CD4, CD5, CD8, CD43, CD45RO and TCRβ has been reported on RS cells in up to 40% of HD.[6] The antigen expression is often of variable intensity and may only involve a small proportion of the RS cells and variants. B lineage markers have been reported at a higher frequency than T cell markers. CD20 detected by the antibody L26 has been reported on RS cells in up to 60% of cases of classic HD.[8] Most reports record levels nearer 20% with the expression being of variable intensity involving only a proportion of the RS cells. CD79a (mb-1), which recognizes surface Ig-associated complex, is a more reliable B cell lineage marker than CD20 which is occasionally expressed on T cells. Korkolopoulou et al[9] identified CD79a staining of RS/HD cells in 16% of NSHD, 19% of MCHD and 4 of 7 cases of LDHD. Usually, less than 10% of neoplastic cells were labelled.

HD and non-Hodgkin's lymphoma

The synchronous and metachronous occurrence of HD and NHL is uncommon, but well recognised.[10] NHL may occur as secondary tumours in patients previously treated for HD presumably as a consequence of DNA damage together with immunosuppression. HD may occur with either B cell or T cell NHL, but is most frequently associated with small lymphocytic lymphoma and follicle centre cell lymphomas. The RS cells that occur in such cases may have an immunophenotype of classic RS cells, or one intermediate between RS cells and B cells. Although uncommon, such cases may have an important bearing on our concepts of the pathogenesis of HD and the origin of RS cells.

Epstein-Barr virus (EBV) and HD

Soon after the discovery of EBV, patients with HD were found to have raised antibody titres against viral capsid antigen, but this was generally attributed to immunosuppression associated with the disease. However, epidemiological studies showed that patients with infectious mononucleosis had a 4-fold increased risk of developing HD.[11] The overall incidence of EBV in HD as determined by detection of transcripts of the EBER genes I and II is 40–50%, with an incidence of 80% in the MCHD subtype.[12] There is a higher incidence of EBV in HD occurring in Oriental and Central/South American populations than in European or North American patients.[13,14] All HD cases found in patients with HIV infection are EBV positive.[15] In RS cells, EBV exhibits a latency pattern II with expression of EBERs, LMP1 and EBNA I. Studies of the EBV terminal repeat region indicate that the virus is clonal in any individual case of HD, supporting a possible aetiological role for the virus.[16,17] Presumably other aetiological factors operate in the EBV negative cases.

Chromosomal abnormalities in HD

Cytogenetic analysis of HD has been limited by the low incidence of RS cells in many cases and difficulties in obtaining metaphase spreads. A combination of FISH and immunocytochemistry has shown numerical chromosome abnormalities in all RS cells studied.[18] Conventional techniques have shown numerical abnormalities in ~40% of cases of HD, but no single non-random chromosomal abnormality is characteristic of the disease.[19] Anaplastic large cell lymphoma, which shares some features of HD, commonly has a t(2;5) translocation, but this abnormality is not characteristic of HD.[20]

VARIABLE REGION GENES IN B CELLS

The genes which encode immunoglobulin in B cells are highly unusual in requiring recombination of three separate elements prior to transcription. This process begins in the pro-B cell with the joining of a D_H-segment gene to one of the J_H genes (Fig. 2). Although there is no membrane Ig at this point, synthesis of the membrane Ig-associated α/β heterodimer (CD79a/b) also begins, and this is expressed until the plasma cell stage.[21] The next event occurs in the pre-B cell and involves combination of one of the available V_H genes to form a V_H–D_H–J_H transcriptional unit, which can be expressed as a μ chain together with a surrogate light chain.[21] The choice of V_H gene is from a germ line repertoire of ~51 potentially functional genes which can be divided into 7

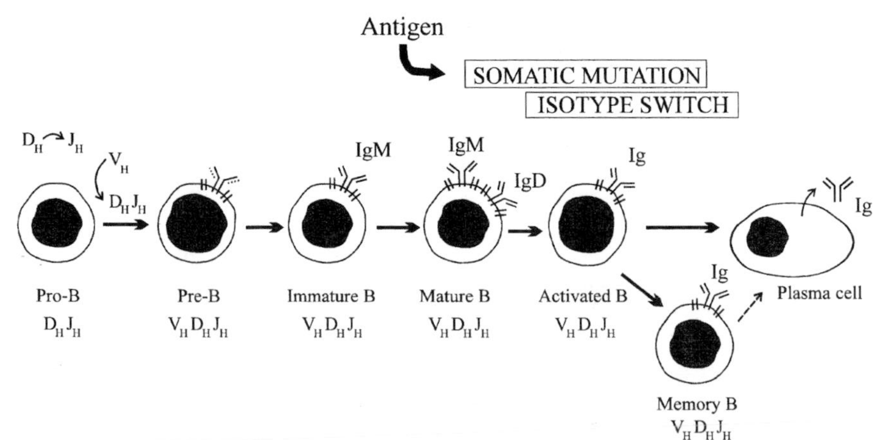

Fig. 2 Changes in immunoglobulin occurring during B cell maturation. During development of B cells from pluripotential stem cells to Ig-secreting plasma cells, Ig genes are recombined and Ig protein synthesized. Following recombination, the pre-B cell expresses Ig heavy chains and a surrogate light chain, together with the Igα/Igβ receptor complex (CD79a/b). Naive B cells express IgM/IgD and, following antigen binding, can undergo further processes of somatic mutation and isotype switching.

families, V_H1–V_H7, varying in size from 1 (V_H6) to 22 (V_H3) gene segments.[22] As maturation continues, a similar joining process occurs for the light chain to create V_L–J_L, and IgM is expressed. One of the features of the joints is that they are often imprecise, with gain and loss of nucleotides, and the D-segment gene may be read in different reading frames, be inverted, or undergo D–D fusion. Non-functional sequences may be produced and, if the second chance provided by the allelic chromosome also fails, the cell will die. The object of the potentially hazardous rearrangement of DNA is to generate a wide range of sequences in the V regions of antibody molecules. It gives rise to a virtually unique sequence in the third complementarity-determining region, CDR3, which is, therefore, a 'clonal signature' of the B cell.

The naive mature IgM+IgD+ B cells (Fig. 2) may then encounter antigen and enter the germinal centre of the lymph node. In this environment, the available range of V region sequences can be extended even further by somatic hypermutation, which introduces mutations across V_H and V_L. If the mutations generate replacement amino acids, they can be selected by antigen, leading to a concentration of optimal amino acids in the contact points CDR1 and CDR2.[23] If mutations are deleterious, or if the cells are not selected, they will die by apoptosis.[24] Antigen-selected B cells will then proliferate and, in the presence of CD4+ T cells and appropriate cytokines, undergo isotype switching.[23] Memory B cells and plasma cells are the final products of this maturation process.

V_H genes in B-cell tumours

Clonality

Since the clonal history of the B cell is evident from the V genes, sequence analysis can place the cell of origin at a defined maturational point, thereby

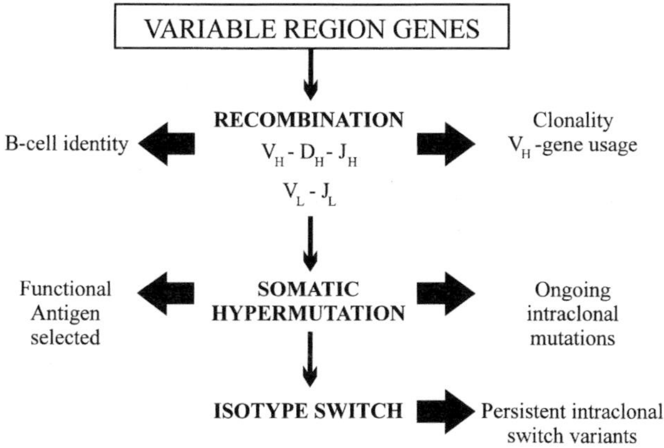

Fig. 3 Changes in immunoglobulin genes relevant for tumour analysis. The three processes of recombination, somatic hypermutation and isotype switching occur during the clonal development of a B cell. Variable region gene analysis can indicate the nature of the cell of origin of a B-cell tumour, and detect events occurring following neoplastic transformation.

providing information which can illuminate conclusions from immunohistochemical techniques. The genetic processes which relate to tumour analysis are summarized in Figure 3. The V_H–D_H–J_H recombination process is a paradigm for a B cell and, if identified, will indicate a B-cell tumour. This has been useful in the analysis of RS cells of HD (see below). Clonality is the next defining feature, and is detected routinely from patient material by 'fingerprint' analysis of the PCR product obtained using a consensus FWR primer (FR3c) together with a consensus primer in J_H (Jc) (Fig. 4).[25] Since the amplification is across the 'clonal signature' sequence, clonality is obvious, with 1/2 bands produced. However, there is a danger that an apparent product may be non-Ig, and sequencing should be used for confirmation. An alternative PCR approach using mixed 5'-primers in the V_H leader (L mix) or

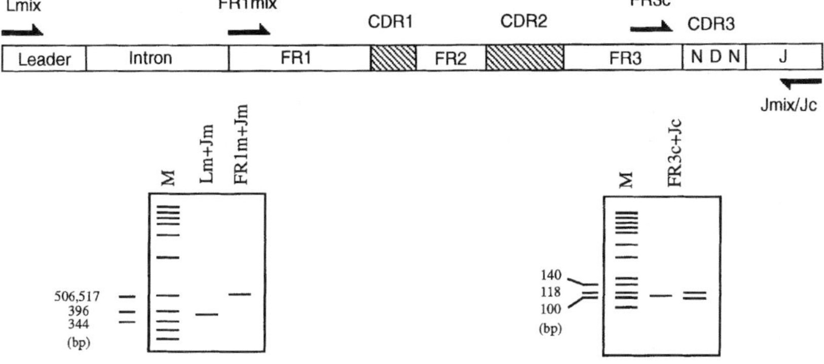

Fig. 4 PCR-based methods used to analyze V_H-genes. Various primer sets are used to amplify V_H gene sequences, and products are separated by gel electrophoresis. Single or double bands obtained from the 'fingerprint' CDR3 region indicate a clonal B-cell population. Longer sequences obtained using primers in the more 5' positions can be cloned and sequenced for analysis of gene usage and somatic mutation events.

```
                                                CDR1                          CDR2                                                             CDR3
V3-53     EVQLVETGGGLIQPGGSLRLSCAASGFTVS  SNYMS  WVRQAPGKGLEWVS  VIYSGGSTYYADSVKG  RFTISRDNSKNTLYLQMNSLRAEDTAVYYCAR
Clone 1   --H---S----V------------------  T-E-T  --------------  I-FG--D---------  ------H---------------T--------T LLRHRHHAQRFPFDN
Clone 2   --H---S----V------------------  T-E-T  --------------  I-FG--D---------  ------H---------------T--------T LLRHRHHAQRFPFDN
Clone 3   --H---S----V------------------  T-E-T  --------------  I-FG--D---------  ------H---------------T--------T LLRHRHHAQRFPFDN
Clone 4   --H---S----V------------------  T-E-T  --------------  I-FG--D---------  ------H---------------T--------T LLRHRHHAQRFPFDN
Clone 5   --H---S----V------------------  T-E-T  --------------  I-FG--D---------  ------H---------------T--------T LLRHRHHAQRFPFDN
Clone 6   --H---S----V------------------  T-E-T  --------------  I-FG--D---------  ------H---------------T--------T LLRHRHHAQRFPFDN

V1-3b     QVQLVQSGAEVKKPGASVKVSCKASGYTFT  SYAMH  WVRQAPGQRLEWMG  WINAGNGNTKYSQKFQG  RVTITGDTSASTAYMELSRLRSEDTAVYYCAR
Clone 7   --------G---------------------  --I--  -L------------  ------E----------  ----S-----------G----N---------- EGATGNVAFDI

V3-49     EVQLVESGGGLVQPGRSLRLSCTASGFTFG  DYAMS  WFRQAPGKGLEWVG  FIRSKAYGGTTEYTASVKG  RFTISRDGSKSIAYLQMNSLKTEDTAVYYCTR
Clone 8   ------------------------------  -----  --------------  -------------------  --------------------S----------- NDYGDISFDH
```

Fig. 5 Detection of tumour-related V_H gene sequences by PCR and cloning. Amplification of cDNA or genomic DNA from a tumour biopsy using the 5′-primers (L mix or FR1 mix in Fig. 4) together with 3′ J mix primers yields V_H sequences which can be cloned in bacteria. Sequencing of random clones can then reveal repeated sequences with identical CDR3s (clones 1–6), which are likely to be derived from tumour cells. Further individual sequences (clones 7 and 8) are from normal B cells in the biopsy.

FWR1 sequence (FR1) (Fig. 4) together with a J_H primer mix, followed by cloning and sequencing, will reveal repeated tumour-related sequences with similar CDR3s (Fig. 5),[26] and, with genomic DNA as source, primers in the constant region can be used. In Figure 5, the repeated identical V_H sequences are characteristic of a B-cell tumour,[26] whereas the two lower distinct sequences are likely to be derived from normal B cells in the biopsy. Although this procedure is highly successful with dispersed cells or frozen biopsy material, there may be problems with paraffin-embedded samples where damaged DNA may provide few sequences, making decisions about derivation from tumour more difficult.

V_H gene usage

Information on the utilization of V_H genes by tumours has revealed some surprising results, with the most dramatic being that a single V_H gene, V_{4-34}, a member of the V_H4 family, is mandatory for encoding the monoclonal IgM anti-red cell autoantibodies found in B cell tumours producing cold agglutinins.[27] The same gene is commonly used in diffuse large cell lymphoma,[25] but has so far never been found in myeloma.[29] These findings must indicate selectivity in the cell of origin of B-cell tumours, and may have implications for pathogenesis.

Somatic hypermutation and isotype switching

Analysis of tumour-derived sequences indicates first if the V_H gene is potentially functional. Alignment of the tumour-derived sequences to the library of germ line genes can then show if the cell has undergone somatic hypermutation (Figs 3 & 5). Recently, this approach revealed an unexpected heterogeneity in chronic lymphocytic leukaemia (CLL), with V_H genes in some cases being unmutated and in other mutated.[30] Interestingly, the unmutated 'naive' pattern is associated with trisomy 12 and atypical morphology.[30] Intraclonal sequence heterogeneity indicates that the tumour clone is still under the influence of the mutation mechanism, known to be activated in the germinal centre.[23] As expected, this pattern is seen in follicular lymphoma[31] and in Burkitt's lymphoma,[32] but not in CLL[30] or myeloma.[29] For some tumours, the pattern of mutation shows clustering of replacement mutations in CDRs, consistent with a role for antigen in selecting, and perhaps driving the B cell.

Isotype switching has obviously occurred in myeloma, but V_H probing has detected transcripts indicative of a co-existing less mature IgM+ precursor cell in at least some cases.[33] Similarly, in IgM+ CLL, clonal variants switched to other isotypes have been found,[34] indicating that tumour cells are not as 'frozen' in differentiation as was first thought.

V_H GENES IN HODGKIN'S DISEASE

There are two major problems in applying V_H gene analysis to HD, the first being heterogeneity of disease, as already outlined. The second is that the putative tumour (RS) cell is present in only small numbers in affected tissues, making conclusions difficult to draw from relatively insensitive techniques, such as Southern blotting, which were applied originally to probe V_H clonality.[35,36]

Lymphocyte predominant HD (LPHD) presents a particular difficulty since it clearly involves B lymphocytes, but the RS variant cell present is quite distinct from classical HD. Application of the more sensitive technique of PCR analysis to whole tissue has yielded variable results.[37] Variability may arise from the problem that electrophoretic bands may be artefactual, or that small clones of normal B cells could generate clonal bands. Using the more refined technology of single cell picking and nested PCR to probe individual cells, only polyclonal populations were detected.[38] However, the large cell lymphomas which develop in a proportion of patients appear to derive from pre-existing B cells in LPHD at least in some cases.[39] The analogy drawn with Sjogren's syndrome where polyclonal B-cell proliferation can progress via oligoclonal populations to a monoclonal lymphoma may be appropriate.[40]

Application of PCR analysis to tissue of classical HD has revealed V_H gene clonality in several studies.[41–43] Although incidence of clonality varies from 23–50% overall, there has been a general consensus that it is higher in the CD20+ cases.[42] These findings have again been extended by single cell isolation or picking to obtain V_H and V_L gene sequences from an array of RS cells from each individual biopsy.[44] Since the investigations are technically demanding, and prone to contamination by surrounding B cells, the results have perhaps inevitably been conflicting.[44–46] However, the weight of evidence supports the clonal B cell nature of RS cells in at least some cases of both NS and MC HD.[44,46] Evidence has also been presented for a mixed population of RS cells of both monoclonal and polyclonal type,[41] which may be reminiscent of a progressive narrowing of clonality seen in patients with lymphoproliferative disease due to immunosuppression following organ transplantation.[40] However, some of the apparently polyclonal cases have since been reassessed as monoclonal, leaving this question open.[47] In fact, the general conclusion that RS cells are derived from clonal B cells has been strongly supported by a recent analysis of 10 cases of classical CD20– HD, which identified clonal V gene sequences in 9/10 cases.[48]

Studies of the clonal sequences derived from RS cells have been too limited to discern preferential usage of particular V_H genes, with members of V_H3, V_H1 and V_H4 identified so far.[44,46,48] Interestingly, somatic mutational changes appear to be common and, in one case, there was evidence for intraclonal variation indicative of ongoing mutational events.[48] These patterns are characteristic of cells which have traversed the germinal centre.[23] However, the majority of identified sequences appear to be non-functional, raising a question over the potential of the RS cell to synthesize immunoglobulin. In fact, only one case has been described so far in which potentially functional V_H and V_L sequences have been found together.[49] A normal B cell with two aberrant V_H gene rearrangements would be eliminated by apoptosis,[24] but a neoplastic B cell may be protected from this fate. However, the high incidence of aberrant V genes in RS cells distinguishes HD from other B cell tumours associated with the germinal centre, such as follicular lymphoma and Burkitt's lymphoma (BL). In both the latter tumour categories, the cell of origin has undergone somatic hypermutation, and mutational activity may persist post transformation. However, the V-genes remain functional and, in the majority, Ig is synthesized and expressed.[32]

Since preparing this article, a paper[50] has appeared describing the presence of clonal populations of germinal centre cells in lymphocyte-predominant HD (LPHD). The clonally related V-gene rearrangements were detected in micromanipulated single RS cells, and appeared to be functional and somatically mutated, with evidence for ongoing mutations.

CONCLUDING REMARKS

Since the presence of a V_H–D_H–J_H transcriptional unit is a paradigm for a B cell, we can conclude that a significant proportion of classical HD cases have RS cells of B cell origin. These classical cases include the NS and MC categories and can be CD20+ or CD20–. In the majority, the B cells are clonal, and V genes are somatically hypermutated, but the encoded Ig is unlikely to be expressed due to aberrant sequences. Accumulation of crippling mutations in B cells may occur in the germinal centre at the centroblast/early centrocyte stage, where there is intense mutational activity prior to antigen selection.[23] It may be that the final neoplastic event leading to HD occurs at this point, distinguishing the cell of origin from the more differentiated surface Ig positive cell of follicular lymphoma or BL. Failure to express Ig should mark a B cell for destruction via apoptosis,[24] but a neoplastic cell may be spared. There could be an influence of EBV on survival, but the actual role of EBV in B cell tumours remains enigmatic.

A major characteristic of HD is the predominant distribution of RS cells in the axial lymph nodes and location of RS cells in a background of reactive or inflammatory cells, features which for many years have distinguished HD from B cell tumours of the germinal centre. The apparent B cell nature of the RS cells indicates a closer relationship with other B cell tumours, but the aberrant nature of V genes suggests that the RS cell may be a 'failed' B cell, clearly different from its close relatives in the aptly named non-Hodgkin's lymphomas.

ACKNOWLEDGEMENTS

This work was supported by the Cancer Research Campaign and the Leukaemia Research Fund, UK. We thank Dr Delin Zhu for help in preparing the figures.

REFERENCES

1. Harris NL, Jaffe ES, Stein H et al. A revised European-American classification of lymphoid neoplasms: a proposal from the International Lymphoma Study Group. Blood 1994; 84: 1361–1392
2. Mason DY, Chan J, de Wolf Peeters C et al. Nodular lymphocyte predominance Hodgkin's disease. A distinct clinicopathological entity. Am J Surg Pathol 1994; 18: 526–530
3. Poppema S. Nodular lymphocyte predominance type of Hodgkin's disease. In: Weiss LM (ed). Pathology of Lymph Nodes. Contemporary Issues in Surgical Pathology, Vol 21. New York: Churchill Livingstone, 1996; 215–228
4. Sundeen JT, Cossman J, Jaffe ES. Lymphocyte predominant Hodgkin's disease nodular subtype with co-existent 'large cell lymphoma': histological progression or composite malignancy? Am J Surg Pathol 1988; 12: 599–606
5. Velardi A, Mingari MC, Moretta L et al. Functional analysis of cloned germinal center CD4+ cells with natural killer cell-related features. Divergence from typical T helper cells. J Immunol 1986; 137: 2808–2812

6. Strickler JG, Burgart LJ, Weiss LM. Classical Hodgkin's disease. In: Weiss LM (ed). Pathology of Lymph Nodes. Contemporary Issues in Surgical Pathology, Vol 21. New York: Churchill Livingstone, 1996; 169–214
7. Colby TV, Warnke RA. The histology of the initial relapse of Hodgkin's disease. Cancer 1980; 45: 289–295
8. Schmid C, Pan L, Diss T, Isaacson PG. Expression of B cell antigens by Hodgkin's and Reed-Sternberg cells. Am J Pathol 1991; 139: 701–709
9. Korkolopoulou P, Cordell J, Jones M et al. The expression of the B-cell marker mb-1(CD79a) in Hodgkin's disease. Histopathology 1994; 24: 511–555
10. Jaffe ES, Zarate-Osorno A, Medeiros LJ. The interrelationship of Hodgkin's disease and non-Hodgkin's lymphomas – lessons learned from composite and sequential malignance. Semin Diagn Pathol 1992; 9: 297–301
11. Kvåle, G Hølby EA, Pederson E. Hodgkin's disease in patients with previous infectious mononucleosis. Int J Cancer 1979; 23: 593–601
12. Hamilton-Dutoit SJ, Palleson G. Detection of Epstein-Barr virus small RNAs in routine paraffin sections using non-isotopic RNA/RNA in situ hybridization. Histopathology 1994; 25: 101–118
13. Chan JKC, Yip TTC, Tasng WYW et al. Detection of Epstein-Barr virus in Hodgkin's disease occurring in an Oriental population. Hum Pathol 1995; 26: 314–328
14. Ambinder RD, Browning PJ, Lorenzana I et al. Epstein-Barr virus and childhood Hodgkin's disease in Honduras and the United States. Blood 1993; 81: 496–504
15. Herndier BG, Sanchez HC, Chang KL et al. High prevalence of Epstein-Barr virus in the Reed-Sternberg cells of HIV-associated Hodgkin's disease. Am J Pathol 1993; 142: 1073–1089
16. Deakon E, Palleson G, Niedobitek G et al. Epstein-Barr virus and Hodgkin's disease: transcriptional analysis of virus latency in malignant cells. J Exp Med 1993; 177: 339–349
17. Gledhill S, Gallagher A, Jones DB et al. Viral involvement in Hodgkin's disease: detection of clonal type A Epstein-Barr viral genomes in tumour samples. Br J Cancer 1991; 64: 227–232
18. Weber-Matthiesen K, Deerberg S, Poetsch M et al. Numerical chromosome aberrations are present within the CD30+ Hodgkin's and Reed-Sternberg cells in 100% of analysed cases of Hodgkin's disease. Blood 1995; 86: 1464–1473
19. Tilly H, Bastard C, Delastre T et al. Cytogenetic studies in untreated Hodgkin's disease. Blood 1991; 77: 1298–1306
20. Wellmann A, Otsuki T, Vogelbruch M et al. Analysis of the t(2;5)(p23;q35) translocation by reverse transcription-polymerase chain reaction in CD30+ anaplastic large-cell lymphomas, in other non-Hodgkin's lymphomas of T-cell phenotype, and in Hodgkin's disease. Blood 1995; 86: 2321–2328
21. van Noesel CJM, van Lier RAW. Architecture of the human B-cell antigen receptors. Blood 1993; 82: 363–373
22. Cook GP, Tomlinson IM. The human immunoglobulin V_H repertoire. Immunol Today 1995; 16: 237–242
23. Kocks C, Rajewsky K. Stable expression and somatic hypermutation of antibody V regions in B cell development pathways. Annu Rev Immunol 1989; 7: 537–559
24. Liu L-J, Joshua DE, Williams GT et al. Mechanism of antigen-driven selection in germinal centres. Nature 1989; 342: 929–931
25. Linke B, Pyttlich J, Tiemann M et al. Identification of structural analysis of rearranged immunoglobulin heavy chain genes in lymphomas and leukemias. Leukemia 1995; 9: 840–847
26. Hawkins RE, Zhu D, Ovecka M et al. Idiotypic vaccination against human B-cell lymphoma. Rescue of variable region gene sequences from biopsy material for assembly as single-chain Fv personal vaccines. Blood 1994; 83: 3279–3288
27. Pascual V, Victor K, Spellerberg M et al. V_H restriction among human cold agglutinins. The V_H4-21 gene segment is required to encode anti-I and anti-i specificities. J Immunol 1992; 149: 2337–2344
28. Hsu FJ, Levy R. Preferential usage of the V_H immunoglobulin gene family by diffuse large cell lymphoma. Blood 1995; 86: 3072–3082
29. Rettig MB, Vescio RA, Cao J et al. V_H gene usage in multiple myeloma: complete absence of the V_H4-21(V4-34) gene. Blood 1996; 87: 2846–2852
30. Oscier DG, Thompsett A, Zhu D, Stevenson FK. Differential rates of somatic hypermutation among subsets of chronic lymphocytic leukemia defined by chromosomal abnormalities. Blood 1997; 89: 4153–4160

31. Zhu D, Hawkins RE, Hamblin TJ, Stevenson FK. Clonal history of a human follicular lymphoma as revealed in the immunoglobulin variable region genes. Br J Haematol 1994; 86: 505–512
32. Chapman CJ, Mockridge CR, Rowe M et al. Analysis of V_H genes used by neoplastic B cells in endemic Burkitt's lymphoma shows somatic hypermutation and intraclonal heterogeneity. Blood 1995; 85: 2176–2181
33. Corradini P, Boccadoro M, Voena C, Pileri A. Evidence for a bone marrow B cell transcribing malignant plasma cell VDJ joined to Cμ sequence in IgG and IgA secreting multiple myelomas. J Exp Med 1993; 178: 1091–1096
34. Efremov DG, Ivanovski M, Batista FD et al. IgM-producing chronic lymphocytic leukemia cells undergo immunoglobulin isotype-switching without acquiring somatic mutations. J Clin Invest 1996; 98: 290-298
35. Weiss LM, Warnke RA, Sklar J. Clonal antigen receptor gene rearrangements and Epstein-Barr viral DNA in tissues of Hodgkin's disease. Hematol Oncol 1988; 6: 233–238
36. Bruiker MG, Poppema S, Buys CH et al. Clonal immunoglobulin gene rearrangements in tissues involved by Hodgkin's disease. Blood 1987; 70: 186–191
37. Weiss LM. Gene analysis and Epstein-Barr viral genome studies of Hodgkin's disease. Int Rev Exp Pathol 1992; 33: 165–184
38. Delabie J, Tierens A, Wu G et al. Lymphocyte predominance Hodgkin's disease: lineage and clonality determination using a single-cell assay. Blood 1994; 84: 3291–3298
39. Wickert RS, Weisenberger DD, Tierens A et al. Clonal relationship between lymphocytic predominance Hodgkin's disease and concurrent or subsequent large cell lymphoma of B lineage. Blood 1995; 86: 2312–2320
40. Stevenson FK. Hodgkin's disease – new insights from immunoglobulin genetics. N Engl J Med 1995; 333: 934–936
41. Tamaru J, Hummel M, Zemlin M et al. Hodgkin's disease with a B-cell phenotype often shows a VDJ rearrangement and somatic mutations in the V_H genes. Blood 1994; 84: 708–715
42. Kamel OW, Chang PP, Hsu FJ et al. Clonal VDJ recombination of the immunoglobulin heavy chain gene by PCR in classical Hodgkin's disease. Am J Clin Pathol 1995; 104: 419–423
43. Orazli A, Jiang B, Lee C-H et al. Correlation between presence of clonal rearrangements of immunoglobulin heavy chain genes and B-cell antigen expression in Hodgkin's disease. Am J Clin Pathol 1995; 104: 413–418
44. Kuppers R, Rajewsky K, Zhao M et al. Hodgkin's disease: Hodgkin and Reed-Sternberg cells picked from histological sections show clonal immunoglobulin gene rearrangements and appear to be derived from B cells at various stages of development. Proc Natl Acad Sci USA 1994; 91: 10962–10966
45. Roth J, Daus H, Trumper L et al. Detection of immunoglobulin heavy-chain gene rearrangements at the single-cell level in malignant lymphomas: no rearrangement is found in Hodgkin and Reed-Sternberg cells. Int J Cancer 1994; 57: 799–804
46. Hummel M, Ziemann K, Lammert H et al. Hodgkin's disease with monoclonal and polyclonal populations of Reed-Sternberg cells. N Engl J Med 1995; 333: 901–906
47. Hummel M, Marafioti T, Stein H. Immunoglobulin V genes in Reed-Sternberg cells. N Engl J Med 1996; 334: 405–406
48. Kanzler H, Kuppers R, Hansmann M-L, Rajewsky K. Hodgkin and Reed-Sternberg cells in Hodgkin's disease represent the outgrowth of a dominant tumor clone derived from (crippled) germinal center B cells. J Exp Med 1996; 184: 1495–1505
49. Yatabe Y, Oka K, Asai J, Mori N. Poor correlation between clonal immunoglobulin gene rearrangement and immunoglobulin gene transcription in Hodgkin's disease. Am J Path 1996; 149: 1351–1361
50. Braeuninger A, Kuppers R, Strickler JG, Wacker H-H, Rajewsky K, Hansmann M-L. Hodgkin and Reed-Sternberg cells in lymphocyte-predominant Hodgkin disease represent clonal populations of germinal center-derived tumor cells. Proc Natl Acad Sci USA 1997; 94: 9337– 9342

6

Molecular genetic changes in prostate cancer

El-Nasir Lalani Andrew Stubbs Gordon W. H. Stamp

Prostate cancer is the commonest cancer in men and the second commonest cause of cancer death in the Western world,[1] and yet it is remarkable how little effort has been expended into the understanding of this disease until relatively recently. Histopathologists have a major role to play in the facilitation of diagnosis and research in modern clinical and research practice and an understanding of the current status of the molecular genetics of the disease is important for the correlation of morphological and scientific data. We anticipate that, in the future, while new diagnostic and therapeutic options will emerge from this work, histological evaluation should remain the 'gold standard' for placing these changes in context and monitoring progression or therapeutic response of the disease.

The incidence of prostate cancer appears to be increasing,[2] although this is partly a consequence of earlier detection,[3] following the introduction of serum assays for prostate specific antigen (PSA) as well as more digital rectal examinations, transrectal ultrasound examinations and increasing use of prostatic needle biopsies as an outpatient procedure. Other factors include the steadily increasing age of populations when the disease is commonest.[4] Variations in diet, particularly saturated fats, may account for demographic differences between Western and Asian populations (in whom the incidence is lowest), but it is at present unclear why African Americans have the highest incidence and mortality rates from this disease.[5]

Dilemmas in diagnosis and therapy

At present, one-half to two-thirds of patients have advanced or metastatic cancer at presentation, and are incurable.[6] Whether PSA (or other) screening

Dr El-Nasir Lalani BSc(Hons) MBChB MRCPath PhD, Senior Lecturer/Honorary Consultant, Imperial College School of Medicine, Hammersmith Hospital, Du Cane Road, London W12 0NN, UK

Dr Andrew Stubbs PhD, Post Doctoral Fellow, Imperial College School of Medicine, Hammersmith Hospital, Du Cane Road, London W12 0NN, UK

Prof. Gordon W.H. Stamp MBChB FRCPath, Imperial College School of Medicine, Hammersmith Hospital, Du Cane Road, London W12 0NN, UK

will enable the identification of cancers at a time when they will be curable is contentious,[6–8] since screening reveals many men with tumours that would never become clinically significant and others which seem localised but with occult metastases which become apparent after radical treatment. The extent of the controversy is demonstrated by one study which postulated that should all men in the UK be screened once and half the detected cancers treated with radical surgery, the predicted operative mortality would exceed the annual death rate from prostate cancer in the same population.[9]

Morphological assessment as the sole basis of assessment?

Conventional histological assessment of prostate cancer is of use but has limitations. The Gleason system, which assesses tumour cytoarchitecture, allows some stratification of indolent and aggressive variants, but over three-quarters of prostate cancers at presentation fall into the intermediate categories where correlation with clinical outcome is weaker.[10] There is also a problem in that biopsy estimation of Gleason grade may be inaccurate. Combining grading with an estimate of tumour volume from imaging or multiple biopsy samples (quadrant or sextant) may give a greater predictive value.[11] For reasons already cited, immunohistochemical study of 'tumour markers' as applied in breast, pancreas or lung have not made any major impact thus far. It is, therefore, essential to identify potential new indicators for progression and metastasis in subgroups of prostate cancers. Conversely it is important to identify changes which may indicate the commonest variety of all, asymptomatic ('histological') prostate cancers which have no, or little, potential to progress, and would be the most prevalent neoplastic alteration in the prostate.

The search for new 'biomarkers' of prostate cancer – why bother?

The disproportionately small research effort into the biology of prostatic carcinoma relative to its morbidity and mortality in the population has recently begun to be redressed to some extent, and information is now emerging about the molecular genetic events which may dictate the progression of this group of cancers. Much of this effort has been directed into alterations in genes described in other solid cancers, e.g. *p16*, *ras*, *p53*, *c erb B-2*, etc., but which have relatively low levels of genetic alteration in prostate cancer. The reasons why tumours arising from different tissues show specific patterns of genetic abnormalities and the mechanisms governing mutational susceptibility in differing cell types are unknown. However, the fact that there are some tissue specific controls over the regulation of cell division and cell death means there is potential for: (i) development of new targeted therapies (gene therapy and immunotherapy); (ii) identification of novel genes which may be fundamental to growth control in the normal and neoplastic prostate; and (iii) development of a diagnostic 'bar code' of genetic mutations in prostate cancer.

There have already been discoveries which indicate that there are genes which are more frequently altered in a proportion of prostatic cancers, and identification of new genes such as PTEN (see later) which may be prostatic epithelial specific. These genetic profiles distinguish prostatic cancers from other solid tumours and may eventually provide a basis for development of screening to identify cancers that have potential for progression from those that will remain latent.

The following article is divided into two sections: (i) methodologies used to identify chromosomal and genetic abnormalities in cancers; and (ii) a review of the current literature on chromosomal abnormalities, oncogenes and tumour suppressor genes TSGs implicated in the development and progression of prostate cancer.

IDENTIFICATION OF GENETIC ABNORMALITIES IN PROSTATE CANCER

THE ROLE OF HISTOPATHOLOGY

Advances made in molecular biology have had a major impact on the practice of surgical pathology[12,13] and pathologists are increasingly being involved in the translation of techniques developed in 'pure' research laboratories to surgically resected or biopsy tissues. Many molecular biological techniques are being adapted for use on routinely fixed paraffin embedded material. Microdissection has increased both specificity and sensitivity for the analysis of DNA, mRNA and protein in samples containing a heterogeneous population of cells. Fixed material is sometimes suboptimal for analysis and the availability of snap-frozen or specially fixed tissues is a major resource in academic pathology institutes.

Methods applicable to human tissue samples

Clues to the presence of a potential genetic abnormality can be obtained from: (i) familial studies; (ii) gene cloning; (iii) gene transfection; (iv) whole or part chromosomal transfer (microcell mediated transfer); and (v) expression studies (immunohistochemical studies, *in situ* hybridisation, etc.). More detailed localisation has been facilitated by advances combining microdissection with molecular biological techniques such as restriction fragment length polymorphism (RFLP) which will detect loss of heterozygosity (LOH), fluorescent *in situ* hybridisation (FISH) for discrimination of gross areas of chromosomal losses or gains and point mutation analysis by allele-specific dinucleotide hybridisation, single strand conformational polymorphism (SSCP) or direct sequencing. Gene amplification, on the other hand, can be detected by Southern blotting, possibly combined with FISH. Comparative genomic hybridisation (CGH) is an additional method for identifying areas of loss between normal and tumour-derived DNAs for the same patient, but is technically demanding. mRNA extracted from a sample, preferably after microdissection to minimise 'normal' contaminants, can be amplified by reverse transcription to make DNA templates followed by PCR amplification, with subsequent sequence analysis.

Microdissection – a research interface

The application of molecular markers to pathological specimens is critically dependent on optimised procedures and the proportion of the sample with the feature of interest, e.g. a specific genetic mutation. Independently arising tumours vary in the combinations of genetic changes they contain and in the precise malignant phenotype they express.[14] Given the heterogeneity of biopsies, and the infiltrative nature of tumours, a low frequency of oncogene/TSG detection could stem from dilution of neoplastic DNA by stromal and/or entrapped non-neoplastic cellular elements. An important consideration in molecular analysis of tissues is the minimisation of the unavoidable contamination of tumour biopsies by such elements.[15] Berthon and colleagues suggest that at least 20% of total DNA from a tumour sample needs to be mutated to score positively in PCR/SSCP analysis. They further suggest that when only one allele is affected greater than 40% of cells present within the specimen used for DNA extraction must be from the tumour.[16] Therefore, the use of precise microdissection techniques is extremely important in analysing molecular markers from fresh and archival material, and is highly dependent on appreciation of tissue cytoarchitecture, the province of histopathologists.

Microsatellite instability

Microsatellites are short DNA motifs up to 6 bases long which show variable number of tandem repeats (usually in the range of 15–35).[17,18] They are highly polymorphic and can accumulate mutations which can then act as markers for genetic linkage analysis. The most common microsatellite is two bases but they can be three, four or five bases in length (short tandem repeats). These repetitive sequences are located mainly within introns and between genes.

DNA repair genes (mismatch repair) maintain the level of microsatellite variation in check, but mutations in the human mismatch repair genes *hMSH2*, *hMLH1*, *hPMS1* and *hPMS2* have been associated with microsatellite instability.[18] In hereditary non-polyposis colorectal carcinoma (HNPCC), many of the tumours exhibit demonstrable microsatellite instability,[19] it does not appear that microsatellite instability is widespread in prostate cancer.

There is in vitro evidence that trinucleotide repeats usually found in the androgen receptor on the X chromosome may also be destabilised in prostate cancer, along with dinucleotide repeats. In prostate cancer, initial studies by Giovanucci et al suggested that shortening of the CAG repeat region in exon 1 of the androgen receptor (AR) gene was associated with advanced and high grade prostate cance.[20] We have found limited CAG polymorphism in prostate cancers with a mode of 19 repeats in over 80% of samples, compared to less than 35% in benign prostates (unpublished observations).

Expansion of trinucleotide repeat regions is associated with several hereditary neurodegenerative disorders, and the greater the expansion, the earlier the onset and severity of disease.[21] In the fragile X syndrome, expansion of trinucleotide repeats causes methylation at CpG residues in the repeat regions and adjacent promotors of the FMRI gene, causing transcription to stop and hence loss of gene expression.[22,23] Alternatively, expanded repeats can be transcribed to give polyglutaminated proteins, as in spino-cerebellar atrophy.

Cytogenetics – gross chromosomal changes

Karyotypic analysis of many primary prostatic cancers has consistently revealed a normal male diploid karyotype (46XY).[24] Cytogenetic changes can broadly be categorised as gains, losses, re-arrangements and transversions. In prostatic carcinoma, chromosomal rearrangements consisting mainly of deletions rather than translocations have been reported. Loss of chromosomes 1, 2, 5, 7, 14, and Y or gains of chromosomes 7, 14, 20, 22 have been reported. Also rearrangements of chromosome arms 2p, 7q and 10q are frequent.[25]

There are several studies which have shown familial clustering in prostate cancer indicating hereditary susceptibility plays a role in a subset of these tumours.[26,27] Segregation analysis of familial prostate cancer suggests the existence of at least one dominant susceptibility locus and predicts that rare high-risk alleles at such loci account in the aggregate for 9% of all prostate cancers and more than 40% of early onset disease.[28]

Loss of heterozygosity – indication of tumour suppressor genes (TSGs)

Several LOH studies have localised candidate TSGs in prostate cancer. In such reports, the most frequent areas of loss are 10q and 16q and less frequently, 13q, 17p and 18q.[29] More recent investigation has highlighted abnormalities of 8p, maximal in 8p12–22. In many cancers there may be losses of alleles detected as LOH by RFLP in up to 20% of the total chromosomes. These consensus areas of deletion, when comparing multiple tumour samples, are still very large, so that searches for specific genes that may be lost can be extremely difficult as many candidate genes may exist within one area. This is one of the problems with identifying candidate genes in areas such as 16q. One way of circumventing this is by applying the technique of representational difference analysis (RDA) which is a means of isolating or identifying the DNA fragments that are present in only one of two sets of genetic information. It utilises the subtractive DNA hybridisation method but differs from conventional methods by using 'representations' of the gene products which reduces the complexity, so that differences in expression are easier to detect. This technology is currently being developed, but potentially can identify regions of LOH and, in particular, areas of homozygous deletions, which for obvious reasons give strong indications of a particular TSG. Thus the potential for identifying homozygous deletions among a high background of heterozygous losses makes RDA an important new approach for the identification of novel TSGs.

CHROMOSOMAL ABERRATIONS, ONCOGENES AND TSGs IN PROSTATE CANCER

CURRENT STATUS OF THE 'GENETIC PROFILE'

In the following section we have highlighted some of the commoner chromosomal aberrations reported in prostate cancer including oncogenes and TSGs. Furthermore, readers' attention is drawn to potential sites considered to harbour TSGs. These potential loci are currently under investigation in several laboratories and may yield specific prostate cancer genes. Under the X chromosome, we have reviewed abnormalities of the androgen receptor in prostate cancer.

Chromosome 1

A genome-wide scan performed in 66 high-risk prostate cancer families provides evidence of linkage to chromosome 1 (1q24–25),[30] indicating a gene conferring susceptibility at this locus, but it is not yet clear how relevant this is to non-hereditary forms of the disease. This locus has been designated HPC1 (hereditary prostate cancer 1). It has previously been demonstrated that the q arm including the 1q24–25 region is increased in copy number in advanced prostate cancer, as demonstrated by CGH. Deletion of region 1q12 has also been reported to be a relatively frequent alteration in prostatic carcinomas.[31]

Chromosome 2

Loss of regions of 2q and regions of 2p has been reported, particularly in advanced androgen-dependent metabolic disease.[26] Interestingly, we have preliminary data indicating selective loss of a region of 2q in prostatic carcinoma cell lines undergoing a transition from androgen dependence to independence (unpublished observations). Further research may uncover TSGs in this region which dictate prostate carcinoma progression.

Chromosome 6

33% of prostate cancers in one series showed LOH at 6q14–21, suggesting the presence of a TSG,[32] a region previously noted to be deleted in ovarian cancers. In the LNCaP (lymph node carcinoma of the prostate) prostatic cell line, a translocation of (6;16)(p21; q22) has been reported.[33] However, cytogenetic and other studies have not indicated a major role for genes on chromosome 6 in the genesis or progression of prostate cancer.

Chromosome 7

Aneusomy (including trisomy of chromosome 7) and its association with higher tumour grade, advanced pathological stage, metastasis and early prostatic carcinoma death have been reported by several groups utilising FISH. Takahashi and colleagues performed PCR analysis of 21 microsatellite loci on 54 paired samples. Chromosome 7 allelic imbalance was found in 30% of the cases of which 28% were losses and 2% gains. The commonest site of allelic loss was at 7q31.1 which correlated with increasing grade and metastasis.[34] Another study indicated allelic imbalance in 46% of cases on 7q.[35] Interestingly, the epidermal growth factor receptor (EGFR) gene is located at 7p13–12 and enhanced expression of EGFR has been reported to correlate with increased grade.[36] Numerical aberration of chromosome 7 is significantly associated with higher Gleason score and metastasis.[37]

Chromosome 8

Allelic loss of the 8p arm in prostate cancer occurs frequently, over 85% in some series,[38–41] and is often accompanied by multiplication of the 8q arm, a likely genetic mechanism underlying these results, which demonstrate gain of chromosome 8. Allelic imbalance of chromosome 8 is associated with advanced disease and high Gleason scores.[38,41] The loss is particularly high in regions 8p11.1–21.1 and somewhat lower at 8p22, indicating these regions contain TSGs.[42] How these alterations correlate with clinical outcome is unclear and it may be that chromosome 8 aberrations are late events[43] being less frequently encountered in prostatic intra-epithelial neoplasia (PIN),[44] in contrast to breast cancers.[45] Further studies are required to confirm this. Experimentally, microcell-mediated transfer of chromosome 8 into the Dunning rat prostate cancer cell line R3327 suppresses the metastatic ability of these cells.[46]

myc genes

The *c-myc* gene is found at 8q24 and is a member of the helix-loop-helix-leucine zipper (HLH-Zip) transcription factors, which dimerise with other members of the family, subsequently permitting DNA binding and may allow the trans–criptional activation domains present within the MYC proteins to modulate expression of genes near the binding sites. There is controversy over *c-myc* being amplified in prostatic carcinomas and there are also conflicting reports of *c-myc* overexpression in prostatic carcinomas, increasing with grade, compared to benign tumours,[47–49] although it has not been found to correlate with survival.[50] One study using FISH found a simple gain of chromosome 8 in 42% of PIN, 25% of primary and 46% of metastatic prostate cancers. Hybridisation specifically for *c-myc* revealed modest increases in copy numbers in 8% PIN, 11% primary carcinomas and 25% of metastases, and substantial increases in 0% PIN, 8% primary and 21% metastatic carcinomas. The latter group strongly correlated with grade.[51]

Chromosome 9

Very few studies have identified any loss or gain of chromosome 9 in prostate cancer but there have been investigations of the *p16* gene which maps to 9p21 (also called *CDK4I* – cyclin-dependent kinase 4 inhibitor, *MTS1* or *ink4*). It is proposed as a genetic target of mutations in certain cancers such as pancreatic adenocarcinoma. Allelic loss of *p16* has been reported in a variety of tumour types, including prostatic carcinoma, some of which are nucleotide sequence changes being accompanied by the loss of the wild type allele, the remainder involving homozygous deletions of both copies. However, there is a very low frequency of genetic abnormality in prostate cancer,[52] contrasting with pancreatic adenocarcinomas (where mutational abnormalities are seen in up to 80% of cases), oesophageal squamous cell carcinoma and familial melanoma, for instance. A mutation at codon 76 has been reported in the human prostatic cancer cell line DU145.[53]

Chromosome 10

In human prostate cancer, deletion of at least one chromosome 10 locus is relatively frequent (37–71%),[54,55] and in one study deletions of 10p (17%) and 10q (14%) (both 40%) have been reported.[56] In vitro studies on a prostatic carcinoma cell line have suggested the presence of a TSG distally on 10p, and which is more frequently deleted in prostatic than other carcinomas.[57] One region of deletion maps to 10p11.2.[55] The MXI1 gene which negatively regulates *c-myc* activity has been found to map to 10q24–25 and, in some cases of prostate cancers, a deletion mutation has been reported. A recent study has also identified a candidate TSG at 10q23, designated *PTEN* (phosphatase and tensin homologue deleted on chromosome ten),[58] which is mutated in prostate, breast and glial cell lines. It has a tyrosine phosphatase domain and shows extensive homology to tensin, a protein interacting with actin filaments at focal adhesions, suggesting it may interfere with cytoskeletal structure by inhibiting protein tyrosine kinases.

Microcell-mediated transfer of a fragment 10pter–q11 suppressed tumourigenesis and enhanced apoptosis[59] and transfer of distal 10p chromosome fragments decreased tumourigenicity in a prostate cancer cell line PPC-1.[60]

Chromosome 11

The 11p11.2 region contains a gene capable of acting as a metastasis suppressor in rat prostatic cancer cell lines.[61] This region contains the membrane glycoprotein KAI 1, which also has a metastasis suppressing activity.[62] KAI 1 is expressed in normal and benign prostatic hyperplasia but is lower in prostate cancer cells.[61] Its role in human prostatic carcinoma is yet to be investigated. The 11pter–q14 region has been claimed to suppress metastatic ability in rat prostate cancer cell lines,[63] although no candidate gene has yet been identified.

Chromosome 12

Microcell mediated transfer has indicated that a gene in the region 12pter–12q13 acts as a tumour suppressor.[64] Previous studies have not implicated chromosome 12 very heavily in the genesis of prostate cancer.

Chromosome 13

The 13q region displays allelic imbalance in up to 30% of primary prostatic carcinomas,[35] a region which contains the retinoblastoma gene (*Rb1*) and *BRCA2* (13q12), but there is little evidence as yet that they have a role in sporadic prostate cancer and further study is needed. It has been suggested that there is another TSG in the region of 13q14.[65] Alterations in the mRNA size of the *BRCA1* gene have been reported to be present in the prostatic cell line DU145 and LOH in the 13q12–13 region was observed in prostate cancers developing in families showing *BRCA2* linkage.

Rb1 TSG

The *Rb1* on chromosome 13q14.2 was the first TSG whose existence was predicted by Knudson. The *Rb1* gene product codes for a 105 kDa nuclear phosphoprotein and functions to suppress cell division by preventing cells in G_1 phase from entering S phase, probably by interacting with transcription factors including the E2F family. Abnormalities of the *Rb1* gene have been found in the DU145 prostate cancer cell line with a point mutation in one allele.[67] The re-introduction of normal *Rb1* gene by retroviral vector transfer into DU145 cell line results in a reduction in its tumourigenicity in nude mice. Limited series of prostatic carcinomas have further shown that there may be lack of expression of Rb1 proteins in a minority of cases,[68] but this is a small proportion compared to other tumours such as breast and other cancers.[69,70]

Chromosome 14

bcl-2 oncogene

The *bcl-2* proto-oncogene was identified in 1984 while studying the t(14;18) translocations which frequently occur in B cell leukemia and non-Hodgkin's follicular lymphomas. The gene is located at chromosome 18q21. The t(14;18) translocation brings the *bcl-2* gene next to the immunoglobulin heavy chain (IgH) loci at chromosome 14. This creates a *bcl-2/igH* fusion gene resulting in overexpression of *bcl-2*. *bcl-2* is referred to as a death suppressor gene. Immunohistochemical studies may demonstrate the protein in tissues and, while it is constitutionally expressed in the basal cell layer, several studies have demonstrated enhanced expression especially in hormone refracory prostate refractory tumours,[71] which suggest it may be connected with development of androgen insensitivity.[72]

c-fos oncogene

The *c-fos* oncogene encodes a protein (fos) that is postulated to act in the intercellular signal transduction pathways in conjunction with jun proteins and seems to facilitate transformation by other oncogenes by binding to specific DNA sequences. It has been claimed that there is a relationship between androgen receptor content and *c-fos* expression,[73,74] androgen deprivation showing a reduction in *c-fos* expression by up to 90% in some prostate carcinoma cell lines. However, no gene amplification for *c-fos* has been demonstrated in prostate cancer.

Chromosome 16

This harbours one of the most frequently deleted regions in prostate cancer (up to 42%) on 16q.[35] Deletions on the long arm of 16q map to 16q 22.1–22.3, 16q 23.2–24.1 and 16q 24.3–qter.[75] The E-cadherin cell:cell adhesion molecule located at 16q22.1 shows decreased expression, especially in poorly differentiated cancers. However, reduced E-cadherin expression has been noted in other cancers and no somatic mutations have been demonstrated in prostatic carcinoma.[75] Furthermore, it appears that there are a number of more important potential TSGs in this region other than E-cadherin itself, possibly in the region of 16q24.[76] The invasive phenotype in prostate cancer may be more associated with the upregulation of other cadherins such as protocadherin 42 and OB-cadherin.[77] A 130 kDa protein (p130) maps to 16q12.2–13 which is a region deleted in some prostate cancers and has been demonstrated to bind to cyclins A and E[78] and thus may be a candidate TSG.

Chromosome 17

p53 TSG

The *p53* tumour suppressor gene is one of the most frequently affected in solid cancers and maps to the 17q13.1 region. It has some similarities with *Rb1* in that it is a nuclear phosphoprotein that appears to arrests cells in G_1. *p53* may function in a protective role, halting division in order to allow repair of genetic damage or, if the latter is too great, directing cells into apoptosis in order to eliminate the possibility of propagating harmful genetic abnormalities[79,80] *p53* function is also lost by a process of allelic deletion and specific point mutations in the remaining gene, eliminating normal function. The situation is complex, in that some of the mutated gene products paradoxically appear to act in a dominant fashion, actively promoting cell division. The analysis of *p53* expression can be difficult. The simplistic idea that the mutated *p53* gene product which is stabilised and has a longer half life, thus rendering it detectable by immunohistochemistry does not necessarily provide an easy evaluation of mutation. This is because over-expressed normal *p53* may be detectable by sensitive immunohistochemical techniques, and some mutated forms of *p53* do not render the product detectable by this technique. Thus, over-expression may be either mutated product or normal product over-expressed in a reactive fashion.

It is more reliable to detect mutations by molecular techniques which include single strand conformational polymorphism (SSCP) or direct DNA sequencing of amplified DNA fragments. Using such approaches several groups have assessed *p53* alterations in prostate cancer compared to those in other human solid cancers but, in general, *p53* alterations appear relatively uncommon falling within the range of 10–20%,[81,82] a figure which contrasts with 50–70% in mammary carcinomas, for example. In addition, prostate cancer does not appear to be a component of the cancer families that have germ line mutations in the *p53* gene. One feature that does emerge is that while *p53* abnormalities are uncommon in early or localised disease, they are much more common in metastatic or advanced local cancers.[83,84] Interestingly, allelic loss of 17p appeared to be highly correlated with increased risk of recurrence,[82] indicating there may be another gene in this region more relevant to prostatic cancer progression.

c-erb 2 oncogene

There is considerable controversy over the expression of *c-erb 2* (also known as *Neu* or *Her-2*) in prostate cancer. *c-erb 2* gene maps to 17q21 and codes for a protein homologous to a truncated form of the epidermal growth factor receptor (EGFR). In many carcinomas, especially breast carcinomas, the major mechanism of *c-erb 2* over-expression is due to genomic DNA amplification without over-production of the mRNA and protein. In a smaller number of cases, over-expression occurs without demonstrable amplification.[85] Amplification of the *c-erb 2* gene in prostate carcinoma appears to be a rare event in contrast to breast carcinomas, but there are other mechanisms where over-expression of the *c-erb 2* gene may occur.

Immunohistochemical studies have given rise to conflicting results almost certainly due to the use of different antibodies.[86–88] Many workers have assumed that cytoplasmic positivity reflects *c-erb 2* over-expression and have, therefore, observed positivity in basal cells in the normal prostate and in up to 80% of prostatic carcinomas. However, other reports using different antibodies and criteria, which include restriction to membrane associated expression, find very few prostatic carcinomas 'positive'. It is important that protein expression in tissue studies should be qualified by intensity, distribution and cellular localisation data rather than positive or negative, to avoid confusion.

It remains to be seen what the functional significance of cytoplasmic versus membrane expression of *c-erb 2* may have, and for the success or otherwise of gene therapy programmes using *c-erb 2* to activate pro drugs.

BRCA1 gene

BRCA1 has been implicated in prostate cancer development by epidemiological and genetic studies, but more recent evidence indicates the region distal to 17q12–21 shows more frequent LOH indicating one or more TSGs may be found.[89] On the other hand, Gao et al claim a region centromeric of *BRCA1* is likely to contain a TSG.[90] Microcell mediated transfer of 17pter–q23 also shows metastasis suppressing activity.[63]

Chromosome 18

Allelic losses of 18q have been identified in 33% of prostate cancers.[35] The deleted in colon cancer (*DCC*) gene is located on chromosome 18q21/22 and reduced expression has been shown in varying numbers of prostate cancers, but its relevance to progression of disease has yet to be elucidated.

Other oncogenes investigated in prostate cancer

ras *genes*

H-ras (11p15,5), *K-ras2* (12p12.1) and *N-ras* (1p13) oncogene abnormalities are relatively rare in prostatic carcinomas, in contrast to say pancreatic cancer, where *K-ras2* mutations are identified in over 85% of cases. Some studies have failed to demonstrate any association between *ras* and grade of cancer in Western populations, although it has been claimed it is important in subgroups of prostate cancers in Far Eastern men. LNCaP cells transfected with a mutated *K-ras* gene subsequently became androgen independent and showed increased anchorage independent colony formation. In addition, transfection of mutated *H-ras* into the rat prostatic cell line results in acquisition of a metastatic phenotype. In human cancers, *H-ras* point mutations are found in less than 5% of prostate cancers but in Japanese males *K-ras* mutations are found in up to 25% in the latent form of prostate cancer. Most of the mutations found in non-progressive latent disease are associated with *K-ras* (A to T transversion code on 61) but clinically manifest cancers are associated with *H-ras* mutations.

X chromosome

Androgen receptor gene abnormalities in prostate cancer

Androgens are required for the development of both the normal prostate and prostate cancer, and the regulation of cellular proliferation in prostate cancer has centred on endocrine therapy. Initially, 70–80% of tumours are sensitive to androgen deprivation, the mechanism of which is probably via a pathway of programmed cell death.[91] However, in patients with advanced disease, most tumours progress to an androgen-independent state with proliferation of cells that do not require androgens for growth.

The mechanism of acquired hormonal insensitivity is unknown,[92] however, in at least some cases, androgen independence has been associated with a lack or mutation of the androgen receptor.[93,94] Proposed mechanisms of progression to androgen independent growth include the loss of androgen receptor (AR) expression,[95] amplification of the AR gene[96] and structural changes in the AR protein.[97]

The AR gene

The human androgen receptor (AR) is a member of the ligand activated steroid thyroid hormone transcription factors.[98] The gene (>90 kb) is located on the X chromosome (Xq11–12) of which the coding region is separated over eight exons (see Figure).[99] The AR cDNA sequence possesses an open reading frame of 2730 bp encoding a protein of 910 amino acids with a molecular mass of 98.5 kDa. There are four functional domains: (i) a highly polymorphic, ~550 bp N-terminal portion which modulates the amplitude[100] and probably the specificity of its target gene effects;[101] (ii) a central 67 bp DNA binding domain (DBD); (iii) an 8 bp nuclear localisation signal; and (iv) a C-terminal 250 hormone binding domain (HBD).

The N-terminal domain is characterised by a high abundance of acidic residues and by the presence of several homopolymeric residues of which expansion of one of the polyglutamine stretches results in decreased translation.[102] The AR's DBD has a 'D-box' on its C-terminal zinc finger for normal dimerisation, and several residues that effect normal transregulatory function after AR-androgen response element (AR-ARE) binding.[103] Once bound, the AR's HBD has transcriptional regulatory properties and contributes to dimerisation and nuclear localisation.[100] Phe_{581} and Arg_{614} are strictly conserved residues of the DBD with Phe_{581} being a key component of the discriminatory N-terminal helix of the DBD and thus concerned with the affinity and specificity of AR-androgen response element (ARE) binding.

AR levels in prostate cancer

Treatment of prostate cancer has focused on androgen ablation therapy and treatment failure is associated with an androgen insensitivity and tumour progression. Biochemical determination of AR levels in both tumour and normal was thought to have a prognostic value or indicative of response to treatment to demonstrate the presence of AR in both cytosol and nuclear fractions of benign and malignant prostatic cells. In one study, a 4-fold decrease in nuclear AR (ARn) was reported in the metastasis compared to the primary tumour.[104] While the total receptor content of both metastatic and primary tissues was similar, the metastatic cells possessed higher levels of cytosolic AR (ARc), a shift which implies 'deactivation' of the receptor.[104] In contrast, Masai et al claimed that, immunocytochemically, AR was exclusively localized in the nuclei of both benign and malignant cells but this may be heterogeneous, especially in poorly differentiated tumours, the proportion of strongly positive cells inversely correlated with Gleason grade.[105] The prognostic value of AR levels, whether total or nuclear, has been difficult to evaluate owing to different assays and to the variability of anti-AR antibodies used in these studies. No correlation between AR positive nuclei and responsiveness to therapy was found in 17 patients with stage D prostatic carcinomas,[106] but a significant correlation between the number of AR positive cells with endocrine response, time-to-progression, and survival has been reported.[107,108] The LNCaP cell line shows androgen responsive growth providing an in vitro AR prostate cancer model.[109] When LNCaP cells were cultured in serum-free conditions (no hormones or other growth factors) then stimulated with either a synthetic androgen or dihydrotestosterone, a 10-fold increase in AR activity was observed.[110] AR protein levels mirror this increase but unexpectedly, AR mRNA levels are decreased.[111] Thus, prostatic tumours may adapt to endocrine treatment by increasing AR protein and activity.[112] In patients with advanced androgen-independent prostate cancer in relapse following androgen ablation therapy, the level of AR mRNA in their bone marrow tissue was similar to the level expressed in LNCaP cells.[113] In contrast, AR mRNA levels were not detectable by PCR in patients who were in complete remission after androgen ablation.[113] These results are consistent with results of immunohistochemical analysis of AR expression in patients with advanced androgen-independent prostatic carcinomas.[112]

Somatic mutation of the AR gene in prostate cancer

Mutations in the three AR functional domains can, in some instances, have dramatic effects on AR function in vitro. LNCaP cells are known to be stimulated by anti-androgens[114] and sequencing of the LNCaP AR gene revealed an A→G transition at codon 877 in exon 8.[94] Transfection of this mutated AR cDNA into COS cells produced a receptor with revealed high binding affinities for progesterone, estradiol, and the non-steroidal anti-androgens.[94,115] The question arising from these data is whether similar mutations exist in vivo. Thus, a mutation which allows tumour cells to activate AR in an androgen depleted medium has been demonstrated in both primary and advanced prostate cancer.[116,117] Other mutations localised to the hormone binding domain (HBD) have similar effects. A Val→Met transition, detected in advanced prostate cancer, is more effectively activated by adrenal androgens (dehydroepiandrosterone and androstenedione), the dihydrotestosterone metabolites (androsterone and androstanediol) and progesterone than the wild type AR.[118]

Earlier studies suggested that the frequency of AR mutations in prostate cancer was low, no mutations being found in exons 2–8 in a series of 18 hormone refractory prostate cancers.[119] In another series of 25 primary prostate tumours, mutations in the AR were discovered in 44%.[120] Thus rapid onset of androgen-independent growth of prostatic carcinomas may be due to selective outgrowth of cells with existing mutated AR rather than the acquisition of new mutations with the onset of treatment.

There are numerous reports of single base pair mutations in the coding region of AR, but there are conflicting data on their frequency (Figure). The reasons for this variation are possibly due to the nature of the extracted DNA, the stage of the tumour, the nature of therapy, or the method of mutation analysis. There are a reported 243 different AR mutations, of these only 10–15% are associated with prostate cancer. These mutations are in the public domain. Furthermore, AR mutations are randomly distributed throughout the coding sequence with no clear hotspots (Figure).[121]

AR gene amplification

Overexpression of genes, due to genomic amplification, is a mechanism by which cancer cells overcome therapeutic interventions.[122] AR gene amplification has been demonstrated in 30% of hormone refractory tumours but not in specimens taken prior to androgen deprivation therapy.[96] Immunohistochemically detectable AR was found in the primary and recurrent tumours by the same group suggesting that AR was transcriptionally active.[96] Amplification was found only after prolonged androgen ablation and

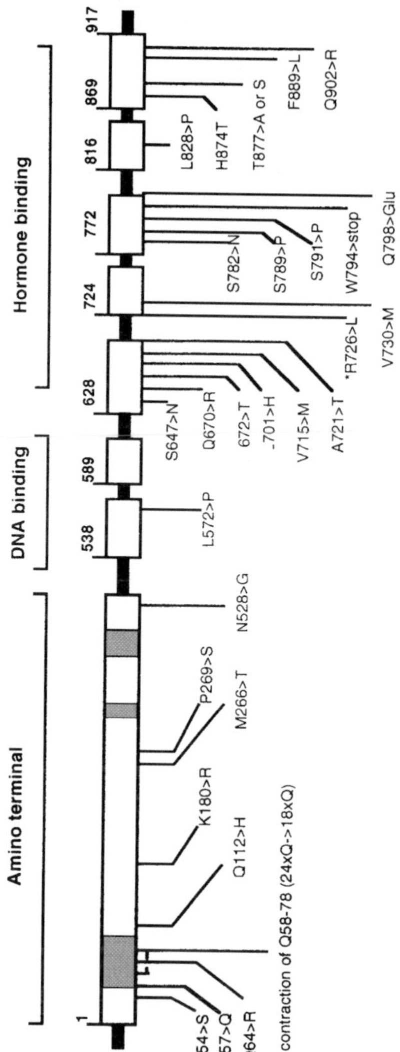

Figure AR gene mutations identified in prostate cancer taken from the AR mutation database.[121] The number of the first amino acid coded by individual exons is shown above each exon (numbered according to Lubahn et al[99]) and the shaded areas in exon 1 indicate the locations of the three homopolymeric regions.

the elevated copy number (up to 4-fold) was associated with enhanced AR transcription.[123,124] Sequence analysis of the amplified HBD revealed that none possessed the promiscuous 877 mutation and that only one possessed a silent mutation.[124] It has been suggested that amplification of AR is most likely to occur in tumours that initially responded to endocrine therapy compared to those with no response to therapy and with a 2-fold increase in the median survival time after recurrence in the former as compared with the latter group.[124] Thus, failure of androgen ablation therapy may be caused by a clonal expansion of androgen-dependent tumour cells that grow in the presence of low serum androgen levels; this adaptation is due to AR gene amplification and the concomitant increased AR expression.

Microsatellite instability of AR exon 1

The transcription activation domain of the AR resides in the N-terminal (encoded by exon 1) which contains the polymorphic trinucleotide repeats CAG and GGC coding for polyglutamine and polyglycine, respectively.[125] The average length of the CAG microsatellite in the population is 21 ±2 (range 11–31)[125] and a modal class of 16 (range 8–17) for GGC.[126] Expansion of the CAG repeats (to 40-52 CAGs) occurs in patients with X-linked spinal and bulbar muscular atrophy.[23] Elimination of the polyglutamine tract results in elevated transcription activation and progressive increase of the CAG caused a linear decrease of transcription activation but not complete elimination of AR transcription activation.[102] It is possible, therefore, that shorter CAG alleles result in more active cell growth, due to increased AR transactivation, even at low levels of androgens during endocrine therapy. Shoenberg et al demonstrated a somatic contraction of the AR CAG repeat (24→18) in a patient unresponsive to antiandrogen therapy.[127] Irvine et al have demonstrated a prevalence of short CAG repeats (< 22 repeats) was greatest (75%) in African American males who have the highest risk of prostate cancer and lowest (49%) in Asians who are at a lower risk of developing prostate cancer. In the 47 patients with < 22 CAG repeats, 43% possessed long GGC alleles (> 16 repeats).[126] Thus linkage disequilibrium occurs between the CAG and the GGC repeats within this patient group, but is absent from subjects without a history of prostate cancer.[105] Stanford et al analyzed the polymorphic (CAG)(n) and (GGN)(n) regions within the androgen receptor gene from 578 participants (301 cases and 277 controls) in a population-based, case control study of prostate cancer in Caucasians aged 40–64 years. They evaluated associations between repeat lengths, the risk of developing prostate cancer and the effects of modifying factors, such as age, body mass index and family history of prostate cancer. The overall age adjusted relative odds of prostate cancer associated with the number of GAG repeats as a continuous variable was 0.97 [95% confidence interval (CI), 0.92 1.03], suggesting that, for each additional CAG repeat, there was a 3% decrease in the risk of developing prostate cancer. The overall results of this study are provocative and support the hypothesis that (CAG)(n) array length is a predictor of risk for prostate cancer.[128]

Androgen-insensitivity without loss or mutation of the androgen receptor

Progression of androgen-independent tumour growth may be a result of several genetic and epigenetic events including mutations in, and altered expression levels of, AR. Mechanisms by which prostate cancer cells circumvent endocrine therapy have thus far focused on: (i) loss of the receptor; (ii) amplification of the wild type AR and clonal expansion of these cells; and (iii) mutations of the AR either resulting in increased transactivation (CAG repeat region; exon 1) and/or loss of specificity for steroid hormones and their antagonists.

However, novel mechanisms not involving loss, mutation or over-expression of the AR have been identified in cell culture systems. Several LNCaP sublines which have either[129] arisen spontaneously or by maintenance of the original line in steroid-depleted medium have resulted in an androgen-independent cell line LNCaP-r (resistant).[130] LNCaP cells are growth stimulated in a biphasic, dose-dependent manner (< 1 nM dihydrotestosterone; DHT).[131] LNCaP-r, which also expresses AR, is not stimulated by DHT (up to 10 nM) and is inhibited by 100 nM DHT.[130] Comparative studies of androgen response patterns and growth rates demonstrate clearly that LNCaP and LNCaP-r are different cell lines[130,132] but the presence of the codon 877 mutation confirms that LNCaP-r is a variant of LNCaP.[132] Thus, although the AR is present and functioning in the LNCaP-r cell line, an alternative pathway is operational circumventing the need for the AR.

PC-3 cells, derived from a bone-metastases of a hormone refractory prostate cancer, are hormone unresponsive. AR transfection studies in PC-3 cells (this cell line does not normally produce an AR transcript) have produced conflicting data. Yuan et al reported a growth inhibition, with dihydrotestosterone (DHT).[133] Deletion of HBD from the construct had no effect on the growth rate of these transfectants. In another study, PC-3 transfected with an identical construct to that used by Yuan et al[133] resulted in androgen-dependent growth stimulated by DHT.[134] These conflicting data have been further compounded by results from a recent study where PC-3 cells were transfected with an episomal AR construct which resulted in growth suppression.[135]

Potential mechanisms for this differential role of androgens in supposedly androgen responsive cell lines (i.e. AR positive) may be due to accessory factors which selectively interact with AR to determine the specificity of AR target gene activation. In a clonal variant of the PC-3 cell line, PC-3^{AR+} (this clone possesses low levels of immunoreactive AR),[136] the level of AR mRNA is similar to that observed in normal androgen responsive genital skin fibroblasts and the level of AR staining (of both amino and carboxy termini) is higher than androgen responsive breast carcinoma cell lines (ZR-75-1, MCF-7 and T47-D). However, these cells did not proliferate in response to the synthetic androgen, mibolerone, and lack specific ligand binding. There are no gross deletions or mutations in either the DBD or HBD which imply a novel mechanism for androgen insensitivity in this prostate cancer cell line.[136] Yeh et al have isolated a novel ligand-dependent AR-associated transcription enhancer (ARA_{70}). In the AR negative prostate cancer cell line, DU-145, ARA_{70} enhances AR transcription (10-fold) in the presence of 0.1 nM DHT or 1 nM testosterone but not with 1 μM of the anti-androgen, hydroxyflutamide.[137] This factor is receptor specific and demonstrates that the tissue specific action of AR is dependent on accessory proteins for the modulation of gene expression by androgens.

To understand the switch from androgen dependence to independence, Klein et al have propagated several locally advanced or metastatic human prostate tumours as xenografts in SCID mice.[138] One of these lines, LAPC-4, established from a tumour which was unresponsive to anti-androgens (androgen independent growth) became androgen dependent in SCID mice. Thus, advanced prostate cancer appears to consist of a heterogeneous population of androgen-dependent and independent cells. LAPC-4 and another line, LAPC-3, both express PSA and wild type AR (in both DBD and HBD) but differ in their androgen dependence. Thus androgen-independence can occur in the absence of mutations in either the DBD or the HBD of the AR gene.[138]

CONCLUSIONS

It is clear that differing cancers reveal distinct patterns of genetic aberration and the currently emerging data indicate that prostatic carcinoma progression is accompanied by particular profiles in the early, late and metastatic stages of the disease. More detailed analysis of these regions will undoubtedly add to diagnosis, therapy selection and provide some of the key answers to understanding of prostate cancer progression. These include why some cancers remain indolent, why the disease is so prevalent in ageing males, why prostate cancer preferentially metastasises to bone and which mechanisms underlie the progression from hormone dependency to independence. We anticipate that pathologists will have a central role in undertaking research which will answer some of these questions and provide a more objective basis for diagnosis and therapy in the future.

REFERENCES

1. Parker SL, Tong T, Bolden S, Wingo PA. Cancer statistics 1996. CA Cancer J Clin 1996; 46: 5–27
2. Boyle P, Maisonneuve P, Napalkov P. Incidence of prostate cancer will double by the year 2030: the argument for. Eur Urol 1996; 29 (Suppl 2): 3–9
3. Waterbor JW, Buescher AJ. Prostate cancer screening (United States). Cancer Causes Control 1995; 6: 267–274
4. Dijkman GA, Debruyne FMJ. Epidemiology of prostate cancer. Eur Urol 1996; 30: 281–295
5. Mettlin C, Natarajan M, Murphy GP. Recent patterns of care of prostate cancer patients in the United States: results from the survey of the American College of Surgeons Commission on Cancer. Int Adv Surg Oncol 1982; 5: 419–424
6. Schroder FH, Boyle P. Screening for prostate cancer – necessity or nonsense? Eur J Cancer 1993; 29A: 656–661
7. Woolf SH. Screening for prostate cancer with prostate-specific antigen. An examination of the evidence [Review]. N Engl J Med 1995; 333: 1401–1405
8. Potosky AL, Miller BA, Albertsen PC, Kramer BS. The role of increasing detection in the rising incidence of prostate cancer. JAMA 1995; 273: 548–552
9. Hall RR. Screening and early detection of prostate cancer will decrease morbidity and mortality from prostate cancer: the argument against. Eur Urol 1996; 29 (Suppl 2): 24–26
10. Isaacs JT. Molecular markers for prostate cancer metastasis: developing diagnostic methods for predicting the aggressiveness of prostate cancer. Am J Pathol 1997; 150: 1511–1522
11. Ravery V, Limot O, Tobolski F et al. Advances in the assessment of clinically localized prostate cancer. Eur Urol 1996; 29: 257–265
12. Arends MJ, Bird CC. Recombinant DNA technology and its diagnostic applications. Histopathology 1992; 21: 303–313
13. Rowley JD, Aster JC, Sklar J. The impact of new DNA diagnostic technology on the management of cancer patients. Survey of diagnostic techniques. Arch Pathol Lab Med 1993; 117: 1104–1109
14. Bishop JM. Molecular themes in oncogenesis. Cell 1996; 64: 235–248
15. Lisitsyn N, Wigler M. Cloning the differences between 2 complex genomes. Science 1993; 259: 946–951
16. Berthon P, Dimitrov T, Stower M, Cussenot O, Maitland NJA. Microdissection approach to detect molecular markers during progression of prostate cancer. Br J Cancer 1995; 72: 946–951
17. Koreth J, O'Leary JJ, McGee JO'D. Microsatellites and PCR genomic analysis. J Pathol 1996; 178: 239–248

18. Karran P. Microsatellite instability and DNA mismatch repair in human cancer. Cancer Biol 1996; 7: 15–24
19. Bishop DT, Hall NR. The genetics of colorectal cancer. Eur J Cancer 1994; 30: 1946–1956
20. Giovanucci E, Stampfer MJ, Krithvas K et al. The CAG repeat within the androgen receptor gene and its relationship to prostate cancer. Proc Natl Acad Sci USA 1997; 94: 3320–3323.
21. Spiegel R, La Spada AR, Kress W, Fischbeck KH, Schmid W. Somatic stability of the expanded CAG trinucleotide repeat in X-linked spinal and bulbar muscular atrophy. Hum Mutat 1996; 8: 32–37
22. La Spada AR, Paulson HL, Fischbeck KH. Trinucleotide repeat expansion in neurological disease. Ann Neurol 1994; 36: 814–822
23. La Spada AR, Wilson EM, Lubhan DB, Harding AE, Fishbeck KH. Androgen receptor gene mutations in X-linked spinal and bulbar muscular atrophy. Nature 1991; 352: 77–79
24. Brothman AR, Peehl DM, Patel AM, McNeal JE. Frequency and pattern of karyotypic abnormalities in human prostate cancer. Cancer Res 1990; 50: 3795–3803
25. Cher ML, Bova GS, Moore DH et al. Genetic alterations in untreated metastases and androgen-independent prostate cancer detected by comparative genomic hybridisation and allelotyping. Cancer Res 1996; 56: 3091–3102
26. Steinberg GD, Carter BS, Beaty TH, Childs B, Walsh PC. Family history and the risk of prostate cancer. Prostate 1990; 17: 337–347
27. Carter BS, Bova GS, Beaty TH et al. Hereditary prostate cancer: epdemiologic and clinical features. J Urol 1993; 150: 797–802
28. Carter BS, Beaty TH, Steinberg GD, Childs B, Walsh PC. Mendelian inheritance of familial prostate cancer. Proc Natl Acad Sci USA 1992; 89: 3367–3371
29. Bova GS, Isaacs WB. Review of allelic loss and gain in prostate cancer. World J Urol 1996; 14: 338–346
30. Smith JR, Freige D, Carpten JD et al. Major susceptibility locus for prostate cancer on chromosome 1 suggested by a genome wide search. Science 1996; 274: 1371–1374
31. Qi H, Dal-Cin P, Van-de-Voorde W et al. del(1)(q12) in adenocarcinomas of the prostate. Cancer Genet Cytogenet 1996; 87: 79-127
32. Cooney KA, Wetzel JC, Consolino CM, Wojno KJ. Identification and characterization of proximal 6q deletions in prostate cancer. Cancer Res 1996; 56: 4150–4153
33. Veronese ML, Bullrich F, Negrini M, Croce CM. The t(6;16)(p21;q22) chromosome translocation in the LNCaP prostate carcinoma cell line results in a tpc/hpr fusion gene. Cancer,Res 1996; 56: 728–732
34. Takahashi S, Shan AL, Ritland SR et al. Frequent loss of heterozygosity at 7q31.1 in primary prostate cancer is associated with tumor aggressiveness and progression. Cancer Res 1995; 55: 4114–4119
35. Latil A, Fournier G, Cussenot O, Lidereau R. Differential chromosome allelic imbalance in the progression of human prostate cancer. J Urol 1996; 156: 2079–2083
36. Morris GL, Dodd JG. Epidermal growth factor receptor mRNA levels in human prostatic tumors and cell lines. J Urol 1990; 143: 1272–1274
37. Matsuura H, Shiraishi T, Yatani R, Kawamura J. Interphase cytogenetics of prostate cancer: fluorescence in situ hybridisation (FISH) analysis of Japanese cases. Br J Cancer 1996; 74: 1699–1704
38. Vocke CD, Pozzatti RO, Bostwick DG et al. Analysis of 99 microdissected prostate carcinomas reveals a high frequency of allelic loss on chromosome 8p12-21. Cancer Res 1996; 56: 24111–24126
39. Macoska JA, Trybus TM, Sakr WA et al. Fluorescence in situ hybridization analysis of 8p allelic loss and chromosome 8 instability in human prostate cancer. Cancer Res 1994; 54: 3824–3830
40. Trapman J, Sleddens HF, van der Weiden MM et al. Loss of heterozygosity of chromosome 8 microsatellite loci implicates a candidate tumor suppressor gene between the loci D8S87 and D8S133 in human prostate cancer. Cancer Res 1994; 54: 6061–6064
41. Bova GS, Carter BS, Bussemakers MJ et al. Homozygous deletion and frequent allelic loss of chromosome 8p22 loci in human prostate cancer. Cancer Res 1993; 53: 3869–3873
42. Cunningham JM, Shan AL, Wick MJ et al. Allelic imbalance and microsatellite instability in prostatic adenocarcinoma. Cancer Res 1996; 56: 4475–4482

43. Macgrogan D, Levy A, Bostwick D, Wagner M, Wells D, Bookstein R. Loss of chromosome arm 8 p loci in prostate cancer: mapping by quantitative allelic imbalance. Genes Chromosom Cancer 1994; 10: 151–154
44. Alers JC, Krijtenburg PJ, Vissers KJ. Bosman FT, van-der-Kwast TH, van-Dekken H. Interphase cytogenetics of prostatic adenocarcinoma and precursor lesions: analysis of 25 radical prostatectomies and 17 adjacent prostatic intraepithelial neoplasias. Genes Chromosom Cancer 1995; 12: 241–250
45. Yaremko ML, Kutza C, Lyzak J, Mick R, Recant WM, Westbrook CA. Loss of heterozygosity from the short arm of chromosome 8 is associated with invasive behaviour in breast cancer. Genes Chromosom Cancer 1996; 16: 189–195
46. Ichikawa T, Nihei N, Kuramochi H et al. Metastasis suppressor genes for prostate cancer. Prostate Suppl 1996; 6: 31–35
47. Jenkins RB, Qian JQ, Lieber MM, Bostwick DG. Detection of *c-myc* oncogene amplification and chromosomal anomalies in metastatic prostate carcinoma by fluorescence *in situ* hybridisation. Cancer Res 1997; 57: 524–531
48. Phillips ME, Ferro MA, Smith PJ, Davies P. Intranuclear androgen receptor deployment and protooncogene expression in human diseased prostate. Urol Int 1987; 42: 115–119
49. Matusik RJ, Fleming WH, Hamel A et al. Expression of the *c-myc* proto-oncogene in prostatic tissue [Review]. Prog Clin Biol Res 1987; 239: 91–112
50. Fox SB, Persad RA, Royds J, Kure RN, Silcocks PB, Collins CC. *p53* and *c-myc* expression in stage A1 prostatic adenocarcinoma: useful prognostic determinants? J Urol 1993; 150: 490–494
51. Qian J, Bostwick DC, Takahashi S et al. Chromosomal anomalies in prostatic intraepithelial neoplasia and carcinoma detected by fluorescence in situ hybridization. Cancer Res 1995; 55: 5480–5484
52. Tamimi Y, Bringuier PP, Smit F, Vanbokhoven A, Debruyne FMJ, Schalken JA. *p16* mutations/deletions are not frequent events in prostate cancer. Br J Cancer 1996; 74: 120–122
53. Jarrard DF, Bova SG, Ewing CM et al. Deletional mutational and methylation analysis of p16/CDNK2/MTS1 activation in primary and metastatic prostate cancer [Abstract]. J Urol 1996; 155: 602A
54. Komiya A, Suzuki H, Ueda T et al. Allelic losses at loci on chromosome 10 are associated with metastasis and progression of human prostate cancer. Genes Chromosom Cancer 1996; 17: 245–253
55. Konig JJ, Teubel W, Romijn JC, Schroder FH, Hagemeijer A. Gain and loss of chromosomes 1, 7, 8, 10, 18, and Y in 46 prostate cancers. Hum Pathol 1996; 27; 720–727
56. Trybus TM, Burgess AC, Wojno KJ, Glover TW, Macoska JA. Distinct areas of allelic loss on chromosomal regions 10p and 10q in human prostate cancer. Cancer Res 1996: 56: 2263–2267
57. Carter BS, Ewing CM, Ward WS et al. Allelic loss of chromosomes 16q and 10q in human prostate cancer. Proc Natl Acad Sci USA 1990; 87: 8751–8755
58. Li J, Yen C, Liaw D et al. PTEN, a putative protein tyrosine phosphatase gene mutated in human brain, breast and prostate cancer. Science 1997; 275: 1943–1947
59. Sanchez Y, Lovell M, Marin MC et al. Tumor suppression and apoptosis of human prostate carcinoma mediated by a genetic locus within chromosome 10pter-q11. Proc Natl Acad Sci USA 1996; 93: 2551–2556
60. Murakami YS, Albertsen H, Brothman AR, Leach RJ, White RL. Suppression of the malignant phenotype of human prostate cancer cell line PPC-1 by introduction of normal fragments of human chromosome 10. Cancer Res 1996; 56: 2157–2160
61. Dong JT, Rinkerschaeffer CW, Ichikawa T, Barrett JC, Isaacs JT. Prostate cancer; biology of metastasis and its clinical implications. World J Urol 1996: 14: 182–189
62. Guo XZ, Friess H, Graber HU et al. KAI 1 expression is up regulated in early pancreatic cancer and decreased in the presence of metastases. Cancer Res 1996; 56: 4876–4880
63. Rinker-Schaeffer CW, Hawkins AL, Ru N et al. Differential suppression of mammary and prostate cancer metastasis by human chromosomes 17 and 11. Cancer Res 1994; 54: 6249–6256
64. Berube NG, Speevak MD, Chevrette M. Suppression of tumorigenicity of human prostate cancer cells by introduction of human chromosome del(12)(q13). Cancer Res 1994; 54: 3077–3081

65. Cooney KA, Wetzel JC, Merajver SD, Macoska JA, Singleton TP, Wojno KJ. Distinct regions of allelic loss on 13q in prostate cancer. Cancer Res 1996; 56: 1142–1145
66. Gudmundsson J, Johannesdottir G, Bergthorsson JT et al. Different tumor types from BRCA2 carriers show wild-type chromosome deletions on 13q12–q13. Cancer Res 1995; 55: 4830–4832
67. Brookstein R, Rio P, Madreperla SA et al. Promoter deletion and loss of retinoblastoma gene expression in human prostate carcinoma. Proc Natl Acad Sci USA 1990; 87: 7762–7766
68. Brooks JD, Bova GS, Isaacs WB. Allelic loss of the retinoblastoma gene in primary human prostatic adenocarcinomas. Prostate 1995; 26: 35–39
69. Varley JM, Armour J, Swallow JE et al. The retinoblastoma gene is frequently altered leading to loss of expression in primary breast tumours [published erratum appears in Oncogene 1990; 5: 245]. Oncogene 1989; 4: 725–729
70. Friend SH, Horowitz JM, Gerber MR et al. Deletions of a DNA sequence in retinoblastomas and mesenchymal tumors: organization of the sequence and its encoded protein [published erratum appears in Proc Natl Acad Sci USA 1988; 85: 2234]. Proc Natl Acad Sci USA 1987; 84: 9059–9063
71. McDonnell TJ, Troncoso P, Brisbay SM, Logothetis CJ, Chung LK, Hsieh JT. *bcl-2* expression in androgen-independent prostate carcinoma [Abstract]. J Urol 1993; 149: 221A
72. Raffo AJ, Perlman H, Chen MW, Day ML, Streitman JS, Buttyan R. Overexpression of *bcl-2* protects prostate cancer cells from apoptosis in vitro and confers resistance to androgen depletion in vivo. Cancer Res 1995; 55: 4438–4445
73. Rijnders AW, van der Korput JA, van Steenbrugge GJ, Romijn JC, Trapman J. Expression of cellular oncogenes in human prostatic carcinoma cell lines. Biochem Biophys Res Commun 1985; 132: 548–554
74. Davies P, Eaton CL, France TD, Phillips ME. Growth factor receptors and oncogene expression in prostate cells. [Review]. Am J Clin Oncol 1988; 11 (Suppl 2): S1–S7
75. Suzuki H, Komiya A, Emi M et al. Three distinct commonly deleted regions of chromosome arm 16q in human primary and metastatic prostate cancers. Genes Chromosomes Cancer 1996; 17: 225–233
76. Cher ML, Ito T, Weidner N, Carroll PR, Jensen RH. Mapping of regions of physical deletion on chromosome 16q in prostate cancer cells by fluorescence *in situ* hybridization (FISH). J Urol 1995; 153: 249–254
77. Morton RA, Foster B, Madewell L, Greenberg NM, Bussemakers JG, Schalken, J. OB cadherin expression in transgenic models of prostate cancer [Abstract]. J Urol 1997; 157: 367A
78. Li Y, Graham C, Lacy S, Duncan AM, Whyte P. The adenovirus E1A-associated 130-kD protein is encoded by a member of the retinoblastoma gene family and physically interacts with cyclins A and E. Genes Dev 1993; 7: 2366–2377
79. Donehower LA, Bradeley A. The tumor suppressor gene *p53*. Biochim Biophys Acta 1993; 1155: 181–205
80. Levine AJ. The tunour suppressor genes. Annu Rev Biochem 1993; 623–651
81. Visakorpi T, Kallioniemi OP, Heikkinen A, Koivula T, Isola J. Small subgroup of aggressive, highly proliferative prostatic carcinomas defined by p53 accumulation. J Natl Cancer Inst 1992; 84: 883–887
82. Brooks JD, Bova GS, Ewing CM et al.An uncertain role for *p53* gene alterations in human prostate cancers. Cancer Res 1996; 56: 3814–3822
83. Navone NM, Troncoso P, Pisters LL et al. p53 protein accumulation and gene mutation in the progression of human prostate carcinoma. J Natl Cancer Inst 1993; 85: 1657–1669
84. Aprikian AG, Sarkis AS, Fair WR, Zhang ZF, Fuks Z, Cordon-Cardo C. Immunohistochemical determination of p53 protein nuclear accumulation in prostatic adenocarcinoma. J Urol 1994; 151: 1276–1280
85. Hynes NE, Gerber HA, Saurer S, Groner B. Over-expression of the c erb B2 protein in human breast tumor cell lines. J Cell Biochem 1989; 39: 167–173
86. Zhau HE, Wan DS, Zhou J, Miller GJ, von Eschenbach AC. Expression of *c-erb B-2/neu* proto-oncogene in human prostatic cancer tissues and cell lines. Mol Carcinog 1992; 5: 320–327
87. Visakorpi T, Kallioniemi OP, Koivula T, Harvey J, Isola J. Expression of epidermal growth factor receptor and ERBB2 (HER-2/Neu) oncoprotein in prostatic carcinomas. Mod Pathol 1992; 5: 643–648

88. Kuhn EJ, Kurnot RA, Sesterhenn IA, Chang EH, Moul JW. Expression of the c-erbB-2 (HER-2/neu) oncoprotein in human prostatic carcinoma [Review]. J Urol 1993; 150: 1427–1433
89. Williams BJ, Jones E, Zhu XL et al. Evidence for a tumor suppressor gene distal to BRCA1 in prostate cancer. J Urol 1996; 155: 720–725
90. Gao X, Zacharek A, Salkowski A et al. Loss of heterozygosity of the BRCA1 and other loci on chromosome 17q in human prostate cancer. Cancer Res 1995; 55: 1002–1005
91. Kyprianou N, Isaacs JT. Identification of a cellular receptor for transforming growth factor-beta in rat ventral prostate and its negative regulation by androgens. Endocrinology 1988; 123: 2124–2131
92. Darbre PD, King RJ. Progression to steroid insensitivity can occur irrespective of the presence of functional steroid receptors. Cell 1987; 51: 521–528
93. Brinkmann AO, Kuiper GG, Ris-Stalpers C et al. Androgen receptor abnormalities [Review]. J Steroid Biochem Mol Biol 1991; 40: 349–352
94. Veldscholte J, Ris-Stalpers C, Kuiper GG et al. A mutation in the ligand binding domain of the androgen receptor of human LNCaP cells affects steroid binding characteristics in response to anti-androgens. Biochem Biophys Res Commun 1990; 17: 534–540
95. Tilley WD, Wilson CM, Marcelli M, McPhaul MJ. Androgen receptor gene expression in human prostate carcinoma cell lines. Cancer Res 1990; 50: 5382–5386
96. Visakorpi T, Hyytinen E, Koivisto P et al. In vivo amplification of the androgen receptor gene and progression of human prostate cancer. Nature Genet 1995; 9: 401–406
97. Klocker H, Culig Z, Kaspar F et al. Androgen signal transduction and prostatic carcinoma [Review]. World J Urol 1994; 12: 99–103
98. O'Malley B. The steroid receptor superfamily: more excitment predicted for the future [Review]. Mol Endocrinol 1990; 4: 363–369
99. Lubahn DB, Joseph DR, Sar M et al. The human androgen receptor: complementary deoxyribonucleic acid cloning, sequence analysis and gene expression in prostate. Mol Endocrinol 1988; 2: 1265–1275
100. Jenster-G, van der Korput HA, van Vroonhoven C, van der Kwast TH, Trapman J, Brinkmann AO. Domains of the human androgen receptor involved in steroid binding, transcriptional activation, and subcellular localization. Mol Endocrinol 1991; 5: 1396–1404
101. Tora L, Gronemeyer H, Turcotte B, Gaub MP, Chambon P. The N-terminal region of the chicken progesterone receptor specifies target gene activation. Nature 1988; 333: 185–188
102. Chamberlain NL, Driver ED, Miesfield RL. The length and location of CAG trinucleotide repeats in the androgen receptor N-terminal domain effect transactivation function. Nucleic Acids Res 1994; 22: 3181–3186
103. Shena M, Feedman LP, Yamamoto KR. Mutations in the glucocorticoid receptor zinc finger region that distinguish interdigitated DNA binding and transcriptional enhancement activities. Genes Dev 1989; 3: 159–161
104. Ekman P, Brolin J. Steroid receptor profile in human prostate cancer metastases as compared with primary prostatic carcinoma. Prostate 1991; 18: 147–153
105. Masai M, Sumiya H, Akimoto S et al. Immunohistochemical study of androgen receptor in benign hyperplastic and cancerous human prostates. Prostate 1990; 17: 293–300
106. Sadi MV, Barrack ER. Image analysis of androgen receptor immunostaining in metastatic prostate cancer: heterogeneity as a predictor of response to hormonal therapy. Cancer 1993; 71: 2574–2580
107. Pertschuk LP, Macchia RL, Feldman JG et al. Immunocytochemical assay for androgen receptors in prostate cancer: a prospective study of 63 cases with long-term follow-up Ann Surg Oncol 1994; 1: 495–503
108. Tilley WD, Lim-Tio SS, Horsfall DJ, Aspinall JO, Marshall VR, Skinner JM. Detection of discrete androgen receptor epitopes in prostate cancer by immunostaining measurement by color video image analysis. Cancer Res 1994; 54: 4096–4102
109. Horoszewicz JS, Leong SS, Kawinski E et al. The LNCaP model of human prostatic carcinoma. Cancer Res 1980; 43: 1809–1818
110. Kokontis J, Talakura K, Hay N, Liao S. Increased androgen receptor activity and altered *c-myc* expression in prostate cancer cells after long term androgen deprivation. Cancer Res 1994; 54: 1566–1573

111. Krongard A, Wilson CM, Wilson JD, Allman DR, McPhail JM. Androgen increases androgen receptor protein while decreasing receptor mRNA in LNCaP cells. Mol Cell Endocrinol 1991; 76: 79–88
112. Hobisch A, Culig Z, Radmayr C, Bartsch G, Klocker H, Hittmair A. Distant metastases from prostatic carcinoma express androgen receptor protein. Cancer Res 1995; 55: 3068–3072
113. Taplin ME, Bubley GJ, Shuster TD et al. Mutation of the androgen-receptor gene in metastatic androgen-independent prostate cancer. N Engl J Med 1995; 332: 1393–1398
114. Olea N, Sakabe K, Soto AM, Sonnenschein C. The proliferative effect of 'anti-androgens' on the androgen-sensitive human prostate tumour cell line LNCaP. Endocrinol 1990; 126: 1457–1463
115. Gaddipatti JP, McLeod DG, Heidenberg HB et al. Frequent detection of codon 877 mutation in the androgen receptor gene in advanced prostate cancers. Cancer Res 1994; 54: 2861–2864
116. Hobisch A, Culig Z, Cato ACB et al. Products of dihydrotestosterone metabolism activate a mutant androgen receptor detected in a late stage prostate carcinoma. Urol Res 1993; 21: 446(Abstract)
117. Suzuki, H, Sato, N, Watabe, Y, Masai, M, Seino, S, Shimazali, J. Androgen receptor gene mutations in human prostate cancer. J Steroid Biochem Mol Biol 1993; 46: 759–765
118. Culig Z, Hobisch A, Cronauer MV et al. Mutant androgen receptor detected in an advanced-stage prostatic carcinoma is activated by adrenal androgens and progesterone. Mol Endocrinol 1993; 7: 1541–1550
119. Ruizeveld de Winter JA, Janssen PJ, Sleddens HM et al. Androgen receptor status in localized and locally progressive hormone refractory human prostate cancer. Am J Pathol 1994; 144: 735–746
120. Tilley WD, Buchanan G, Hickey TE, Bentel JM. Mutations in the androgen receptor gene are associated with progression of human prostate cancer to androgen independence. Clin Cancer Res 1996; 2: 277–285
121. Gottilieb B, Trifiro M, Lumbroso R, Vasiliou DM, Pinsky L. The androgen receptor gene mutations database. Nucleic Acid Res 1996 24: 151–154
122. Kellens RE. Gene Amplification in Mammalian Cells. A Comprehensive Guide. New York: Marcel Dekker, 1993
123. Koivisto P, Visakorpi T, Kallioniemi OP. Androgen receptor gene amplification: a novel molecular mechanism for endocrine therapy resistance in human prostate cancer. Scand J Clin Lab Invest 1996; 56: 57–63
124. Koivisto, P, Kononen J, Palmberg C et al. Androgen receptor gene amplification: a possible molecular mechanism for androgen deprivation therapy failure in prostate cancer. Cancer Res 1997; 57: 314–319
125. Edwards A, Hammond HA, Jin L, Caskey CT, Chakrabarty R. Genetic variation at five trimeric and tetrameric tandem repeat loci in four human population groups, Genomics 1992; 12: 241–253
126. Irvine RA, Yu MC, Ross RK, Coetzee GA. The CAG and GGC microsatellites of the androgen receptor gene are in linkage disequilibrium in men with prostate cancer. Cancer Res 1995; 55: 1937–1940
127. Shoenberg MP, Hakmi JM, Wang S et al. Microsatellite mutation (CAG24–18) in the androgen receptor gene in human prostate cancer. Biochem Biophys Res Commun 1994; 198: 74–80
128. Stanford JL, Just JJ, Gibbs M et al. Polymorphic repeats in the androgen receptor gene: molecular markers of prostate cancer risk. Cancer Res 1997; 57: 1194–1198
129. van Steenbrugge GJ, van Uffelen CJC, Bolt J, Schröder FH. The human prostatic cancer cell line LNCaP and its derived sublines: an in vitro model for the study of androgen sensitivity. J Steroid Biochem Mol Biol 1991; 40: 201–214
130. Hasenson M, Hartley-Asp B, Kihlfors C, Lundi A, Gustafsson JA, Pousette A. Effect of hormones on growth and ATP content of a human prostatic carcinoma cell line LNCaP-R. Prostate 1985; 7: 183–194
131. Berns EMJ, de Boer W, Mulder E. Androgen-dependent growth regulation and release of specific protein(s) by the androgen receptor containing human prostate tumour cell line LNCaP. Prostate 1986; 9: 247–259

132. Joly-Pharaboz MO, Soave MC, Nicholas B et al. Androgens inhibit the proliferation of a variant of the human prostate cancer cell line LNCaP. J Steroid Biochem Mol Biol 1995; 55: 67–76
133. Yuan S, Trachtenberg J, Mills GB, Brown TJ, Xu F, Keating A. Androgen-induced inhibition of cell proliferation in an androgen-insensitive prostate cancer cell line (PC-3) transfected with human androgen receptor complimentary DNA. Cancer Res 1993; 53: 1304–1311
134. Hansen NM, Chang C, Chodak GW, Rukstalis DB. Modulation of hormone sensitivity in PC3 cells by transfection of the normal androgen receptor. Surg Forum 1991; 43: 745–748
135. Heisle LE, Evangelou A, Lew AM, Trachtenberg J, Elsholtz HP, Brown TJ. Androgen-dependent cell cycle arrest and apoptotic death in PC-3 prostatic cell cultures expressing a full-length human androgen receptor. Mol Cell Endocrinol 1997; 126: 59–73
136. Tilley WD, Bental JM, Aspinall JO, Hall RE, Horsfall DJ. Evidence for a novel mechanism of androgen resistance in the human prostate cancer cell line PC3. Steroids 1995; 60: 180–186
137. Yeh S, Chang C. Cloning and characterisation of a specific coactivator, ARA_{70}, for the androgen receptor in human prostate cells. Proc Natl Acad Sci USA 1996; 93: 5517–5521
138. Klein KA, Reiter RE, Redula J et al. Progression of metastatic human prostate cancer to androgen independent in immunodeficient SCID mice. Nature Med 1997; 3: 402–408

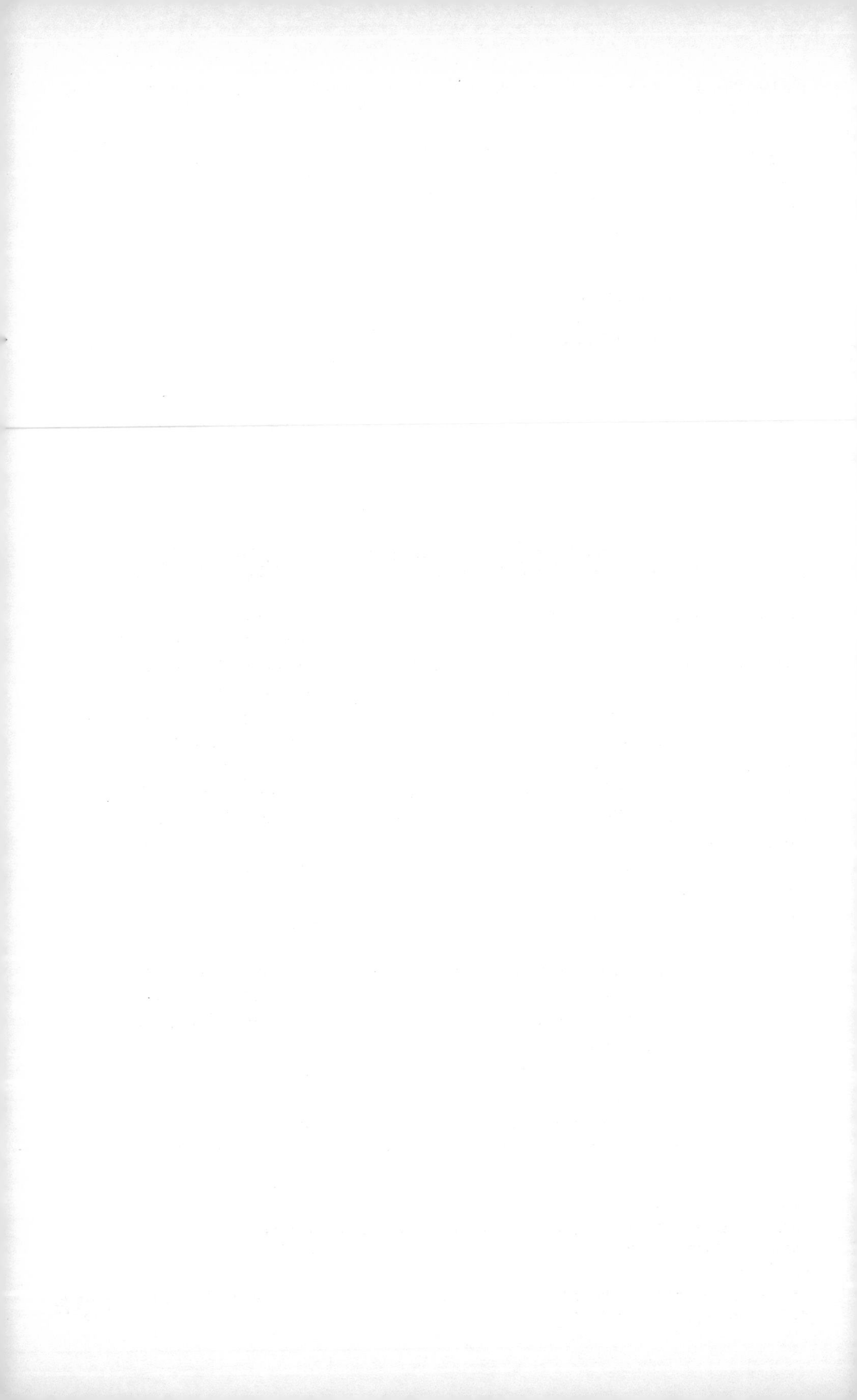

7

Prostate cancer – current developments

C. S. Foster Y. Ke

BACKGROUND

Prostate cancer is the second leading cause of male death from malignant diseases in Europe and in the US. Throughout the Western world, the incidence is greater than 30% in men over 50 years of age, rising to 80% by age 80 years. At diagnosis, approximately 75% of patients already have locally extensive or metastatic disease.[1] For these patients prognosis is poor, the 5-year survival being less than 15%, the majority dying from metastatic disease. Currently, no independent markers are available with which to predict the behaviour of any individual prostate cancer or to determine the host's response to his malignancy.[2] A possible mechanism by which prostatic carcinoma cells may evade immune surveillance is through loss in expression of Class I and Class II MHC determinants during progression from *in situ* neoplasia to metastatic cancer.[3] Proliferation indices do not predict those tumours which will behave aggressively, although they may correlate with the retrospective behaviour of prostate cancer as a group.[4]

At diagnosis, prostate cancer is frequently a systemic disease – even though early metastases may be undetectable by current techniques. Failure to prevent or eliminate metastatic disease is the fundamental problem underlying the presently inadequate management of prostate cancer. Novel methods which will seek-out and destroy individual metastatic tumour cells in any part of the body without damaging host tissues are now required. Ionizing radiation is inappropriate for treating widely-disseminated metastases, and currently employed cytotoxic chemotherapeutic regimens are inadequate to tackle this

Prof. C. S. Foster MD PhD FRCPath, Professor and Director of Anatomic Pathology, Department of Cellular and Molecular Pathology, Duncan Building, University of Liverpool, PO Box 147, Liverpool L69 3GA, UK

Dr Y Ke, Department of Cellular and Molecular Pathology, Duncan Building, University of Liverpool, PO Box 147, Liverpool L69 3GA, UK

disease. Although prostate cancer is regarded as a 'chemotherapy-resistant' neoplasm, expression of high levels of multidrug resistance protein P-170 by rat prostate cancers have been demonstrated to modulate the more aggressive metastatic phenotype of this disease.[5,6] Hormonal manipulation is ineffective long-term and is often associated with significant morbidity.

Progression of somatic cells into a tumourigenic state is influenced by multiple molecular factors including oncogenes, tumour suppressor genes and angiogenic factors. Possible genetic therapies for prostate cancer include development of agents to target oncogenes and intracellular signalling pathways. Nucleic acid-based targeting of abnormal transcriptional or translational processes involved in neoplasia is attractive because of the specificity involved in nucleic acid pairing, and because this offers potential therapy at an early stage of gene expression. Fundamental to such an approach is the prerequisite to identify and characterize those genes involved during initial stages of tumourigenesis or in determining the metastatic phenotype of human prostate cancer.

Identification of cellular features which accurately predict the behaviour of prostate cancer occurring within a specific patient is a major challenge facing contemporary urological pathology. Traditionally, diagnostic histopathologists have attempted to forecast the behaviour of a carcinoma by comparing morphological features of the neoplasm with those of its normal tissue counterpart. Although this approach has identified some features common to prostate cancers **as a group**, it has been singularly inadequate at predicting the behaviour of individual cancers at the time of their original diagnosis. Paradoxically, primary prostatic carcinomas which are morphologically indistinguishable according to currently available criteria, and discovered incidentally, are not equally lethal but exhibit an extensive range of behavioural phenotypes for which reliable diagnostic markers are not yet available. Thus, a fundamental dilemma in the current management of prostatic cancer is that it is not yet possible to identify clinically important cancers while they are confined to the prostate gland and before either local invasion or metastatic spread has occurred. Conversely, clinically unimportant cancers which have not yet developed a potentially metastatic phenotype do not require aggressive treatment – and from which patients should be spared to lessen overall morbidity. Anatomically-localized prostatic neoplasms are frequently not benign. Unfortunately, conventional therapy is of only short-term value in controlling phenotypically metastatic primary tumours – whether confined within the prostate or spread to tissues beyond the anatomical limits of the gland. For many patients with **potentially** metastatic disease, although progression might be slow, it will remain inexorable until such a time that biologically appropriate therapeutic approaches are developed to curb the otherwise inevitable malignant behaviour.

During recent years, unassisted histopathological criteria have been supported by the development of a variety of molecular biological techniques with which to identify phenotypically metastatic prostate cancer cells. Throughout these studies, changes within the genome have been consistently and progressively linked with a variety of human neoplasms. Until recently, such changes might have been considered to occur in the three interrelated groups of 'growth factors', 'oncogenes' and 'tumour-suppressor' genes.

Recently, a fourth group of 'metastasis genes' has been added to the list, subsequent to identification of novel gene sequences capable of transforming formerly benign epithelial cells into the metastatic phenotype following transfection of genomic DNA from malignant epithelial cells. Currently, studies originating from diametrically-opposed ends of the prostate cancer spectrum (i.e. from the earliest identifiable focus of *in situ* neoplasia to aggressively invasive metastatic cancer cells) are converging to define the precise cellular and molecular biological factors which determine the origin and eventual behavioural phenotype of a precancerous lesion. Identification of genes which, through mutation and modified expression, not only allow accurate prediction of the manner in which a neoplasm is likely to progress, but also provide novel targets for molecular genetic intervention and therapeutic control of potentially metastatic prostate cancers at the time of initial diagnosis when the early neoplasm is confined within the anatomical boundaries of the prostate gland, is being performed in several different laboratories. This review of the major areas of prostate cancer pathology in which important progress is currently being made will now concentrate on the three interrelated topics of: (i) stem cells; (ii) prostatic intra-epithelial neoplasia; and (iii) molecular genetic events in early prostate cancer. Since the scope of these subjects is vast, not all of the data currently available can be considered in the space available and omission of a particular topic, class of molecules, or group of genes should not be taken as an indication that they are not important to the pathogenesis of prostate cancer. Instead, this article will concentrate on **processes**, supported by the most significant recent advances in the particular field.

PROSTATIC EPITHELIAL STEM CELLS

It is a biological axiom that to maintain integrity of any tissue, loss of parenchymal cells must be compensated by an equivalent replacement with cells of identical phenotype. Such replacement may occur either by mitosis within a population of already-differentiated cells or by *de novo* replacement through selective differentiation following mitotic proliferation of a precursor stem cell population. Such stem cells may be either completely undifferentiated, or partially differentiated with a restricted repertoire of residual potential differentiation. In mature glandular epithelial tissues such as breast, pancreas and prostate, both types of cellular recruitment occur. Given that the composition of normal prostatic epithelium includes the complex interaction of the three phenotypically distinct cell types of elongate fusiform basal cells, small polygonal neuroendocrine cells and cuboidal/columnar luminal (secretory) cells, it is now become apparent how these individual cell lineages share a common origin and are also related in a precursor–progeny sequence in which basal epithelial cells play a fundamental role in normal prostatic growth as well as in the development of prostate cancer.

Studies performed during the past decade have identified some of the phenotypic characteristics of these putative epithelial stem cells now considered to be located in the inconspicuous basal cell layer around the periphery of prostatic terminal ducts, ductules and acini. These elongate cells contain scant cytoplasm and separate the underlying basement membrane from overlying luminal epithelial cells.[7] Basal cells have been identified to develop following the androgenic stimulation of immature prostatic epithelium which occurs at puberty.[8] However, the observation that basal cells develop only during postnatal prostatic parenchymal differentiation suggests that these should be regarded as 'second-order' while their progenitor (embryological) cell of origin (i.e. 'first-order') stem cells continue to exist. This is not a semantic concept without practical application, but an important problem which is fundamental to understanding the aetiopathogenesis of prostate cancer, particularly since strong evidence now indicates that the particular genetic events leading to prostatic neoplasia and to prostate cancer occur within this population of basal cells. It is those genetic events (whether mutational, genetic imprinting or other) which occur within the embryological 'first-order' stem cells and predispose an individual to prostate cancer. Thereafter, such genetic modifications are transmitted to all prostatic epithelial progeny throughout the subsequent lifetime of that individual. Conversely, second-order stem cells, in which genetic events of a potentially malignant nature are induced postnatally, may be replaced by obliteration followed by proliferation of non-defective first-order stem cells, and hence their effects eradicated.[9]

There are several compelling lines of evidence to support the notion that the basal cell layer contains the prostatic epithelial stem cell population.[10] Using double-label techniques for phenotypic markers, Bonkhoff et al showed the three basic epithelial cell types to be linked in a precursor–progeny relationship. Among the various prostatic cell types, basal cells have the greatest capacity to differentiate into all epithelial cell lineages through intermediate phenotypes.[11] The proliferative compartment of both normal and hyperplastic epithelium resides in the basal cell layer. Approximately 70% of proliferating epithelial cells are phenotypically basal. The remaining 30% of proliferating cells belong to the secretory epithelium (differentiation compartment), whereas chromogranin A-expressing endocrine-paracrine cells comprise a postmitotic cell population.[12,13]

With respect to the physiological replenishment of cells occurring within normal prostatic epithelium, basal cells are the most capable of dividing and differentiating into other cell types, such as secretory cells.[7,8,14] Although both basal cells and secretory cells retain the ability to divide, the usual proliferative compartment is the basal cell layer.[15] Transition forms have been reported between basal cells, secretory luminal and neuroendocrine cells, although rarely – and only in tissue culture.[15,16] Prostate-specific antigen (PSA) and prostatic acid phosphatase (PAP) immunoreactivity is present in a subset of basal cells, suggesting that basal cells can acquire the immunophenotype of secretory cells.[17] Basal cells also retain the ability to undergo metaplasia, including squamous differentiation in prostatic infarction and myoepithelial differentiation in sclerosing adenosis. Other evidence supporting the stem cell origin of basal cells includes identification of the apoptosis-suppressing *bcl-2* oncoprotein exclusively in basal cells[18] and the androgen independence but androgen responsiveness of basal cells as documented by the presence of 5-alpha-reductase-isoenzyme-2 and the nuclear androgen receptor.[19] Evidence of the stem cell role for basal cells in prostate tissue is provided by the differential expression of the oncoprotein Bcl-2 which blocks programmed cell death in both stem cell and proliferation compartments of normal tissues.[20,21] In the prostate, Bcl-2 expression is restricted to the basal cell layer, whereas the secretory epithelium generally lacks this oncoprotein in both normal and hyperplastic conditions.[10,18] Down-regulation of Bcl-2 within the differentiation compartment suggests that secretory luminal cells undergo programmed cell death after terminal differentiation and are replaced by generative basal cells.[10] Accordingly, the proliferative compartment of the prostatic epithelium is able to accumulate biologically active dihydrotestosterone, which binds with high affinity to the appropriate androgen receptor. Since subsets of basal cells are androgen-responsive, it is likely that the effect of androgen on these particular cells induces differentiation towards secretory luminal cell types.[10] Immunohistochemically, the elongate basal cells which contain the stem cell population are distinct from the argentaffinic neuroendocrine cells, which comprise the third discrete lineage of prostatic epithelial differentiation. Based on current knowledge, these three basic epithelial cell types are clearly differentiated by their marker expression and hormonal regulation. The luminal secretory epithelium requires continuous support by androgens for its maintenance and widely expresses nuclear androgen receptor, prostatic specific antigen (PSA) and cytokeratins 8 and 19, similar to that reported in common prostate cancer.[22] Basal cells may focally and transiently express nuclear receptors for oestrogens (ER) and progesterone (PR), but consistently lack nuclear androgen receptor. With the exception of the small defined population already described, basal cells lack PSA but strongly express high molecular weight cytokeratins which may be identified immunohistochemically using antibodies such as 34β-E12 or AE1/AE3.[23] The endocrine-paracrine cell, the third epithelial phenotype of prostatic epithelium, is characterized by endocrine markers such as chromogranin A.

In addition to androgens and oestrogens, nonsteroidal growth factors are implicated in the control of basal cells. Epidermal growth factor (EGF) is required by prostatic epithelial cells for in vitro proliferation.[22] In the human prostate, EGF is produced by secretory luminal cells, whereas the basal cell layer (proliferative compartment) strongly expresses the EGF receptor. Insulin-like growth factor-1 (IGF-1), nerve growth factor (NGF) and members of the fibroblast growth factor family, particularly basic FGF, also affect proliferation since the pertinent receptors are expressed by cells within the basal layer (Fig. 1). With respect to EGF and its receptor (EGFr), these form a positive feedback loop in the non-neoplastic prostate, but which becomes disrupted during neoplasia as evidenced by loss of the majority of EGFr from the tumour cells and failure to maintain an appropriate intracellular topographical distribution for the EGFr which is retained. While basic FGF is expressed only by basal epithelial cells in the normal prostate, acidic FGF is not expressed at immunohistochemically-identifiable levels until the epithelial cells have started to develop early morphological features of dysplasia (Fig. 1).

Based on the data outlined above, the prostatic epithelium is composed of two functional compartments.[10] The proliferative compartment is androgen-independent and is localised in the basal cell layer. The secretory epithelium represents the differentiation compartment which is androgen-dependent but has a limited proliferative potential.[15] The growth rate within the proliferative

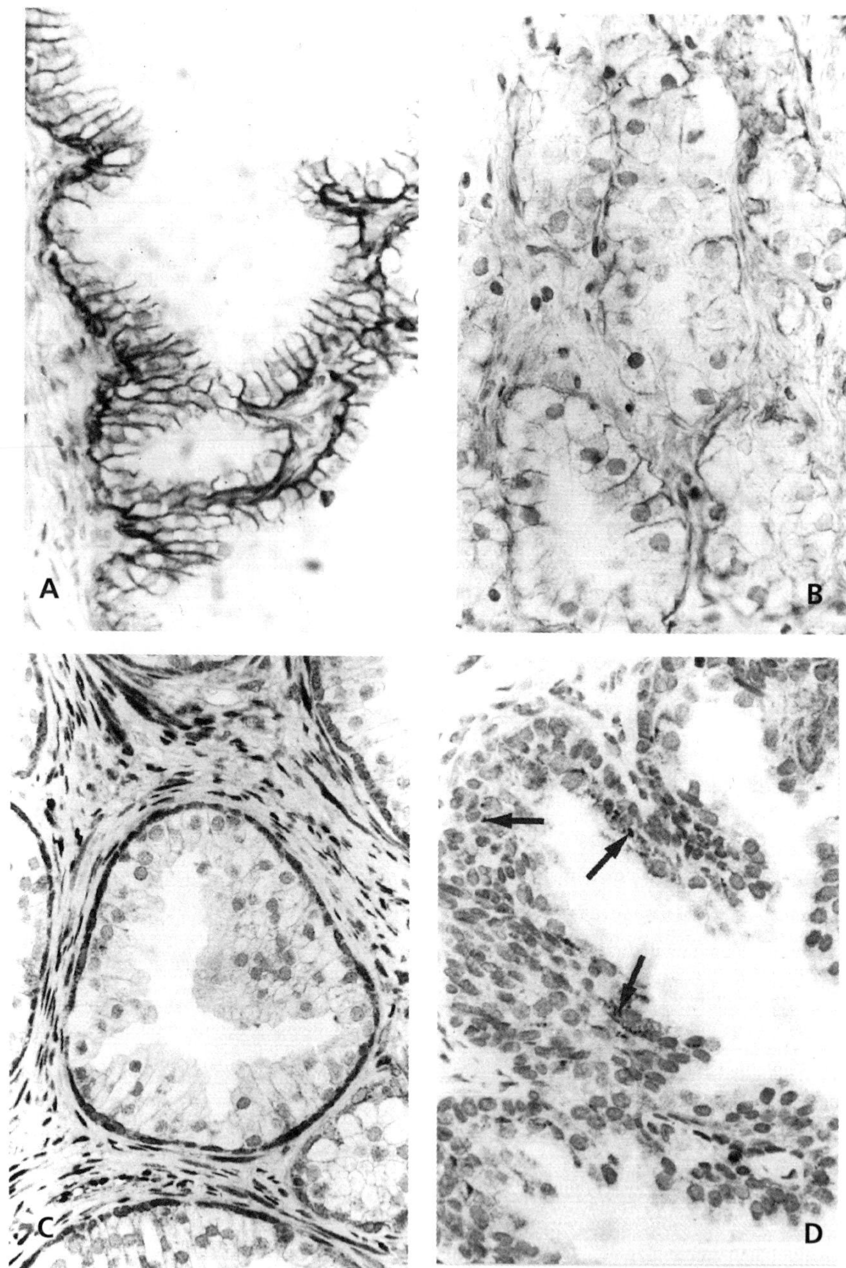

Fig. 1 (**A**) Expression of EGFr restricted to plasma membranes of basal epithelial cells and to basolateral membranes of luminal (secretory) epithelial cells in human normal (non-neoplastic) prostate. (**B**) Well differentiated prostatic adenocarcinoma (Gleason grade 2) in which malignant pseudo-acini are composed of neoplastic cells without a basal cell layer. Expression of EGFr is highly attenuated. (**C**) Expression of basic FGF restricted to the basal cell layer of human non-neoplastic epithelium, and to a population of stromal cells. Luminal epithelial cells do not express this growth peptide. (**D**) Atypical epithelial hyperplasia amounting to high grade PIN in which small amounts of acidic FGF are expressed by neoplastic epithelial cells (arrows). This is the very earliest stage at which such neoplastic cells can be recognised to be committed to inevitable malignant progression.

compartment is regulated by EGF and other growth factors (IGF, NGF, FGF) affecting proliferation, and by Bcl-2 which blocks programmed cell death.[10] Thus, the proliferative compartment (basal cell layer) contain a small stem cell population which gives rise to all epithelial cell lineages via intermediate phenotypes. These differentiation processes within the prostatic cell system are most probably regulated in a balanced vectorial manner by a combination of circulating steroid hormones together with a local non-steroidal paracrine effect. Oestrogens cause basal cell hyperplasia in vivo, indicating that the differentiation process from basal to secretory luminal cells is arrested by oestrogens. Conversely, androgens induce differentiation towards a secretory luminal-cell phenotype. Accordingly, turnover of the secretory epithelium largely depends upon the number of androgen-responsive target cells within the proliferative basal cell layer compartment, which is mediated by balanced trophic stimulation, either simultaneously or sequentially, with oestrogen and androgen.

PROSTATIC INTRAEPITHELIAL NEOPLASIA (PIN)

First reported as a distinct pathological entity in 1987, prostatic intraepithelial neoplasia (PIN) refers to the appearances occurring in the middle region of the spectrum extending between morphologically normal and frankly malignant prostatic epithelium.[24] Originally classified into three groups, the consensus view endorsed by an international conference held at the Mayo Clinic in 1995 was that PIN should be considered only as either 'low' (formerly '1') or 'high' (formerly '2' or '3') grade.[25] It is characterized by a range of architectural and cytological factors which include progressive loss of the epithelial two-cell arrangement with eventual disappearance of basal cells.[26] During this process, the overall proliferative rate of the affected epithelium may remain constant, or become increased, as the balance between cellular proliferation and atrophy by apoptosis becomes deranged. While hyperplasia is not *per se* an obligatory characteristic of PIN, it is a frequent accompaniment. However, there is no absolute requirement for the original steady-state within the epithelium to become altered while mutational events shift the affected populations of cells from normality through dysplasia to absolute neoplasia (carcinoma *in situ*) and, eventually, to invasive malignancy. Thereafter, as apoptotic regulatory mechanisms fail, there is a common tendency for numbers of malignant cells to increase by geometric progression. However, this is uncommon and hyperplasia is recognised as an important component in the three architectural patterns (Fig. 2) of tufting, micropapillary and cribriform.[27] The fourth pattern (flat) is explained by a retained balance between hyperplasia and atrophy. Prostatic intraepithelial neoplasia is not detectable by transrectal ultrasonography, MRI scanning or any technique other than microscopic examination.[28] With respect to diagnostic criteria, the cytological hallmarks of PIN are nuclear and nucleolar enlargement. In the most severe foci, nuclei are usually uniformly enlarged, although condensed hyperchromatic forms may also be found. Increased variability of nuclear morphology is associated with low-grade intraepithelial neoplasia.

The importance of diagnosing PIN is its high predictive value as a prognostic marker for the occurrence of adenocarcinoma. Evidence to support this

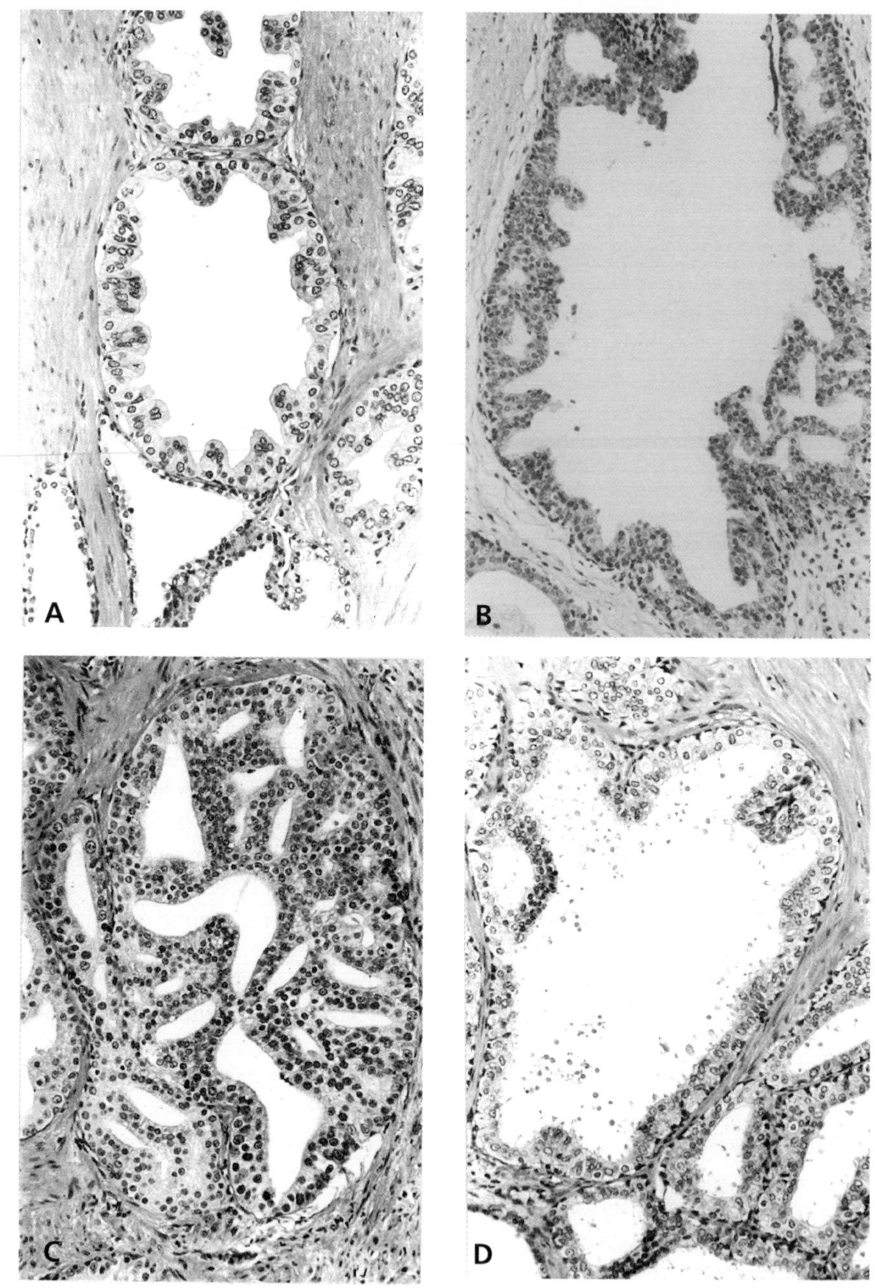

Fig. 2 Morphological appearances of high grade PIN. (**A**) tufting; (**B**) micropapillary; (**C**) cribriform and (**D**) flat. Note the distinctive appearance of the characteristic 'budding' from the luminal plasma membrane in (D).

circumstantial association as a functional relationship has been obtained from several sources. Davidson compared 100 patient needle-biopsies of high-grade PIN with 112 control biopsies matched for clinical stage, patient age and serum PSA.[29] In subsequent biopsies of both cohorts of patients, adenocarcinoma

Table 1 PIN as a predictor of prostate cancer

PIN Grade	Patients with PIN	% Developing cancer	Time interval (years)	Reference
High	32	41	1.5	Markham 1989[102]
Low	23	13	1.5	
High	104	39	#	Park et al 1989[103]
High	10	100	#	Brawer et al 1991[104]
Low	11	18	#	
High	33	73	#	Berner et al 1993[105]
				Weinstein et al 1993[106]
High	81	40.5	1.0	Bostwick et al 1995[30]
High	100	35	6	Davidson et al 1995[29]
High	37	51	0.5	*Keetch et al 1995[107]
Low	21	19	0.5	

*This was a highly selective study in which the likelihood of finding cancer was enhanced by abnormal PSA/digital rectal examination/transrectal ultrasonographic findings.
#Time-interval between diagnosis of PIN and re-biopsy with diagnosis of cancer either not stated or immediate and, therefore, of no significant duration.

appeared in 35% of those with PIN when compared to 13% of the controls. Of the parameters measured, PIN provided the highest risk-ratio. Only thereafter were patient age and serum PSA concentrations the next most significant predictors of cancer. Conversely, the **amount** of PIN on biopsy, the architectural pattern of PIN, patient ethnic origin, digital rectal examination findings and transrectal ultrasound results were not candidate predictors. With respect to an initial diagnosis of PIN, the likelihood of detecting prostate cancer in successive biopsies performed on an individual patient was greater in those undergoing more than one biopsy on any single occasion (44%) than in those in which only one biopsy was performed (32%). This high predictive value of PIN for prostate cancer has been substantiated in the findings of eight published studies involving a total of 371 patients (Table 1).

High grade PIN is currently identified in up to 16% of contemporary needle biopsies, separately from that encountered in transurethral resection specimens,[30] thus further emphasizing the differences between peripheral prostatic tissue sampled by needle biopsy and control tissues taken on TURP. All surgical pathologists reporting prostatic biopsies should routinely search for PIN, grade it according to conventional criteria, and report it to the submitting urologists as a benign but potentially premalignant entity in order to ensure close follow-up of affected patients. When PIN is encountered in TURP specimens, all residual chippings should be embedded and examined microscopically. To differentiate high grade PIN from *in situ* or invasive cancer, the presence of basal cells may be confirmed immunohistochemically using antibodies such as AE1/AE3 or 34β-E12 which recognise high molecular weight cytokeratins.[23] Where basal cells are preserved as an intact or fragmented basal layer in PIN, absence of basal cells is an important marker raising a high suspicion of prostate cancer. While identification of PIN, whether of low- or high-grade should not dictate or influence therapeutic decisions,[25] follow-up at between 3–6 monthly intervals for a minimum of 2 years is recommended and thereafter at 12 monthly intervals for life.[31]

MOLECULAR GENETIC EVENTS IN PROSTATE CANCER

ONCOGENE ACTIVATION

Point mutation of a cellular gene (proto-oncogene) such as *c-ras* into the corresponding oncogene is one common and important mechanism of neoplastic transformation.[32] However, in human prostate cancer, the role of cellular oncogenes remains poorly defined. Studies of oncogene activation and product expression have been singularly disappointing. An early study by Viola et al examined expression of the *ras*-p21 protein product using the mouse monoclonal antibody RAP-5 which identifies amino acid sequence 10–17 of ^{Ha}-*ras*, ^{Ki}-*ras* and N-*ras* p21.[33] Although good correlation was found between Gleason grade and/or degree of nuclear anaplasia with expression of this oncogene product peptide sequence for prostate cancers as a **group**, no correlation was reported with individual tumour behaviour. Conversely, Peehl et al reported data conflicting with those of Viola et al by employing the NIH3T3 transfection assay to show only one of eight prostate carcinomas examined contained transforming sequences homologous with ^{Ki}-*ras* and suggested that activation of oncogenes detectable by the 3T3 assay is not a frequent occurrence in this malignancy.[34] More recently, Carter et al examined 24 primary human prostate carcinomas together with five prostatic cell-lines for mutations at codons 12, 13 and 61 of ^{Ha}-*ras*, ^{Ki}-*ras* and N-*ras* genes.[35] Wild-type and mutant alleles in genomic DNA extracted from tissues and cell lines were amplified using PCR. In the material studied, only two mutations were detected: one was an A→G transition causing a glutamine to arginine amino acid substitution at codon 61 of the ^{Ha}-*ras* gene in one of 24 primary prostatic carcinomas. The second was a G→T transversion causing a glycine to valine amino acid substitution at codon 12 of the ^{Ha}-*ras* gene in prostate tumour cell line (TSU-PR1). Data from another study revealed heterogeneous expression of *ras* oncogene p21 protein to occur in 25% of prostate cancer cells within a single primary tumour expressing that protein.[36] In all other prostate cancers hitherto reported, amplification of genomic sequences of ^{Ha}-*ras*, ^{Ki}-*ras*, *c-myc*, *N-myc*, *c-sis*, or *c-fos* has not been found. Considering the consensus finding of a consistently elevated growth fraction in all prostatic carcinomas examined, absence of activated *c-myc* is surprising. Comparable data have been reported from studies of the Dunning R3327 rat prostatic adenocarcinoma model, although searches for transforming sequences of DNA homologous to those of known oncogenes, using the 3T3-transfection assay, have been unsuccessful.[37] Information from several sources indicates that no presently known oncogenes are specifically or consistently activated in either human or rodent prostate cancer. All studies suggest that, currently, there is no known oncogene marker with which to enhance detection of prostatic malignancy or to identify prostate cancers which might have developed by a particular route or which will behave in a predictable phenotypic manner.

Table 2 Prostate tumour suppressor gene sequences

Chromosomal location	Gene	% Prostate cancers	Identification technique	Reference
8p 22		< 20		Vocke 1996[108]
8p 12.21		80		
10pter-q11	PAC 1			Sanchez 1996[109]
13q		~33		Cooney 1996[110]
8p 22				MacGrogan 1996[111]
				Bova 1996[112]
17p				Kunimi 1996[113]
6q 14-21				Cooney 1996[114]
10p			Chromosome transfer	Murakami 1996[115]
10p & 10q		29	LOH	Ittmann 1996[116]
17p		8		
17q		41		
7q12-21	BRCA1	70	FISH	Williams 1996[117]
17q21	BRCA1	50	LOH	Gao 1995 [118]
8p21		43	LOH	Kagan 1995[119]
8p22		46	PCR	Macoska 1995[120]
10q23-25	Mxi1	62	SSCP	Gray 1995[121]
9p21	CDKN2	2	SSCP	Komiya 1995[122]
9p21	CDKN2	60	Methylation analysis	Herman 1995[123]
9p21	CDKN2		Microsatellite analysis	Cairns 1995[124]
8p22-p21.3		57	Deletion mapping	Suzuki 1995[125]
17q12-22			Chromosome transfer	Murakami 1995[98]
8p12-21		> 90	LOH	Emmert-Buck 1995[126]
10q24-25	Mxl1		FISH	Eagle 1995[127]
11p11.2	Kal1		Gene transfer	Dong 1995[51]
17q21	BRCA1	52	LOH	Goa 1995[128]
8p		46	Microsatellite analysis	MacGrogan 1994[129]
8p		36–69	Microsatellite analysis	Trapman 1994[130]
8q		11–25		
	Krev-1		Gene transfer	Burney 1994[131]
12pter-12q13			Gene transfer	Berube 1994[132]

TUMOUR SUPPRESSOR GENES

A second group of cellular genes recognized to be important modulators of the malignant phenotype are the 'tumour-suppressor' genes. Table 2 summarizes the current status of these genes, and their putative chromosomal locations, presently recognized to be responsible for suppressing either the neoplastic or the metastatic phenotype within prostatic epithelium. Although the normal functions of these gene sequences are not well defined, it is likely that they are involved in promoting cellular differentiation in addition to mediating arrest of cellular proliferation by growth inhibitory cytokines.[38] With respect to the well characterised tumour suppressor genes RB and p53, loss of heterozygosity (LOH) involving the long arm of chromosome 13 has been reported to occur in as many as one-third of primary prostate cancers. A third tumour-suppressor gene (KAI1) which appears to be active in some prostate cancers, has been located on human chromosome 11p11.2.

Candidate tumour suppressor genes on 13q which may be important in the development of prostate cancer include the retinoblastoma susceptibility gene (RB) and a gene associated with inherited breast cancer (BRCA2). The RB gene was first localised to chromosome 13q14.1 by cytogenetic studies,[39] cloned by Friend et al[40] and was the original tumour-suppressor gene to be identified.[41] In defined subsets of all human epithelial neoplasms, in addition to all retinoblastomas, mutational inactivation of RB is to be found. Exogenous copies of wild-type RB have been shown to suppress tumourigenicity in several different types of tumour cells with endogenous RB mutations. One study confirmed the presence of RB mutations in a population human prostate cancers, which supports the probability that mutation of a gene responsible for tumour suppression might be an important step in the genesis of at least some prostate cancers.[42] Another study found loss of heterozygosity in 24 (60%) of 40 informative patients with prostate cancer. Loss of RB occurred with a similar frequency in early-stage and low-grade cancers as in more advanced cancers, although loss of RB was also found in one patient with morphological features of benign prostatic hyperplasia (BPH). Expression of pRB, the protein product of RB, was completely absent from seven cancers and markedly reduced in the other two, while nuclear pRB expression was always present in areas of BPH, whether adjacent to cancer containing tissue or with BPH alone. The study suggested loss of RB to be an early event in prostatic tumourigenesis. Using LOH analysis, 19 (48%) of 40 prostate cancer cases demonstrated allelic loss with at least one marker. Furthermore, 13 (33%) of 40 cases had evidence of allelic loss involving a region of 13q14 containing RB. To test the hypothesis that RB is the targeted tumour suppressor gene in this region, 37 of 40 cases were further assessed for expression of pRB. This analysis, revealed that 8 (22%) of 37 prostate tumours demonstrated no pRB expression. However, allelic loss at RB, assessed with an intragenic marker, did not correlate with absent pRB expression. Taken together, these data support the findings that allelic loss of a common region of 13q14 occurs in approximately one-third of prostate cancers. Lack of correlation of LOH at RB with absent pRB expression suggests the existence of another tumour suppressor gene in this region to be important in prostate cancer. Thereafter, full expression of metastatic potential is likely to reside with other attributes of the neoplastic cells.

Wild-type p53 protein is a nuclear protein which regulates entry into, and progression through, the cell-cycle.[43] The protein exhibits many properties consistent with its being the product of a tumour suppressor gene.[44] Although present at low levels in most adult murine tissues, it was the original studies by Finlay et al which first suggested increased levels of p53 protein to be associated either with an abnormal mutated protein or stabilization of the protein in a complex with other proteins.[45] In normal and transformed cells, p53 protein may be present in different cellular compartments.[46] In non-transformed cells, it occurs within the cytoplasm in association with the cytoskeleton. In transformed cells the protein is usually located in the nucleus. Point-mutations occurring in a highly-conserved region of the gene are known

Table 3 Expression of tumour suppressor gene p53 by primary and metastatic prostate cancers

Group of tumours	Tumour type	Number in series	p53 (%)
Group 1	Benign hyperplasia	n = 13	7 (54)
Group 2	Primary carcinomas (UK)	*n* = 21	10 (47)
Group 3	Primary carcinomas (USA)	*n* = 32	5 (16)
	Lymph node metastases (USA)	*n* = 32	6 (19)
Group 4	Lymph node metastases (USA)	*n* = 19	4 (21)

to activate p53 in the primary rat embryo fibroblast transfection assay for dominant oncogenes,[47] whereas the wild-type protein has a tumour-suppressor action.[48] Abrogation of wild-type p53 expression, a common finding in many malignancies, could eliminate these activities. Identification of increased levels of detectable protein within tissues thus provides a marker for mutated p53.

In this laboratory, expression of p53 in a wide range of benign and malignant prostatic tissues has been examined immunohistochemically using rabbit polyclonal antibody CM-1.[49] The data are summarized in Table 3. Essentially, four distinct groups of prostatic tissues were examined: benign prostatic hyperplasias with no morphological evidence of dysplasia (PIN) or associated neoplasia (Group 1); primary prostatic carcinomas from within the UK (Group 2); primary prostatic carcinomas together with their corresponding lymph node metastases, collected at the Veterans Administration Cancer Center, Temple, TX, USA (Groups 3 and 4, respectively). Within Group 2 (UK tissues), 47% of primary prostatic carcinomas revealed expression of p53 protein by at least 5% of tumour cells. In contrast, only 16% of the primary carcinomas in Group 3 (US tissues) exhibited p53 protein expression. In neither group was there correlation with tumour grade. Examination of corresponding lymph node metastases revealed the proportions of prostate cancers exhibiting p53 expression to be similar to that of the primary carcinomas obtained in the UK. The reason for the disparity in expression of p53 between primary prostate cancers obtained from the UK and the US is not immediately apparent. Explanations include possible differences in the aetiopathogenesis of this disease between the two countries and different stages of the disease at detection. However, it is possible that patients attending a Veterans Administration hospital in the US are subjected to a more rigorous level of screening than are patients in the UK, who present either randomly or only when symptomatic (whether for prostatic or other disease) and, therefore, have their prostate cancers detected at a significantly earlier stage than those in the UK. If this is correct, then it might also explain the high incidence of mutated p53 found in morphologically benign hyperplastic tissues in the UK. Nevertheless, despite these caveats, less than 50% of all malignant prostatic disease examined in this combined series contained tumour cells expressing mutated p53 protein – a finding strongly suggesting that inactivation of this tumour-suppressor gene is unlikely to be a consistent or important event during initiation of the majority of human prostate cancers. This view is supported by a recently published study which analysed genetic mutations producing nuclear accumulation of p53 protein in 100 prostatic adenocarcinomas. PCR-SSCP methodology revealed p53 mutation and accumulation in only 5 carcinomas with involvement of exons 5 and 7 for one tumour each and exon 6 for three tumours.[50] These data further confirm growing opinion that p53 mutations are infrequent and, when they do occur, appear late in the progression of prostatic carcinogenesis. These findings, obtained using molecular techniques, also cast some doubt on previous unsupported immunohistochemical studies which indicated a higher expression of p53 protein, particularly in early prostate cancers.

KAI1 is a metastasis-suppressor gene isolated by *Alu*-PCR techniques from human chromosome 11p11.2 and shown to suppress metastasis when introduced into the Dunning rat AT6.1 prostate cancer cells. The protein product of the gene is reported to be reduced in human cell lines derived from metastatic prostate cancers.[51] KAI1 encodes a 267 amino acid peptide sequence containing four hydrophobic domains, probably transmembrane, together with a large, putatively extracellular, hydrophilic domain containing three potential N-glycosylation sites. Evolutionarily conserved and distributed widely in human normal tissues, KAI1 encodes one member of a structurally distinct family of leukocyte surface glycoproteins with likely, but hitherto undefined, biological functions. A characteristic structural feature of this family is that all members contain four transmembrane domains and a large extracellular N-glycosylation domain. Although the precise functions of these protein are unconfirmed, their membrane localization and extensive glycosylation suggest that they function in cell–cell interactions and cell–extracellular matrix interactions,[52] both of which are important in invasion and metastasis. In particular, the N-glycosylation of these molecules is consistent with their presumed role in metastasis suppression because the association between processing of N-linked oligosaccharides and metastatic phenotype is well documented. In addition to *KAI1*, expression of genes *MRP-1* and *ME491*, two other members of this family, has been correlated with metastasis.

METASTASIS GENES

Genes for adhesion molecules

The term 'adhesion molecules' refers to a highly diverse and enlarging collection of molecules synthesized by cells (particularly epithelial cells) which provide a structural and functional interface with the extracellular environment. Although the particular functions of these molecules are as varied as their structures, their common role is to promote and to maintain cellular attachment. The consequence is that information (on position, orientation, environment, etc.) is received and interpreted by these cells, thus causing constant modulation of their cellular phenotype. Many studies have shown altered expression, particularly loss of adhesion molecules during progression from normal prostatic epithelium to invasive prostate cancer. However, expression of the CD44 group of adhesion molecules appears to be particularly associated with development of the metastatic phenotype in this disease.

Changes in the expression of a wide range of adhesion molecules (including the integrins, E-cadherin, C-CAM and tenascin) have been implicated in the pathogenesis and behavioural phenotypes of different epithelial neoplasms, including prostate cancer. While novel data on these molecules have been obtained, involvement of the CD44 group of molecules has received particular attention. CD44 is a cell surface adhesion molecule involved in cell–cell and cell–matrix interaction.[53] The CD44 gene contains 20 exons and several CD44 isoforms that are variants of a common standard hematopoietic form (CD44s) which have been identified by sequence analysis. Potentially, ten of these exons can be alternatively spliced.[54,55] Epithelial cells contain exons 12–14 inserted into the CD44's transcripts, and this isoform is designated as CD44E. Other CD44 variants (CV44v) differ in the middle region located on the external side of the cell membrane. CD44vs are variably expressed by epithelial cells[56,57] and have attracted considerable attention because they are involved in tumour progression.[58] Studies in animal models and on human cell lines have suggested a correlation between up-regulation of particular variants and metastasis. Transfection of CD44v6 (CD44 isoform containing v6) confers metastatic potential to non-metastasizing pancreatic carcinoma cells in rats.[59,60] Co-injection of variant specific monoclonal antibodies with metastatic cells leads to retardation or complete blockage of metastatic spread in vivo.[61] Spliced variants containing CD44v6 are over expressed by aggressive non-Hodgkin's lymphomas and also by some human carcinomas.[62] CD44v6 is increasingly expressed during human colorectal and gastric tumour progression. CD44 variants v4, v6 and v9 investigated by methods are also, but variously, expressed by other types of human malignancies including lung, endometrial, ovarian, and urothelial[63] carcinomas and skin tumours, whereas v5 is up-regulated in melanomas. Abnormal expression of CD44v6 occurs in more than 80% of locally invasive and metastasizing human prostate cancers. However, of particular diagnostic importance is the finding of high levels of CD44v6 protein expression in significant numbers of morphologically benign prostatic biopsies containing atypical basal cell hyperplasia or PIN of both low- and high-grade (Fig. 3). Thus, early expression of CD44v6 may be a marker of inevitable neoplastic disease progression or be the first marker (yet found) which accurately identifies the metastatic phenotype of prostate cancer, but at a time before the neoplastic cells have taken on the full morphological panoply of malignancy.

Calcium binding proteins

The two proteins osteopontin and p9Ka occupy a functional domain between external and intracellular environments. Using molecular and cell-biological techniques, both molecules have been identified to be specifically involved in promoting the metastatic dissemination of rat and human prostate cancers. Osteopontin is a reversibly phosphorylated acidic adhesive glycoprotein secreted by bone and by glandular luminal epithelial cells. In the latter, it is concentrated at the apical surfaces.[64,65] It is a calcium-binding protein shown to promote cell attachment and spreading through its Gly-Arg-Gly-Asp-Ser binding domain.[66] Cell attachment to osteopontin has been shown to be mediated, in part, through cell-surface integrin $\alpha_V\beta_3$,[67] which is also a receptor for other adhesive agents including vitronectin, fibrinogen, von Willebrand factor, thrombospondin and fibronectin. Osteopontin expression is increased following neoplastic transformation and correlates with the metastatic

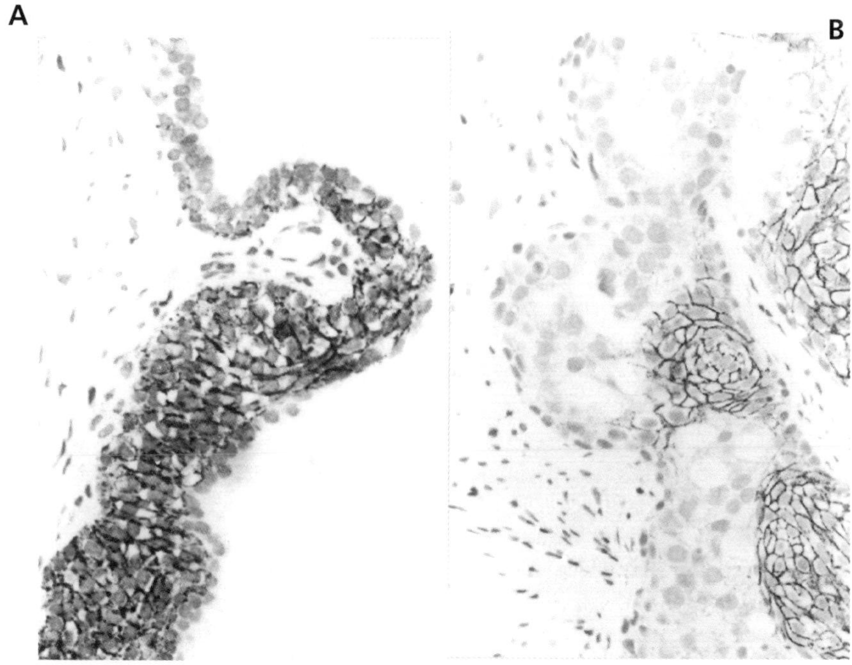

Fig. 3 Expression of CD44v6 by early neoplastic human prostatic epithelium. (**A**) A focus of atypical epithelial cell hyperplasia in which basal cells and luminal cells have become morphologically indistinguishable. CD44v6 is expressed by all cells within this focus of abnormal proliferation, but not by adjacent non-neoplastic epithelium. (**B**) CD44v6 expressed by foci of proliferating epithelial cells in a region of high grade PIN. Although morphologically, and possibly aetiologically, distinct from the appearance in (A), expression of this determinant may be regarded as a reliable hallmark of malignant behaviour.

potential of mouse transformed cell lines. Recent studies in our laboratory have confirmed a direct correlation between osteopontin mRNA expression and metastatic potential of different cell types within the Dunning model of rat prostate cancer. In human tissues, immunohistochemistry has confirmed high levels of osteopontin protein expression in invasive prostate cancer cells (Fig. 4). While clearly demonstrating both mRNA and protein expression in neoplastic epithelial cells of both rat and human prostate cancers, our data do not support the findings of Brown et al who localized osteopontin only to the infiltrating macrophage population of breast and prostate cancers – but not to the epithelial cells.

In contrast to osteopontin, which is at least partially secreted, the protein p9Ka is a strictly intracellular molecule belonging to the S100 class of Ca^{2+}-binding molecules. Barraclough first identified the molecule by subtractive hybridization performed between rat mammary epithelial cells of differing metastatic potential.[68] This protein is not only selectively enhanced in metastatic carcinomas, but transfection of its gene to previously benign epithelial cells has been shown to transfer and to promote the metastatic phenotype. In our laboratory, direct correlation has been confirmed between expression of p9Ka mRNA and protein with the metastatic phenotype of Dunning rat prostate cancer cells.[69] Rat p9Ka gene contains three exons of 37,

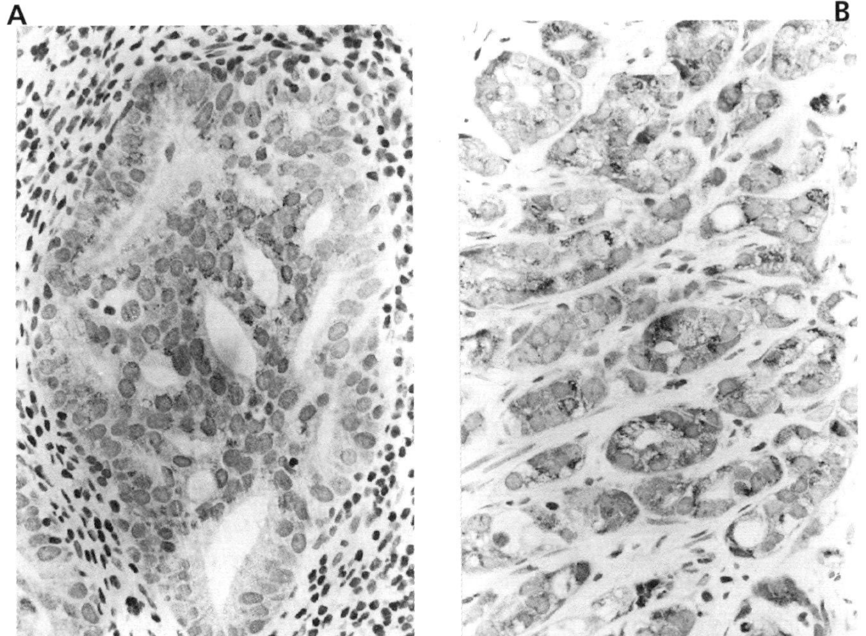

Fig. 4 Expression of osteopontin. (**A**) High grade (cribriforming) PIN expressing osteopontin predominantly within the central, but not peripheral, epithelial cells comprising the lesion. (**B**) Heterogeneous expression of osteopontin within poorly differentiated invasive (metastatic) prostate cancer cells. Despite its role as a cell-adhesion molecule in malignant epithelium, this protein is characteristically expressed within the cytoplasm and not along plasma membranes.

156 and 295 nucleotide pairs with two intervening sequences of 1172 and 675 nucleotide pairs. The nucleotide sequence of the p9Ka gene contains a potential coding region of 101 amino acids, including the initiating methionine residue.[70] Regions of this derived amino acid sequence correspond exactly to the primary sequence of proteolytic fragments of purified natural p9Ka. Studies of homology have revealed p9Ka to exhibit 27% amino acid sequence similarity to rat vitamin D-dependent intestinal calcium-binding protein;[71] greater than 40% similarity to members of the S-100 family of EF-hand-containing proteins, including subunits of S-100,[72] and the growth-regulated calcyclin;[73] and 32% similarity with p11, the small subunit of annexin II.[74] In common with all these proteins, p9Ka contains two EF-hand calcium-binding sites. The C-terminal loop (residues 62–730) of p9Ka corresponds to an almost perfect EF-hand sequence,[75] whereas, the N-terminal, potential calcium-binding region, is a variant EF-hand loop typical of that found in the S-100 family of proteins.[76]

Immunofluorescence studies have indicated that recombinant p9Ka binds to sites on at least two intracellular polypeptides and that it is located on cytoskeletal components in a pattern identical with the distribution of actin filaments, when stained with phalloidin.[77] These observations are supported by more recent data concerning other S-100 like Ca^{2+} binding proteins which have been shown to modulate the organization of epithelial cytoskeletal filaments through Ca^{2+}-dependent mechanisms, thus influencing events associated with differentiation and inflammatory activation.[78] Thus the primary function of p9Ka appears to be that of a molecular organiser specifically activated via differential Ca^{2+} binding. The ion binding properties of p9Ka have been studied using both natural p9Ka purified by high performance liquid chromatography[79] and recombinant p9Ka produced in *Escherichia coli* cells.[77] The affinity of p9Ka for Ca^{2+} determined in vivo is less than that of high affinity, regulatory calcium-binding proteins such as calmodulin,[77] calcium storage proteins such as parvalbumin[80] and the calcium ion-transporting vitamin D-dependent intestinal calcium ion-binding protein.[81] However, p9Ka has an affinity for Ca^{2+} in the same range as that of other closely related small Ca^{2+}-binding proteins of the S-100 protein family, for which calcium binding has been determined.[82] Binding of Ca^{2+} by p9Ka in vitro is strongly antagonized by physiological concentrations of Na^+, K^+ or Mg^{2+},[77] a property which p9Ka shares with other S-100 type-proteins. If the binding affinities measured in vitro reflect those in vivo, it is likely that p9Ka preferentially binds Ca^{2+} in locations in which these ions are either elevated above normal levels, or where the K^+ concentration is low. Ca^{2+} concentrations regulate a wide range of biological functions – such as cell motility, stimulus-secretion coupling, and carbohydrate metabolism – through a class of calcium-binding proteins. Abnormal changes in Ca^{2+} metabolism result in impaired, or failed, regulation of various dependent intracellular processes – and, thus, have serious consequences as evidenced by changed cellular behaviour. Although enhanced expression of p9Ka promotes metastasis by affecting Ca^{2+} levels or fluxes within cells, it is not yet known whether this is by a direct effect on a specific metabolic process or through an indirect mechanism.

Novel genes promoting the metastatic phenotype

Previous work on the metastatic process has indicated that failure to identify 'metastasis-associated' genes is a serious omission within the general field of cancer biology. The reasons are understandable: first, it has been technically easier, and less speculative, to search for known oncogenes or for mutations in tumour suppressor genes. Second, no appropriate or reliable in vivo models, with which to identify metastasis-associated (particularly 'metastasis-promoting') gene sequences have been available until recently. During early studies of tumourigenesis, the technique of DNA transfection, together with cell-selection using a drug-resistant plasmid, identified a series of activated cellular oncogenes in the chemically-transformed mouse fibroblast NIH3T3 cell line and in a variety of human tumour cell lines.[32,83–86] When inoculated into immunocompetent hosts, such transformants from localised non-metastasizing fibrosarcomas whereas the parental cells fail to do so.[87]

Recovery of donor DNA fragments from within the genome of cells established from metastatic tumours was a major logistical difficulty to be overcome in DNA transfection experiments. During earlier studies, human DNA transfected into 3T3 cells was recovered through identification of human-specific *Alu* sequences.[88,89] While several oncogenes have been identified by this method, the significant risk involved in this strategy is that *Alu* sequences are not contained in every fragment of human DNA (only 50% according to probability and depending on the sizes of the fragments). Recent

```
 ↓***********PCR primer sequence************↓
5'-AAT CCA AGC TTG CGG CCG ATC AGG CCG AAT ATG CGG CCG CAT TAT-3'
    3-A GGT TCG AAC GCC GGC TAG TCC GGC TTA TAG GCC GGC GTA ATA TCG A-5
         Hind III (1)              Sfi I                        Not I           Hind III (Def)
```

Fig. 5 Nucleotide structure of the short synthetic DNA sequences used to 'flank' malignant genomic DNA transfected into recipient benign cells. The sequences are constructed to contain unique restriction sites and to act as PCR primaries during subsequent recovery of transfected sequences (*see* Chen et al[90]).

work in our laboratory to identify 'metastasis-promoting' genes in breast and prostate cancers has employed the specific strategy of 'flanking' all fragments of donor DNA with short synthetic DNA oligonucleotide sequences (Fig. 5) before transfection.[90] These identification sequences of DNA were engineered in such a manner that they could be ligated to the fragments of genomic DNA released by digestion with *Hind III*, and also were able to ligate to both ends of the fragments when cut-back by *Hind III*. This approach has provided a powerful strategy for recovering specific fragments of donor DNA from within the genome of cells derived from metastases.

To validate DNA transfection as a method of assaying for gene sequences responsible for the metastatic phenotype of prostate cancer, a syngeneic carcinogen induced rat mammary epithelial cell-line (RAMA 37) was developed in this laboratory.[91] The model yields benign encapsulated epithelial tumours, with no metastatic behaviour, when inoculated into syngeneic rats. Generation of metastatic variants of RAMA 37 cells has been used as the in vivo assay to identify the metastatic capability of genomic DNA and cDNAs from rat and human mammary epithelial cells.[68,92] The RAMA 37 model is unique and is also more suitable than either of the only other two cell-systems (NIH3T3 cells or Dunning G cells) that might be used as recipients for epithelial DNA. The former are mouse fibroblasts while the latter are not totally benign,[93] and, therefore, would not provide a reliable essay with which to detect the metastatic phenotype. During the past 2 years, the work performed in this laboratory has unequivocally demonstrated that the RAMA 37 cell-line is a reliable system with which to identify DNA sequences able to induce the metastatic phenotype. Using this approach, we have identified a novel series of gene sequences which promote the metastatic phenotype of rat prostate cancer.[94] Homologous sequences from the human disease are presently being confirmed.

The second approach to the identification of 'metastasis genes' is based upon the technique known as 'mRNA differential display PCR' devised by Liang and Pardee.[95] In this process, mRNA is compared from two cells which are genotypically equivalent, although not necessarily identical, and which express distinct phenotypes (e.g. normal or benign with metastatic malignant). The method involves reverse transcription of mRNAs with an oligo-dT primer anchored to the beginning of the poly(A) tail, followed by the PCR reaction in the presence of a second 10mer arbitrary primer in the sequences. Amplified cDNA subpopulations of 3′ termini of the mRNA, as defined by this pair of primers, are distributed on a DNA sequencing gel. By changing primer combinations, 15 000 individual mRNA species from a mammalian cell line may be visualized using approximately 200 primer pairs. This provided

Fig. 6 'Differential display' identification of genes expressed by normal and malignant prostatic epithelial cells. This figure gives an example of a PCR amplification reaction performed on total RNA samples in the presence of [^{35}S]-labelled dATP. The primer pair used for this reaction are: 5′-AAGCTTTTTTTTTTTG-3′ and 5′-AAGCTTGATTGCC-3′.**Lane 1**: PNT-2 (normal prostatic cell-line). **Lane 2**: PC-3 (malignant cell-line). **Lane 3**: Du145 (malignant cell-line). Arrow indicates the position of F24 cDNA.

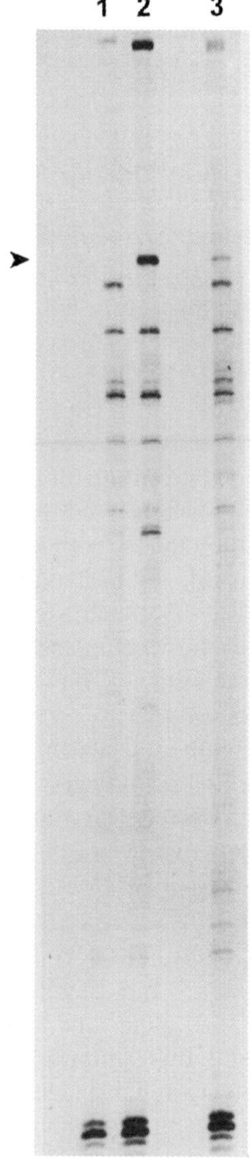

fingerprinting for mRNA and allows the mRNA samples to be analyzed side-by-side. Genes expressed at elevated levels in malignant cells may be 'metastasis-promoting' genes, whereas genes highly expressed in non-neoplastic parental cells are likely to be 'metastasis-suppressor' genes. The technique has been used to isolate cDNAs differentially expressed by androgen-dependent and androgen-independent human prostate carcinoma cells.[96] However, until recently, it was not possible to compare the mRNA patterns between malignant prostate cells and their normal counterparts because of the lack of a well characterized human normal prostate epithelial cell line, despite the fact that a number of human malignant prostatic carcinoma cell lines have been established. Generation and characterization of a human normal prostatic epithelial and fibroblast cell model by Berthon et al has provided an excellent system with which to study the molecular pathology of human prostate cancer. In this model, successful immortalization of human prostate cells was achieved with SV40 expressing both large *T* and small *t* oncogenes.[97] During the past year, our laboratory has employed differential display techniques to perform some fundamental experiments in our ongoing study of the molecular pathology of human prostate cancer. Fifty-two cDNA fragments differentially-expressed in prostate cancer have been isolated. Northern blot analyses of these candidate 'tumour-promoting' genes showed that while some were false positives, or that their expression levels were too low to be significant, others are hitherto unreported gene sequences. Our preliminary analyses has focused on a single gene (F24) expressed at very high levels by malignant cell lines PC-3 and Du-145, but not by the normal cell line, PNT-2. Preliminary sequence analyses together with a search of the gene data bank has revealed the isolated cDNA fragment to comprise a nucleotide sequence which does not correspond to any currently known gene (Fig. 6).

Chromosome-transfer studies have confirmed human chromosome 17q12-22 to contain a novel tumour suppressor gene in this region.[98] Hybridization of non-metastatic Dunning AT2.1 cells with highly metastatic prostate carcinoma AT3.1 cells[99] led to the discovery of a small metastasis-suppressor gene and its human counterpart (KAI1) located on human chromosome 11p11.2 51. Conversely, following differential display analysis of cell lines with distinct behavioural phenotypes from within the Dunning rat prostatic carcinoma model, the protein thymosin β15 was identified to be selectively elevated in the metastatic carcinoma cells,[100] and, hence, its gene regarded as a second possible 'metastasis gene'. A third putative metastasis associated gene located on human chromosome 1 has been provisionally identified following linkage analysis.[101] However, as yet, there are no experimental data to locate, or even to support the existence, of a particular metastasis gene at this site.

CONCLUSIONS

Metastatic malignant disease is the single most important cause of increasing morbidity, progressive treatment failure and subsequent mortality of prostate cancer, in common with the majority of human cancers. Throughout the past two decades, analysis of a range of cellular parameters considered likely to be associated with neoplastic transformation and increasing metastatic potential has been singularly disappointing since no correlation with the behaviour of **individual** prostate cancers has become evident, and no events identified at the molecular genetic level have been shown to correlate with the occurrence of human prostate cancer or with any individual behavioural phenotype of the established disease. Recently, however, novel information from the diverse fields of carbohydrate chemistry, protein expression and molecular genetic techniques has begun to converge and to provide an understanding of the cell-biology of metastatic disease not hitherto attained. In this respect, separation of the field into subjects such as 'oncogenes', 'ion binding proteins' and 'adhesion molecules' is distinctly artificial, although inevitable in a reductionist environment.

However, advances in the fields of glycobiology (made several years ago), and adhesion molecules (made very recently) are now clearly uniting to explain the cell-biological factors governing the metastatic behaviour of malignant epithelial cells. Within the overall study of malignant disease, advances made in field prostate cancer research, principally through the use of cell lines not available in other tissue systems together with unique molecular biological approaches, in beginning to pinpoint the particular early genetic damages which determine the metastatic behavioural phenotype of a primary prostatic neoplasm. Some of the important advances have been outlined in this review. It is anticipated that the rate of these advances will continue to accelerate significantly with the expectation that biologically appropriate therapies for the management of patients with prostate cancer may soon be developed.

ACKNOWLEDGEMENTS

The Stanley Thomas Johnson Foundation (Switzerland), Pfizer Research International, the Albert McMaster Fund of the British Medical Association, The Prostate Cancer Cure Foundation and the North West Cancer Research Campaign (UK) have provided funding through which recent data have been obtained in this laboratory and which is now included in this review. We are grateful to Mr Alan Williams for photographic assistance and to Mrs Jill Gosney for typing and editing the manuscript.

REFERENCES

1. Foster CS. Predictive factors in prostatic hyperplasia and neoplasia. Hum Pathol 1990; 21: 575–577
2. Foster CS, Abel PD. Clinical and molecular techniques for diagnosis and monitoring of prostatic cancer. Hum Pathol 1992; 23: 395–401
3. Sharpe JC, Abel PD, Gilbertson JA, Brawn P, Foster CS. Modulated expression of human leukocyte antigen class I and class II determinants in hyperplastic and malignant human prostatic epithelium. Br J Urol 1994; 74: 609–616
4. McLoughlin J, Foster CS, Price P, Williams G, Abel PD. Evaluation of KI-67 monoclonal antibody as prognostic indicator for prostatic carcinoma. Br J Urol 1993; 72: 92–97
5. Bashir I, Sikora K, Foster CS. Multidrug resistance and behavioral phenotype of cancer cells. Cell Biol Int 1993; 17: 907–917
6. Bashir I, Sikora K, Abel P, Foster CS. Establishment and in vivo characterization of multidrug resistant Dunning R3327 rat prostate carcinoma cell lines. Int J Cancer 1994; 57: 719–726
7. Dermer GB. Basal cell proliferation in benign prostatic hyperplasia. Cancer 1978; 41: 1857–1862
8. Wernert N, Seitz G. Immunohistochemical investigation in different cytokeratins and vimentin in the prostate from the fetal period up to adulthood and in prostate carcinoma. Pathol Res Pract 1987; 182: 617–626
9. Aumuller G. Morphologic and endocrine aspects of prostatic function. Prostate 1983; 4: 195–214
10. Bonkhoff H, Remberger K. Differentiation pathways and histogenetic aspects of normal and abnormal prostatic growth: a stem cell model. Prostate 1996; 28: 98–106
11. Bonkhoff H, Stein U, Remberger K. Multidirectional differentiation in the normal, hyperplastic and neoplastic human prostate: simultaneous demonstration of cell specific epithelial markers. Hum Pathol 1994; 25: 42–46
12. Bonkhoff H, Wernert N, Dhom G, Remberger K. Relation of endocrine-paracrine cells to cell proliferation in normal hyperplastic and neoplastic human prostate. Prostate 1991; 18: 91–98

13. Bonkhoff H, Stein U, Remberger K. Endocrine-paracrine cell types in the prostate and prostatic adenocarcinomas are postmitotic cells. Hum Pathol 1995; 26: 167–170
14. Cleary KR, Choi HY, Ayala AG. Basal cell hyperplasia of the prostate. Am J Clin Pathol 1983; 80: 850–854
15. Bonkhoff H, Stein U, Remberger K. The proliferative function of basal cells in the normal and hyperplastic human prostate. Prostate 1994; 24: 114–118
16. Heatfield BM, Sanefuji H, Trump BF. Long-term explant culture of normal human prostate. Methods Cell Biol 1980; 21: 171–194
17. Devaraj LT, Bostwick DG. Atypical basal cell hyperplasia of the prostate. Immunophenotypic profile and proposed classification of basal cell proliferations. Am J Surg Pathol 1993; 17: 645–659
18. Colombel M, Symmans G, Gil S et al. Detection of the apoptosis-suppressing oncoprotein bcl-2 in hormone-refractory human prostate cancer. Am J Pathol 1993; 143: 390–400
19. Bonkhoff H, Stein U, Aumuller G, Remberger K. Differential expression of 5-alpha-reductase isoenzymes in the human prostate and prostatic carcinomas. Prostate 1996; 29: 261–267
20. Hockenberry D, Zutter M, Hickey W, Nahm M, Korsmeyer SJ. bcl-2 protein is topographically restricted to tissues characterized by apoptotic cell death. Proc Natl Acad Sci USA 1991; 88: 6961–6965
21. Long-Lu Q, Abel P, Foster CS, Lalani EN. *bcl-2*: role in epithelial differentiation and oncogenesis. Hum Pathol 1996; 27: 102–110
22. Ware JL. Prostate cancer progression. Implications of histopathology. Am J Pathol 1994; 145: 893–993
23. Allsbrook WC, Pfeiffer EA. Histochemistry of the prostate. In: Foster CS, Bostwick DG. (eds) Pathology of the Prostate. Philadelphia: W B Saunders, 1997; Ch. 15, pp 282–303
24. Bostwick DG, Brawer MK. Prostatic intra-epithelial neoplasia and early invasion in prostate cancer. Cancer 1987; 59: 788–794
25. Montironi R, Bostwick D, Bonkhoff H et al. Workgroup 1: Origins of prostate cancer. Cancer 1996; 78: 362–365
26. Bostwick DG. Progression of prostatic intraepithelial neoplasia to early invasive adenocarcinoma. Eur Urol 1996; 30: 145–152
27. Bostwick DG, Amin MB, Dundore P, Marsh W, Schultz DS. Architectural patterns of high grade prostatic intraepithelial neoplasia. Hum Pathol 1993; 24: 298–310
28. Lee F, Torp-Pedersen ST, Caroll JT, Siders DB, Christensen-Day C, Mitchell AE. Use of transrectal ultrasound and prostate-specific antigen in diagnosis of prostatic intraepithelial neoplasia. Urology 1989; 24: 4–8
29. Davidson D, Bostwick DG, Qian J et al. Prostatic intraepithelial neoplasia is a risk factor for adenocarcinoma: predictive accuracy in needle biopsies. J Urol 1995; 154: 1295–1299
30. Bostwick DG, Qian J, Frankel K. The incidence of high grade prostatic intraepithelial neoplasia in needle biopsies. J Urol 1995; 154: 1791–1794
31. Bostwick DG. High grade prostatic intraepithelial neoplasia: the most likely precursor of prostate cancer. Cancer 1995; 75: 1823–1836
32. Shih C, Shilo B, Goldford MP, Dannenberg S, Weinberg RA. Passage of phenotypes of chemically transformed cells via transfection of DNA and chromatin. Proc Natl Acad Sci USA 1979; 76: 5714–5718
33. Viola MV, Fromwitz F, Oravez S et al. Expression of *ras* oncogene p21 in prostate cancer. N Engl J Med 1986; 314: 133–137
34. Peehl DM, Wehner N, Stamey TA. Activated Ki-*ras* oncogene in human prostatic adenocarcinoma. Prostate 1987; 10: 281–289
35. Carter BS, Epstein JI, Isaacs WB. *ras* gene mutations in human prostate cancer. Cancer Res 1990; 50: 6830–6832
36. Fan K. Heterogeneous subpopulations of human prostatic adenocarcinoma cells. Potential usefulness of P21 protein as a predictor of bone metastasis. J Urol 1988; 139: 318–322

37. Cooke DB, Quarmby VE, Mickey DD, Isaacs JT, French FS. Oncogene expression in prostate cancer: Dunning R3327 rat dorsal prostatic adenocarcinoma system. Prostate 1988; 13: 263–272
38. Stanbridge EJA. Human tumor suppressor genes. Annu Rev Genet 1990; 24: 615–657
39. Yunis JJ, Ramsay N. Retinoblastoma and subband deletion of chromosome 13. Am J Dis Child 1978; 132: 161–163
40. Friend SH, Bernards R, Rogelj S et al. A human DNA segment with properties of the gene that predisposes to retinoblastoma and osteosarcoma. Nature 1986; 323: 643–646
41. Benedict WF, Xu HJ, Hu SX, Takahashi R. Role of the retinoblastoma gene in the initiation and progression of human cancer. J Clin Invest 1990; 85: 988–993
42. Bookstein R, Rio P, Madreperla SA et al. Promoter deletion and loss of retinoblastoma gene expression in human prostate carcinoma. Proc Natl Acad Sci USA 1990; 87: 7762–7766
43. Mercer WE, Avignolo C, Baserga R. Role of the p53 protein in cell proliferation as studied by microinjection of monoclonal antibodies. Mol Cell Biol 1984; 4: 276–281
44. Levine AJ, Momand J. Tumor suppressor genes: the p53 and retinoblastoma sensitivity genes and gene products. Biochim Biophys Acta 1990; 1032: 119–136
45. Finlay CA, Hinds PW, Tan TH, Eliyahu D, Oren M, Levine AJ. Activating mutations for transformation by p53 produce a gene product that forms an hsc 70-p53 complex with an altered half life. Mol Cell Biol 1988; 8: 531–539
46. Rotter V, Abutbul H, Ben-Ze'ev A. p53 transformation-related protein accumulates in the nucleus of transformed fibroblasts in association with the chromatin and is found in the cytoplasm of non-transformed fibroblasts. EMBO J 1983; 2: 1041–1047
47. Hinds P, Finlay C, Levine AJ. Mutation is required to activate the p53 gene for cooperation with the *ras* oncogene and transformation. J Virol 1989; 63: 739–746
48. Finlay CA, Hinds PW, Levine AJ. The p53 proto-oncogene can act as a suppressor of transformation. Cell 1989; 57: 1083–1093
49. Foster CS, McLoughlin J, Bashir I, Abel PD. Markers of the metastatic phenotype in prostate cancer. Hum Pathol 1992; 23: 381–394
50. Mottaz AE, Markwalder R, Fey MF et al. Abnormal p53 expression is rare in clinically localized human prostate cancer: comparison between immunohistochemical and molecular detection of p53 mutations. Prostate 1997; 31: 209–215
51. Dong JT, Lamb PW, Rinker-Schaeffer CW et al. KAI 1, a metastasis suppressor gene for prostate cancer on human chromosome 11p11.2. Science 1995; 286: 884–886
52. Sharon N, Lis H. Lectins as cell recognition molecules. Science 1989; 246: 227–234
53. Charpin C, Garcia S, Bouvier C et al. Automated and quantitative immunocytochemical assays of CD44v6 in breast carcinomas. Hum Pathol 1997; 28: 289–296
54. Arch R, Wirth K, Hofmann M et al. Participation in normal immune responses of a metastasis-inducing splice variant of CD44. Science 1992; 257: 682–685
55. Screaton GR, Bell MV, Jackson DG, Cornelis FB, Gerth U, Bell JI. Genomic structure of DNA coding the lymphocyte homing reception CD44 reveals at least 12 alternatively spliced exons. Proc Natl Acad Sci USA 1992; 89: 12160–12164
56. Mackay CR, Terpe HJ, Stauder R, Marston WL, Stark H, Gunthert U. Expression and modulation of CD44 variant isoforms in humans. J Cell Biol 1994; 124: 71–82
57. Terpe HJ, Stark H, Prehm P, Gunthert U. CD44 variant isoforms are preferentially expressed in basal epithelia of non-malignant human fetal and adult tissues. Histochemistry 1994; 101: 79–89
58. Sy MS, Guo YJ, Stamenkovic I. Distinct effects of two CD44 isoforms on tumour growth in vivo. J Exp Med 1991; 174: 859–866
59. Gunthert U, Hofmann M, Rudy W et al. A new variant of glycoprotein CD44 confers metastatic potential to rat carcinoma cells. Cells 1991; 65: 13–24
60. Rudy W, Hofmann R, Schwartz-Albiez R et al. Two major CD44 proteins expressed on a metastatic rat tumor cell line are derived from different splice variants: each one individually suffices to confer metastatic behavior. Cancer Res 1993; 53: 1262–1268
61. Seiter S, Arch R, Reber S et al. Prevention of tumor metastasis formation by anti-variant CD44. J Exp Med 1993; 177: 443–455

62. Koopman G, Heider KH, Horst E et al. Activated human lymphocytes and aggressive non-Hodgkin's lymphomas express a homologue of the rat metastasis-associated variant of CD44. J Exp Med 1993; 177: 897–904
63. Hong RL, Pu YS, Hsieh TS, Chu JS, Lee WJ. Expressions of E-cadherin and exon V6-containing isoforms of CD44 and their prognostic values in human transitional cell carcinoma. J Urol 1995; 153: 2025–2028
64. Nomura S, Willis AJ, Edwards DR, Heath JK, Hogan BLM. Developmental expression of 2ar (osteopontin) and SPARC (osteonectin) RNA as revealed by in situ hybridization. J Cell Biol 1988; 106: 441–450
65. Brown LF, Berse B, Van De Water L et al. Expression and distribution of osteopontin in human tissues: widespread association with luminal epithelial surfaces. Mol Cell Biol 1992; 3: 1169–1180
66. Oldberg A, Franzen A, Heinegard D. Cloning and sequence analysis of rat bone sialoprotein (osteopontin) cDNA reveals an Arg-Gly-Asp cell-binding sequence. Proc Natl Acad Sci USA 1986; 83: 8819–8823
67. Ross FP, Chappell J, Alvarez JI et al. Interactions between the bone matrix proteins osteopontin and bone sialoprotein and the osteoclast integrin alpha-v-beta-3 potentiate bone resorption. J Biol Chem 1993; 268: 9901–9907
68. Davies BR, Davies MPA, Gibbs FEM, Barraclough R, Rudland PS. Induction of the metastatic phenotype by transfection of a benign rat mammary epithelial cell-line with the gene for p9Ka, a rat calcium-binding protein, but not with the oncogene EJ-*ras*-1. Oncogene 1993; 8: 999–1008
69. Ke Y, Jing C, Barraclough R, Smith P, Davies MPA, Foster CS. Elevated expression of calcium-binding protein p9Ka is associated with increasing malignant characteristics of rat prostate carcinoma cells. Int J Cancer 1997; 71: 832–837
70. Barraclough R, Savin J, Dube SY, Rudland PS. Molecular cloning and sequence of the gene for p9Ka: a cultured myoepithelial cell protein with strong homology to S-100, a calcium-binding protein. J Mol Biol 1987; 198: 13–20
71. Desplan C, Heidmann O, Lillie JW, Auffray C, Thomasset M. Sequence of rat intestinal vitamin D-dependent calcium-binding protein derived from cDNA clone evolutionary implications. J Biol Chem 1983; 258: 3502–3505
72. Kuwano R, Maeda T, Usui H et al. Molecular-cloning of cDNA of s100-alpha subunit messenger RNA. FEBS Lett 1986; 202: 97–101
73. Calabretta B, Battini R, Kraczmarek L, Deriel JK, Baserga R. Molecular-cloning of the cDNA for a growth factor-inducible gene with strong homology to S-100, a calcium-binding protein. J Biol Chem 1986; 261: 2628–2632
74. Gerke V, Weber K. The regulatory chain in the p36-kd substrate complex of viral tyrosine-specific protein-kinases is related in sequence to the S-100 protein of glial-cells. EMBO J 1985; 4: 2917–2920
75. Tufty RM, Kretsinger RH. Troponin and parvalbumin calcium-binding regions predicted in myosin light chain and T4 lysozyme. Science 1975; 187: 167–169
76. Krestsinger RH, Tolbert D, Nakayama S, Pearson W. The EF-hand, homologs and analogs. In: Heizmann CW. (ed). Novel calcium-binding proteins: fundamental and clinical implications. Berlin: Springer, 1991; 17–37.
77. Gibbs FEM, Wilkinson MC, Rudland PS, Barraclough R. Interactions in vitro of p9Ka, the rat S-100 related, metastasis-inducing, calcium-binding protein. J Biol Chem 1994; 269: 18992–18999
78. Goebeler M, Roth J, Van Den Bos C, Ader G, Sorg C. Increase of calcium levels in epithelial cells induces translocation of calcium-binding proteins migration inhibitory factor-related protein 8 (MRP8) and MRP14 to keratin intermediate filaments. Biochem J 1995; 309: 419–424
79. Barraclough B, Gibbs F, Smith JA, Haynes GA, Rudland PS. Calcium ion-binding by the potential calcium ion-binding protein, p9Ka. Biochem Biophys Res Commun 1990; 169: 660–666
80. Pechere JF. Calcium-binding proteins and calcium function. Amsterdam: Elsevier, 1977
81. Van Eldik LJ, Zendegui JG, Marshak OR, Watterson DM. Calcium-binding proteins and the molecular basis of calcium action. Int Rev Cytol 1982; 77: 1–61

82. Hilt D, Kligman D. The S-100 protein family: a biochemical and functional overview. In: Heizmann CW. (ed). Novel calcium-binding proteins: fundamentals and clinical implications. Berlin: Springer, 1991; 65–103
83. Cooper GM, Okenquist S, Silverman L. Transforming activity of DNA of chemically transformed and normal cells. Nature 1980; 284: 181–188
84. Shih C, Padhy LC, Murray M, Weinberg RA. Transforming genes of carcinomas and neuroblastomas introduced into mouse fibroblasts. Nature 1981; 290: 261–264
85. Krontiris TG, Cooper GM. Transforming activity of human-tumor DNAs. Proc Natl Acad Sci USA 1981; 78: 1181–1184
86. Reitsma PH, Rothberg PG, Astrin SM et al. Regulation of *myc* gene expression inHL-60 leukemia-cells by a vitamin-D metabolite. Nature 1983; 303: 396–400
87. Land H, Parada LF, Weinberg RA. Tumorigenic conversion of primary embryo fibroblasts requires at least 2 cooperating oncogenes. Nature 1983; 304: 596–602
88. Hayle AJ, Darling DL, Taylor AR, Train D. Transfection of metastatic capability with total genomic DNA from human and mouse metastatic tumor cell-lines. Differentiation 1993; 54: 177–189
89. Gate CC, Belloni DR, Marin-Padilla M. Acquisition and enhanced expression of the metastatic phenotype following transfections of genomic mouse tumor DNA containing human SCLC gene sequences. Clin Exp Metastasis 1995; 13: 203–217
90. Chen H, Ke Y, Oates AO, Barraclough R, Rudland PS. Isolation of and the effector for metastasis-inducing DNAs from a human metastatic carcinoma cell line. Oncogene 1997; 14: 1581–1588
91. Rudland PS. Stem-cells and the development of mammary cancers in experimental rats and in humans. Cancer Metastasis Rev 1987; 6: 55–83
92. Davies BR, Fernig DG, Barraclough R, Rudland PS. Effect on tumorigenicity and metastasis of transfection of a diploid benign rat mammary epithelial-cell line with DNA corresponding to the messenger-RNA for basis fibroblast growth-factor. Int J Cancer 1996; 65: 104–111
93. Isaacs JT, Isaacs WB, Feitz WFJ, Scheres J. Establishment and characterization of seven Dunning rat prostatic cancer cell-lines and their use in developing methods for predicting metastatic abilities of prostatic cancer. Prostate 1986; 9: 261–281
94. Ke Y, Beesley C, Smith P, Barraclough R, Rudland P, Foster CS. Generation of metastatic variants by transfection of a nonmetastatic rat epithelial cell-line with genomic DNA from rat prostatic carcinoma cells. Br J Cancer 1998; 77: 287–296
95. Liang P, Pardee AB. Differential display of eukaryotic messenger RNA by means of the polymerase chain reaction. Science 1992; 257: 967–971
96. Blok LJ, Kumar MV, Tindall DJ. Isolation of cDNAs that are differentially expressed between androgen-dependent and androgen-independent prostate carcinoma cells using differential display PCR. Prostate 1995; 26: 213–224
97. Berthon P, Cussenot O, Hopwood L, Le Duc A, Maitland NJ. Functional expression of SV40 in normal human prostatic epithelial and fibroblastic cells: differentiation pattern of non-tumorigenic cell lines. Int J Oncol 1995; 6: 333–343
98. Murakami YS, Brothman AR, Leach RJ, White RL. Suppression of malignant phenotype in a human prostate cancer cell-line by fragments of normal chromosomal region 17q. Cancer Res 1995; 55: 3389–3394
99. Ichikawa T, Ichikawa Y, Isaacs JT. Genetic factors and suppression of metastatic ability of prostatic cancer. Cancer Res 1991; 51: 3788–3792
100. Bao L, Loda M, Janmey PA, Stewart R, Anand-Apte B, Zetter BR. Thymosin beta 15: a novel regulator of tumor cell motility upregulated in metastatic prostate cancer. Nat Med 1996; 2: 1322–1328
101. Smith JR, Freije D, Carpten JD et al. Major susceptibility locus for prostate cancer on chromosome 1 suggested by a genome-wide search. Science 1996; 274: 1371–1374
102. Markham CW. Detection and correlation with invasive cancer in fine-needle biopsy. Urology 1989; 24: 57–61
103. Park C, Galang C, Johenning P, Marksem J, Tannenbaum M. Follow-up aspiration biopsies for dysplasia of the prostate. Lab Invest 1989; 60: 70A
104. Brawer MK, Bigler SA, Sohlberg OE, Nagle RB, Lange PH. Significance of prostatic intraepithelial neoplasia on prostate needle biopsy. Urology 1991; 38: 103–107

105. Berner A, Danielsen HE, Pettersen EO, Fossa SD, Reith A, Nesland JM. DNA distribution in the prostate: normal gland, benign and premalignant lesions and subsequent adenocarcinomas. Anal Quant Cytol Histol 1993; 15: 247–252
106. Weinstein MH, Epstein JI. Significance of high grade prostatic intraepithelial neoplasia on needle biopsy. Hum Pathol 1993; 24: 624–629
107. Keetch DW, Humphrey P, Stahl D, Smith DS, Catelona WJ. Morphometric analysis and clinical follow-up of isolated prostatic intraepithelial neoplasia in needle biopsy of the prostate. J Urol 1995; 154: 347–351
108. Vocke CD, Pozzatti RO, Bostwick DG et al. Analysis of 99 microdisected prostate carcinomas reveals a high frequency of allelic loss on chromosome 8p12-21. Cancer Res 1996; 56: 2411–2416
109. Sanchez Y, Lovell M, Marin MC et al. Tumor suppression and apoptosis of human prostate carcinoma mediated by a genetic locus with human chromosome 10pter-q11. Proc Natl Acad Sci USA 1996; 93: 2551–2556
110. Cooney KA, Wetzel JC, Merajver SD, Macoska JA, Singleton TP, Wojno KJ. Distinct regions of allelic loss on 13q in prostate cancer. Cancer Res 1996; 56: 1142–1145
111. MacGrogan D, Levy A, Bova GS, Isaacs WB, Bookstein R. Structure and methylation-associated silencing of a gene with a homozygously deleted region of human chromosome band 8p22. Genomics 1996; 35: 55–65
112. Bova GS, MacGrogan D, Levy A, Pin SS, Bookstein R, Isaacs WB. Physical mapping of chromosome 8p22 markers and their homozygous deletion in a metastatic prostate cancer. Genomics 1996; 35: 46–54
113. Kunimi K, Amano T, Uchibayashi T. Point mutation of the p53 gene is an infrequent event in untreated prostate cancer. Cancer Detect Prev 1996; 20: 218–222
114. Cooney KA, Wetzel JC, Consolino CM, Wojno KJ. Identification and characterization of proximal 6q deletions in prostate cancer. Cancer Res 1996; 56: 4150–4153
115. Murakami YS, Albertsen H, Brothman AR, Leach RJ, White RL. Suppression of the malignant phenotype of human prostate cancer cell line PPC-1 by introduction of normal fragments of human chromosome 10. Cancer Res 1996; 56: 2157–2160
116. Ittmann MM. Loss of heterozygosity on chromosome 10 and 17 in clinically localized prostate carcinoma. Prostate 1996; 28: 275–281
117. Williams BJ, Jones E, Zhu XL et al. Evidence for a tumor suppressor gene distal to BRCA1 in prostate cancer. J Urol 1996; 155: 720–725
118. Gao X, Zacharek A, Grignon DJ et al. Localization of potential tumor suppressor loci to a Mb region on chromosome 17q in human prostate cancer. Oncogene 1995; 11: 1241–1247
119. Kagan J, Stein J, Babaian RJ et al. Homozygous deletions at 8p22 and 8p21 in prostate cancer implicate these regions as the sites for candidate tumor suppressor genes. Oncogene 1995; 16: 2121–2126
120. Macoska JA, Trybus TM, Benson PD et al. Evidence for three tumor suppressor gene loci on chromosome 8p in human prostate cancer. Cancer Res 1995; 55: 5390–5395
121. Gray IC, Phillips SM, Lee SJ, Neoptolemos JP, Weissenbach J, Spurr NK. Loss of the chromosomal region 10q23-25 in prostate cancer. Cancer Res 1995; 55: 4800–4803
122. Komiya A, Suzuki H, Aida S, Yatani R, Shimazaki J. Mutational analysis of CDKN2 (CDK41/MTS1) gene in tissues and cell lines of human prostate cancer. Jpn J Cancer Res 1995; 86: 622–625
123. Herman JG, Merlo A, Mao L et al. Inactivation of the CDKN2/p 16/MTS1 gene is frequently associated with aberrant DNA methylation in all common human cancers. Cancer Res 1995; 55: 4525–4530
124. Cairns P, Polascik TJ, Eby Y et al. Frequency of homozygous deletion at p16/CDKN2 in primary human tumours. Nat Genet 1995; 11: 210–212
125. Suzuki H, Emi M, Komiya A et al. Localization of a tumor suppressor gene associated with progression of human prostate cancer with a 1.2 Mb region of 8p22-p21.3. Genes Chromosomes Cancer 1995; 13: 168–174
126. Emmert-Buck MR, Vocke CD, Pozzatti RO et al. Allelic loss on chromosome 8p12-21 in microdissected intraepithelial neoplasia. Cancer Res 1995; 55: 2959–2962

127. Eagle LR, Yin X, Brothman AR, Williams BJ, Atkin NB, Prochownik EV. Mutation of the MXI1 gene in prostate cancer. Nat Genet 1995; 9: 249–255
128. Gao X, Zacharek A, Salkowski A et al. Loss of heterozygosity of the BRCA1 and other loci on chromosome 17q in human prostate cancer. Cancer Res 1995; 55: 1002–1005
129. MacGrogan D, Levy A, Bostwick D, Wagner M, Wells D, Bookstein R. Loss of chromosome arm 8p loci in prostate cancer: mapping by quantitative allelic imbalance. Gene Chromosomes Cancer 1994; 10: 151–159
130. Trapman J, Sleddens HF, van-der-Weiden MM et al. Loss of heterozygosity of chromosome 8 microsatellite loci implicates a candidate tumor suppressor gene between the loci D8S87. Cancer Res 1994; 54: 6061–6064
131. Burney TL, Rockove S, Eiseman JL, Jacobs SC, Kyprianou N. Partial growth suppression of human prostate cancer cells by the Krev-1 suppressor gene. Prostate 1994; 25: 177–188
132. Berube NG, Speevak MD, Chevrette M. Suppression of tumorigenicity of human prostate cancer cells by introduction of human chromosome del(12)(q13). Cancer Res 1994; 54: 3077–3081

8

Current developments in lung cancer

P. S. Hasleton

The aim of this chapter is not to review the recent molecular biological studies carried out on carcinoma of the lung and mesothelioma.[1] It will attempt to highlight some current problems in the pathology of neuroendocrine tumours, adenocarcinoma and the related entity of atypical alveolar hyperplasia and some recent work on malignant mesothelioma.

INCIDENCE

The different geographical incidences of lung cancer still provides much interest. A recent study of SEER (Surveillance Program, Epidemiology and End-Results) conducted at the National Cancer Institute between 1969 and 1971 showed a rise in age adjusted lung cancer incidence from 37.8 to 68.2 per 100 000. Lung cancer rates in both white and black males reached a peak around 1984 and then subsequently declined. Among white and black males, squamous cell carcinoma, small cell carcinoma and large cell carcinoma declined after peaks in the 1980s. The rate for adenocarcinoma in males peaked at the end of that decade. However, the incidence of squamous, adeno- and small cell carcinoma is rising in black and white females.[2] Previously, in the US, the most frequent histological type was squamous cell carcinoma. However, during the mid-1980s the rate for adenocarcinoma surpassed that for the squamous cell variant. This trend appears similar in Japan but is not apparently reflected in the UK, where a study in the South East of Scotland[3] showed 48% squamous cell carcinoma, 24% small cell and 13% adenocarcinoma. The significance of these figures, however, could be disputed since, in the UK, only approximately 60% of patients receive histological proof of the diagnosis.

Dr P. S. Hasleton, Department of Pathology, South Manchester University Hospitals NHS Trust, Wythenshawe Hospital, Southmoor Road, Manchester M23 9LT, UK

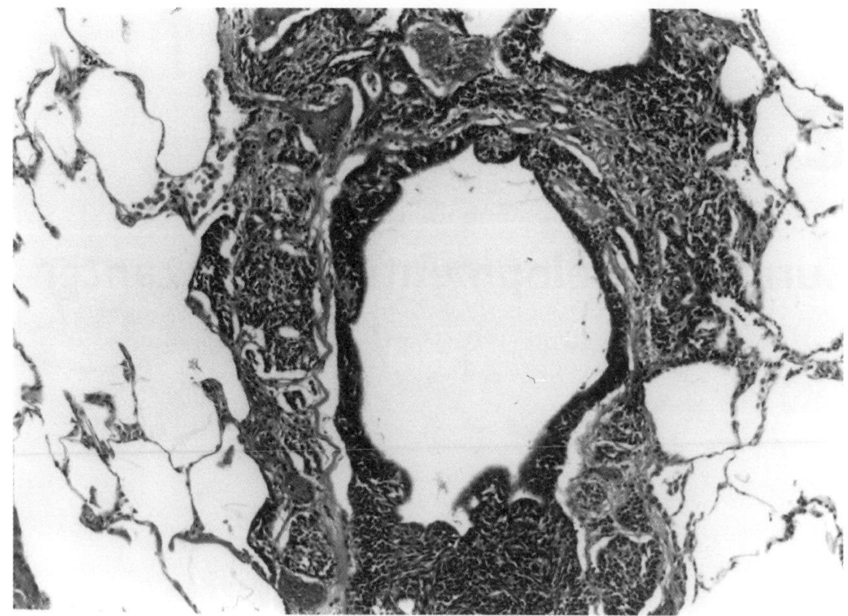

Fig. 1 Neuroendocrine proliferation inside a bronchiole as well as outside it. Note there is no marked inflammation or interstitial pulmonary fibrosis. Stain: haematoxylin and eosin, × 125.

NEUROENDOCRINE PROLIFERATIONS AND TUMOURS

Neuroendocrine cell hyper- and hypoplasia

Armas et al[4] described neuroendocrine hyperplasia which simulated interstitial pulmonary fibrosis. The thickening of the alveolar wall and the intra-alveolar proliferation were due to neuroendocrine cells and mild to moderate interstitial fibrosis. This case was not associated with tumourlets or marked interstitial fibrosis. The neuroendocrine hyperplasia was thought to precede the fibrosis since there was multicentric involvement of the lung with lesions having well-delineated borders and normal intervening parenchyma. Areas of mild interstitial fibrosis without neuroendocrine hyperplasia were not seen. The authors regarded this as a pulmonary neuroendocrine cell (PNEC) dysplasia, but it is not known if it is a hyperplasia or a dysplasia. The malignant potential is unknown. The importance of this case is that neuroendocrine cells may proliferate in the absence of pre-existing lung disease. The cells did not express any peptide hormones. It is, therefore, just possible, despite the lack of hormone production, that the neuroendocrine cells could stimulate the fibrosis, rather than vice versa. This author favours the concept that the tumourlets and most neuroendocrine proliferations arise secondary to fibrosis or inflammation and the lesion described above with neuroendocrine cell proliferation and fibrosis is a different entity. Rarely there may be a neuroendocrine proliferation inside and around bronchioles (Fig. 1) causing lung disease severe enough to require transplantation.

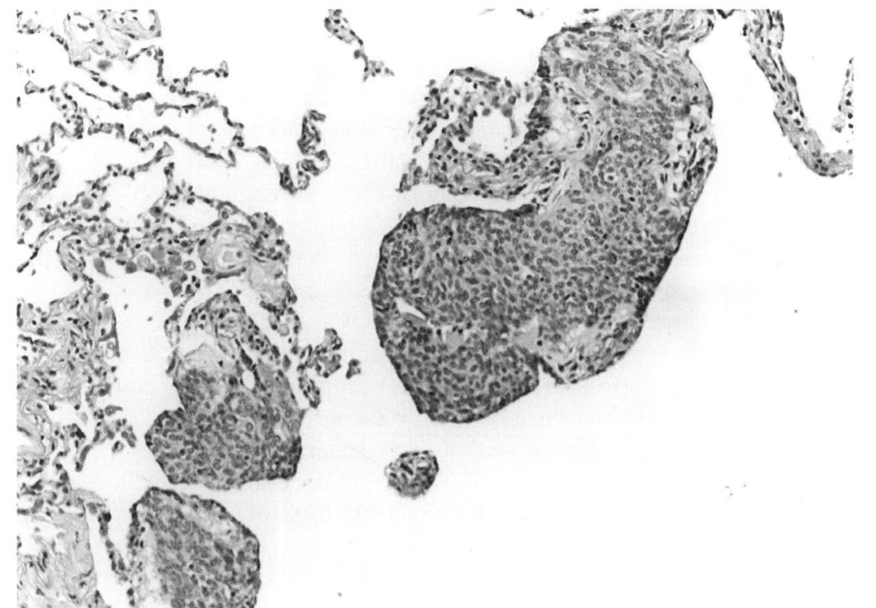

Fig. 2 Lung tissue in the same lobe as a peripheral carcinoid. There is a focal but definite increase in neuroendocrine cells, with a normal alveolar wall. Stain: haematoxylin and eosin, × 125.

Pulmonary neuroendocrine hyperplasia has been shown by immunolabelling lung tissue immediately adjacent to peripheral carcinoids in 19 out of 25 lungs resected for peripheral carcinoids.[5] Eight cases showed bronchiolitis obliterans. The changes in pulmonary endocrine cells were focal and involved less than 20% of terminal and respiratory bronchioles assessed. There were hyperplastic changes including a linear increase of pulmonary endocrine cells along the basement membrane (Fig. 2) and a cluster of pulmonary endocrine cells in the bronchial epithelium.

A recent study of central carcinoid tumours[6] compared tumour resection margins and airways adjacent to 28 typical carcinoid tumours with those from pulmonary adeno-, squamous (SQCC) and small cell carcinomas (SCLC). Unused adult donor lungs acted as further controls. Pulmonary neuroendocrine cells (PNEC) were identified by antibodies against PGP 9.5, bombesin, chromogranin and calcitonin. The number of immunoreactive cells in the bronchial epithelium was expressed per mm length of epithelium and per 10 000 epithelial cells.

The Tukey test suggested that more PNEC were expressed in resection margins of normal lungs in comparison to those with TC, SQCC and SCLC. However, in large airway epithelium adjacent to typical carcinoids, the number of PNEC was less than in normal bronchi but higher than in tumour-free resection margins. There was no significant difference between normal lungs and those with adenocarcinoma.

Carcinoid tumours, SQCC and SCLC are probably producing factors with an inhibitory paracrine effect on the local pulmonary neuroendocrine population. This does not explain why adenocarcinomas are not suppressing the pulmonary neuroendocrine cell population.

General characteristics of neuroendocrine tumours

Neuroendocrine pulmonary tumours share some common immunohistochemical, ultrastructural and morphologic characteristics. The main categories are typical carcinoid, atypical carcinoid, large cell neuroendocrine carcinoma and small cell carcinoma. 30% of non-small cell carcinomas show neuroendocrine features with positivity for synaptophysin and chromogranin and dense core granules ultrastructurally. The prognosis of such tumours is unknown or if they are more or less responsive to chemotherapy than tumours lacking neuroendocrine differentiation. A larger number of cases must be studied.

All carcinoid tumours whether typical, atypical or large cell neuroendocrine tend to have a male predominance.[7] 71% of patients with typical carcinoids were non-smokers. The corresponding figures for atypical carcinoids and large cell neuroendocrine tumours were 33% and 3%, respectively.

Carcinoid tumours may be central or peripheral. The peripheral tumours have been regarded as being atypical. This might be because they have a spindle cell pattern. They cause problems in differential diagnosis, being confused with nerve sheath tumours, leiomyomas or, rarely, spindle cell squamous carcinomas. Most peripheral carcinoids show no evidence of nuclear pleomorphism or mitotic activity and are benign. Central carcinoids are commoner and, for some unknown reason, are more frequently right-sided.

Endocrine manifestations include the carcinoid syndrome. In pulmonary carcinoids, it presents usually with left-sided valvular lesions and is rare, having an incidence of 1–7%. It is unknown why pulmonary carcinoids manifest so rarely as the carcinoid syndrome. It may be because the peptides or kinins produced by these tumours are rapidly inactivated by the endothelial cells of the lung. The syndrome is more common in pulmonary carcinoid tumours with metastases.[8] Immunocytochemical studies demonstrate many peptides and other mediators in these tumours. However, this technique may be exquisitely sensitive or the total amount of mediator produced may be too small in most cases to cause valvular disease.

The histology of typical carcinoids is very varied and is dealt with elsewhere.[9,10] A summary of different histological features seen in pulmonary carcinoid tumours is given in the Table.

Apoptosis in bronchopulmonary carcinoids

Typical bronchial carcinoid tumours have two cell populations. The predominant cell type consists of small uniform cells with regular central nuclei and a faintly eosinophilic cytoplasm (Fig. 3). The second population are smaller cells with little cytoplasm and hyperchromatic nuclei, which ultrastructurally are apoptotic cells.[11] Morphometric analysis of individual cell death in bronchial carcinoid tumours shows the proportion of dead or apoptotic tumour cells does not differ significantly between typical and atypical carcinoids (17% and 13%, respectively). In diploid tumours, the percentage of apoptotic cells is 18%, whereas in aneuploid the figure is 12%. Individual cell death appears to play no part in the association with poor prognosis in atypical carcinoids. These figures are all the more remarkable since squamous cell carcinoma of the cervix or bronchus have apoptotic indices ranging between 1.5% and 10%.[12]

Table Histological variations of bronchopulmonary carcinoid tumours

Trabecular
Insular
Undifferentiated growth pattern
Atypical carcinoid
Papillary
Goblet cell
Melanin-containing
Spindle cell
Signet ring cell
Bronchoalveolar carcinoma pattern
Carcinoid containing bone
Carcinoid with an amyloid component

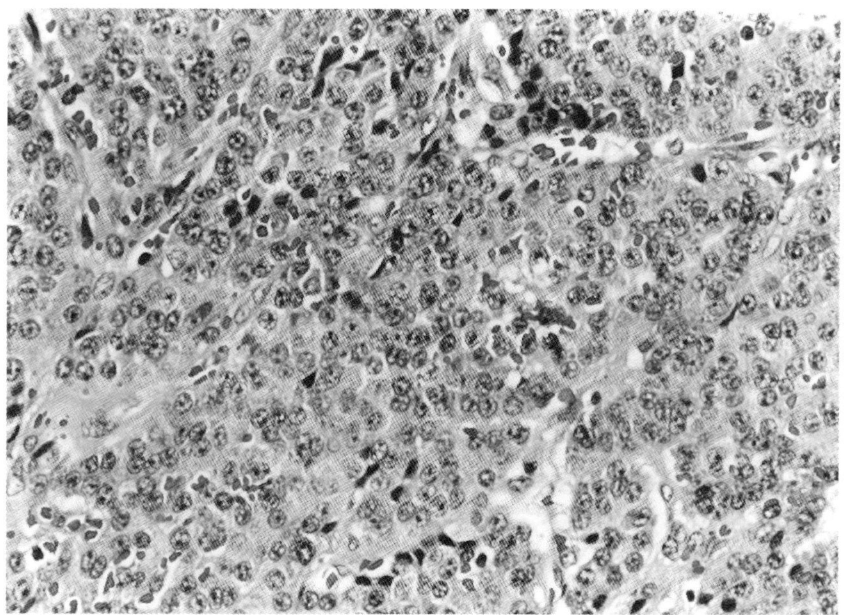

Fig. 3 Typical carcinoid tumour with a population of small, dark, hyperchromatic apoptotic cells. Stain: haematoxylin and eosin, × 313.

A recent study[13] looked at expression of proliferating nuclear antigen by Ki-67 immunostaining of 31 typical and 16 atypical carcinoids. Ki 67 reacts with a nuclear antigen expressed by proliferating cells and measures the growth fraction in individual tissues and tumours. The proliferation status was significantly higher in histologically typical than atypical carcinoids. Using a 4% cut-off, the authors observed a significant difference for the 4 year survival rate. A semi-quantitative analysis of the proliferation index by Ki 67 immunostaining identifies high risk subsets of patients with atypical carcinoids. Such carcinoid tumours, while rare, can be relatively easily diagnosed by light microscopy.

Ploidy status

A few typical carcinoids tumours show tumour in adjacent lymph nodes. This usually implies a poor prognosis but this is not necessarily the case in typical carcinoids. Cases have been documented surviving many years. In a study of ploidy in bronchopulmonary carcinoid tumours, two cases with lymph node metastases and a typical architecture were DNA aneuploid.[14]

Ploidy has limited value for determining prognosis in bronchopulmonary carcinoid tumours. In a study of 53 patients, those with diploid tumours tended to survive longer than those with DNA aneuploidy, but the difference was of borderline statistical significance. The incidence of DNA aneuploidy in tumours with lymph node metastases was significantly higher than in those without. The most powerful predictor of prognosis in a Cox multivariant analysis was the histological growth pattern. The other variables of independent significance were the presence of involved lymph nodes and nuclear pleomorphism. Another flow cytometric study showed that aneuploidy was more common in tumours 3 cm or greater in diameter.[15]

One group studied 60 typical carcinoids, of which 58 showed euploid DNA histograms, compared with only 50% (20 of the 40) atypical carcinoids.[16] Deaths from tumour were exclusively observed among patients with atypical or DNA aneuploid tumours. As documented above, the presence of lymph node metastases alone was not associated with poor prognosis as long as the primary tumour or the related metastases showed a diploid DNA content. This study was also remarkable for the large number of peripheral tumours. There was a significant difference in survival between cases with diploid and aneuploid cell patterns. The cut-off point in tumour size in this study was 1.4 cm. None of the 20 patients with a pulmonary carcinoid measuring 1.4 cm in diameter died from their tumour, whereas all 8 tumour-related deaths the tumour measured more than 1.4 cm.

These authors summarised the total number of carcinoids studied by ploidy. Of the 296 typical carcinoids examined, 91% (270) had a diploid DNA content. Only 3/46 typical carcinoids (7%) had a diploid DNA. In several smaller collections of tumours, the number of diploid atypical carcinoids exceeded the aneuploid. In a literature review, the number of diploid atypical carcinoids was 36%.

The occurrence of diploidy among atypical carcinoids raises the question whether flow cytometric analysis is of prognostic value for this tumour. It is useful as a prediction for outcome but of no value in the diagnosis of atypical carcinoids. There is a significant correlation between aneuploidy in atypical carcinoids and large tumour size, irrespective of the presence of metastatic disease.

Immunocytochemistry in the diagnosis of pulmonary carcinoid tumours

Most bronchopulmonary carcinoid tumours cause little diagnostic difficulty. The need for special stains arises with unusual growth patterns, such as spindle or papillary carcinoids. Special stains are used more frequently in atypical and especially large cell neuroendocrine tumours of the lung.

Stains used in the diagnosis of neuroendocrine tumours fall into several groups. Silver stains used to be the method of choice and, in one series, 73%

were positive with Grimelius.[17] Such stains have been largely replaced by immunocytochemistry. Protein gene product 9.5 and neuron specific enolase (NSE) are non-specific.[18,19] A marker rarely used but able to detect many carcinoids is human prealbumin (transthyretin). It was not seen in diffusely in squamous, adeno- or small cell carcinomas. The distribution and intensity of staining varies in some series using Leu 7.[20] In the series of neuroendocrine tumours reported by Loy et al,[19] 100% of cases were positive with synaptophysin and 37% were positive with chromogranin A. This group looked at carcinomas without morphologic features of neuroendocrine differentiation and found that synaptophysin was positive in 62% and chromogranin A in 17%. They concluded that many of the commercially available antibodies used as neuroendocrine markers were non-specific in the diagnosis of neuroendocrine tumours. Immunohistochemistry provides no advantage over light microscopy for the classification or prediction of prognosis in pulmonary neuroendocrine tumours.[20] There are fewer neuroendocrine positive cells in atypical or large cell neuroendocrine carcinomas, further detracting from their usefulness.

The most useful markers, if they are to be used as a panel, are transthyretin, chromogranin A and synaptophysin. The problem still exists that in comparing any study with the literature, different authors have used different antibodies and methodology.

Atypical carcinoids

A large series of large cell neuroendocrine carcinomas were studied by Travis et al.[7] However, a group of pulmonary pathologists from around the world could only assemble a total of 23 atypical carcinoids. These patients were 6 years older than those with typical carcinoids (mean age 56 years). They had a male predominance (59%), 67% smoked and stage I and II tumours accounted for 83% of cases. Several series of atypical carcinoids have been described.[21–23] The first and probably the best description is by Arrigoni et al.[21] The other two studies had a total of 56 cases. The symptoms were the same as in typical carcinoid. 35 tumours were central and 21 peripheral. There was no predilection for right or left side. The series of Travis et al[20] is unusual in that 4/6 cases had Cushing's syndrome. Between 33 and 80% of the cases were smokers.

The cut surface of the tumour was yellow and of variable consistency with ill-defined margins. None of the tumours showed necrosis macroscopically. Histologically, the tumours have a well defined carcinoid pattern and the necrosis is often small and punctate. The average mitotic counts are 3–4/10 high power fields[20] and no greater than 10/10 high power fields. The tumour cells were uniform with a moderate nuclear/cytoplasmic ratio and a fine-to-slight coarse nuclear chromatin. Faint nucleoli were seen in two cases. Mitoses are absent or rare in typical carcinoids. Nuclear pleomorphism and hyperchromatism are usually absent in typical carcinoids but present in atypical. Regional lymph node metastases are seen in almost 50% of cases in atypical carcinoids but, as noted above, may be identified in 15% of typical carcinoids. In small bronchial biopsies, atypical carcinoids may be diagnosed as small cell carcinoma. This is due to sampling, but could result in inappropriate chemotherapy. Since the numbers of atypical carcinoids treated with chemotherapy are relatively small,

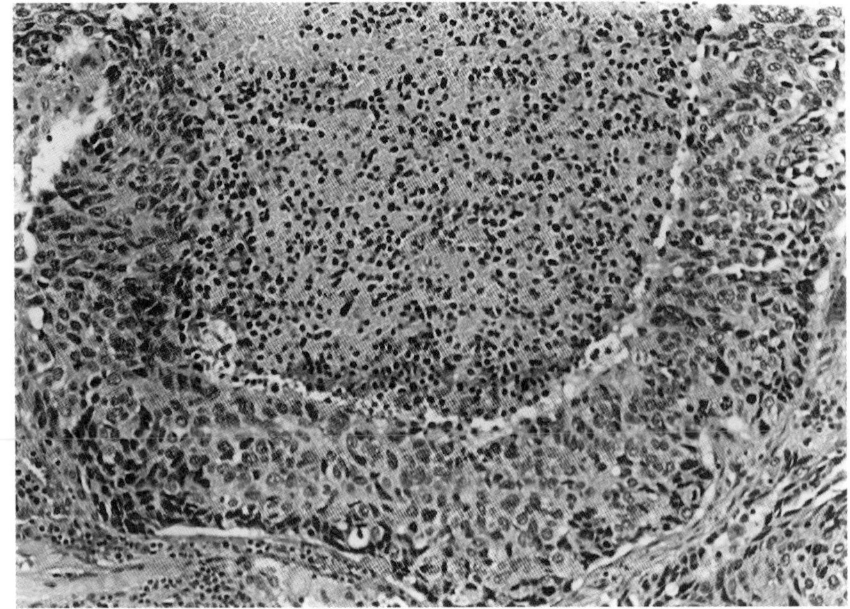

Fig. 4 Large cell neuroendocrine carcinoma with a large area of necrosis and a tendency to peripheral pallisading. Stain: haematoxylin and eosin, × 125.

no rational chemotherapeutic regime has been identified for this tumour. At the moment surgery appears the treatment of choice.

Large cell neuroendocrine carcinoma

Large cell neuroendocrine carcinoma has only recently been identified and is a high grade tumour[20,24] 97% of these patients smoked. The 5 year survival is 34%, a figure not significantly different from small cell carcinoma. The patients were generally older than those with typical and atypical carcinoids (mean age 60 years). None of the patients in the series of Travis et al[20] had any endocrine manifestations. 57% of large cell neuroendocrine tumours were stages I and II in the 49 cases collected by Travis et al.[7]

The tumours averaged 3.2 cm in diameter, were tan, firm circumscribed masses with foci of haemorrhage and necrosis. Histologically, there were organoid, trabecular and pallisaded patterns. Necrosis was prominent (Fig. 4), sometimes with large infarct-like areas.

The tumour cells are large and polygonal rather than fusiform, with a low nuclear/cytoplasmic ratio and a high mitotic rate. The mitotic count was high, averaging 66 per 10 high power fields in the series of Travis et al,[20] but sometimes exceeded 100. The nuclear chromatin is coarsely granular and nucleoli may be prominent. There is peripheral pallisading and varying degrees of necrosis. DNA encrustation of vessel walls may be present. Immunohistochemistry is little help in differentiating large cell neuroendocrine carcinoma from either atypical carcinoid or non-small cell carcinoma with neuroendocrine features.

Small cell carcinoma will not be considered in this chapter. It usually provides little diagnostic difficulty for most histopathologists. In recent

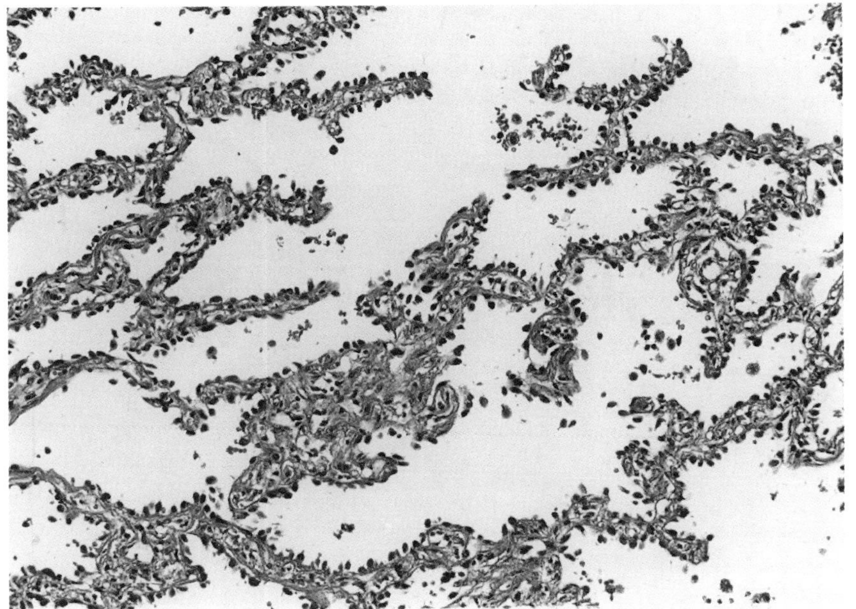

Fig. 5 Atypical adenomatous hyperplasia with a slightly thickened alveolar wall, lined by small hyperchromatic peg-shaped cells. There was an adenocarcinoma in another lobe. Stain: haematoxylin and eosin, × 125.

Medical Research Council trials only 5% of cases of small cell carcinoma were misdiagnosed.

Atypical adenomatous hyperplasia

This condition was first described by the late Roberta Miller in 1990.[25] Since then, it has been designated various names including bronchioloalveolar cell adenoma, atypical adenomatous hyperplasia (AAH), atypical alveolar cell hyperplasia and atypical broncho-alveolar cell hyperplasia. None of these names is ideal and the original name coined by Miller of bronchioloalveolar cell adenoma is likely to cause confusion with an alveolar adenoma, which is a benign multicystic neoplasm that recapitulates both alveolar epithelium and mesenchyme. Alveolar adenoma is usually a solitary, multicystic, circumscribed nodule, 1--2 cm in diameter. The cysts are separated by delicate stroma lined by flattened cells. The term adenoma could cause confusion with mucinous cystadenoma or other true bronchial mucus gland adenomas. Pulmonary pathologists have wrestled with this problem, but the term atypical adenomatous hyperplasia (AAH) is at the moment preferred.

AAH are usually found incidentally in up to 10% of surgically resected lungs, removed for lung cancer. The lesions are usually found in patients with adenocarcinoma, especially bronchioloalveolar carcinoma. However, in one recent study,[26] AAH co-existed with squamous carcinoma of the lung, metastatic colonic and renal cell adenocarcinomas. In this series, when smoking history was available, 14/20 were non-smokers.

AAH has been defined[25] as a small lesion, usually 5 mm or less. Any bronchioloalveolar cell tumour larger than 5 mm and showing marked nuclear

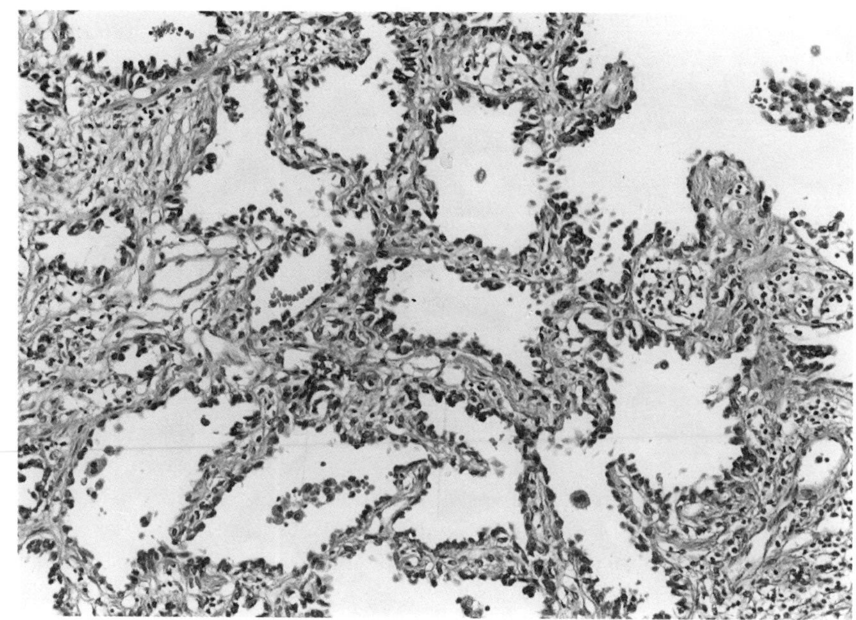

Fig. 6 Bronchioloalveolar carcinoma with a thickened alveolar wall and lined by hyperchromatic epithelial cells. Morphologically the cells are similar to those seen in AAH, but the lesion here was several cm in diameter. Apart from the size of the tumour and the slightly higher cell density, this lesion is similar to that in Figure 5. Stain: haematoxylin and eosin, × 125.

atypia should probably be classified as bronchioloalveolar carcinoma.[27] However, unless other techniques (*vide infra*) are used, it may be difficult histologically to distinguish a bronchoalveolar carcinoma from AAH.

Histologically, there is a uniform proliferation of cuboidal, low columnar or pyramidal epithelial cells, which grow along the alveolar septa. The septa are thickened by varying degrees (Fig. 5). Characteristically, there are no admixed, ciliated or mucus-secreting cells. The lesions have been divided into low- and high-grade AAH.[26] In low grade AAH, the cell density is low and they are arranged in a single layer, either intermittently or continuously on the alvoelar septa. There are minimal variations in size, shape and hyperchromatism in the small nuclei. In high grade AAH, the cell density is increased, with larger nuclei, showing increased variation in size, shape and nuclear hyperchromatism. It is difficult to distinguish this lesion from early bronchioloalveolar carcinoma (BAC). These authors thought that BAC exhibited more nuclear atypia, hyperchromatism and a higher cell density (Fig. 6).

To clarify this problem, Kitamura et al studied nuclear area and p53 and carcinoembryonic antigen (CEA) expression.[26] The mean nuclear areas increased from low grade AAH (32.44 μm^2) through high grade (45.85 μm^2) to early BAC (52.10 μm^2) and overt BAC (56.60 μm^2). The only significant differences were in the values for mean nuclear areas between low grade AAH and the other three categories and high grade AAH and early BAC. 95% of low grade AAH were negative for p53, the corresponding figure was 31% in overt BAC.[26] Kerr et al[28] found higher values, with 58% of cases of AAH positive for this antibody.

As stated above, any tumour above 5 mm, showing marked nuclear atypia is best classed as bronchioloalveolar carcinoma. The cut-off value of 40 μm for mean nuclear area distinguished effectively between low and high grade AAH.

The prognostic significance of AAH was addressed by the Vancouver group.[29] They studied 37 lungs, distended and fixed with Bouin's fixative. Specimens were sectioned at 1–1.5 cm intervals to correspond with the plane of section of the CT scan. Pre-operative chest radiographs and CT of the thorax, when available, were reviewed retrospectively by two radiologists to evaluate the sensitivity of those modalities in detecting co-existing small nodules and bronchogenic carcinoma. Patients were followed up for at least 18 months postsurgery. Patients were also included that had died within this period. 50% of the patients in this study had bronchioloalveolar carcinoma. 11/24 available scans showed one or more nodules ranging from 4–10 mm in diameter in the same lobe as the carcinoma (n = 3), in a lobe remote from the primary carcinoma (n = 3) or in the same lobe containing the carcinoma plus lobe remote from it (n = 5). AAH was retrospectively detected in more than 46% of patients in whom they were detected pathologically. There was no significant difference in the age, follow-up interval or survival rate for the 13 patients with no radiological detectable nodules pre-operatively as against those with nodules detected on their CT scan.

This good prognosis of some BAC has been recently highlighted.[30] These authors described five types of pulmonary adenocarcinoma. The localised BAC was distinguishable from AAH by increased cellularity, cell atypia and a size greater than 1 cm in greatest dimension. However, they retained alveolar structures. Fibrotic foci in the tumours were absent. It was considered an *in situ* peripheral adenocarcinoma and had 100% 5-year survival, similar to AAH.

Mesothelioma

A recent update on the pathology of malignant mesothelioma has been published.[31] Stains commonly used to differentiate adenocarcinoma from epithelial mesothelioma are diastase/PAS, which are positive in adenocarcinoma but negative in **most** cases of mesothelioma. In epithelial mesotheliomas, of the antibodies – CAM 5.2, AE1/3, CK5/6, CEA (carcinoembryonic antigen), Leu M1, B72.3 and Ber EP4 – the last four are negative, whereas CAM 5.2, CK5/6 and AE1/3 are usually positive.

Newer antibodies include calretinin, a calcium-binding protein of 29 kDa, a member of a large family of EF-hand proteins, to which S100 protein belongs. Two different polyclonal antisera to calretinin consistently immunostained mesothelial cells and malignant epithelial mesothelioma in paraffin embedded tissue sections as well as in cytology proliferations. Only one sarcomatoid mesothelioma was studied and showed moderate immunoreactivity. Squamous cell carcinoma of lung and head and neck may be positive, but these tumours will usually cause little diagnostic difficulty.[32] E- and N-cadhedrin may distinguish pleural mesotheliomas from pulmonary adenocarcinomas.[33]

Finally, a fascinating piece of work regarding possible aetiology has come from the Penarth group.[34] DNA sequences and immunoreactivity associated with Simian virus 40 transforming factors, LT antigens (SV40LTAg) have been identified in fresh frozen tissue in a high proportion of recent cases of pleural mesothelioma from the US, Italy and Germany.[35,36] SV 40 is not normally infective in man but it is known to transform human cells and tissue culture. A large cohort of Western people were accidently inoculated parenterly, through polio vaccine contaminated with live SV, given between 1959 and 1961. This study from Cardiff detected SV40LTAg-DNA in both recently diagnosed and in archival tissue from British mesotheliomas in the perivaccination period. Thus, apart from asbestos as the commonest cause of mesothelioma, a possible viral factor has to be added to the aetiological table. This could be another reason for the current continuing rise in the incidence of mesothelioma in Britain.[37]

ADDENDUM

A recent study[38] of Simian virus 40 and pleural mesothelioma in humans did not show an association between SV40 and mesothelioma. The findings, these authors felt, called into question an association with this virus.

REFERENCES

1. Sundaresan V, Rabbitts PH. Genetics of lung tumours. In: Hasleton PS, ed Spencer's Pathology of the Lung, 5th Edn. New York: McGraw Hill, 1996
2. Travis WD, Lubin J, Reis L, Devesa S. United States lung carcinoma incidence trends: declining for most histologic types among males, increasing among females. Cancer 1996; 77: 2464–2470
3. Edinburgh Lung Group. Patients presenting with lung cancer in South East Scotland. Thorax 1987; 42: 853–857
4. Armas OA, White DA, Erlandson RA, Rosai J. Diffuse idiopathic pulmonary neuroendocrine cell proliferation presenting as interstitial lung disease. Am J Surg Pathol 1995; 19: 963–970
5. Miller RR, Muller NL. Neuroendocrine cell hyperplasia and obliterative bronchiolitis in patients with peripheral carcinoid tumours. Am J Surg Pathol 1995; 19: 653–658
6. Bostanci AG, Hasleton PS. Neuroendocrine cell population in bronchial resection margins from different lung tumours [Abstract]. J Pathol 1997; 181 (Suppl): 30A
7. Travis WD, Hasleton PS, Brambilla E et al. IASLC Panel. Neuroendocrine (NE) tumors of the lung: prognostic factors in 152 cases. Abstract IASLC meeting, Dublin, August 1997
8. McCaughan BC, Martini N, Baines MS. Bronchial carcinoids: review of 124 cases. J Thorac Cardiovasc Surg 1985; 89: 8–17
9. Dail DH, Hammar SP. eds Pulmonary Pathology, 2nd Edn. New York: Springer-Verlag, 1994; 1214–1221
10. Hasleton PS. In: Hasleton PS, ed Spencer's Pathology of the Lung, 5th Edn. New York: McGraw Hill, 1996; 896-911
11. Al-Saffar N, Moore JV, Hasleton PS. A morphometric analysis of individual cell death in bronchial carcinoids. Cell Tissue Kinet 1990; 23: 325–330
12. Moore JV, Hasleton PS, Buckley CH. Tumour cords in 52 bronchial and cervical cell squamous cell carcinomas: inferences for their cellular kinetics and radiobiology. Br J Cancer 1985; 51: 407–413
13. Costes V, Marty-Ane C, Picot MC et al. Typical and atypical bronchopulmonary carcinoid tumours: a clinico-pathologic and Ki-67-labelling study. Hum Pathol 1995; 26: 740–745
14. Jones DJ, Hasleton PS, Moore M. DNA ploidy in bronchopulmonary carcinoid tumours. Thorax 1988; 43: 195–199
15. El-Naggar A, Balance W, Abdul-Karim F et al. Typical and atypical bronchopulmonary carcinoids: a clinicopathologic and flow cytometric study. Am J Clin Pathol 1991; 95: 828–834

16. Padberg B-C, Woenckhaus J, Hilger G et al. DNA cytophotometry and prognosis in typical and atypical bronchopulmonary carcinoids: a clinicomorphologic study of 100 neuroendocrine lung tumours. Am J Surg Pathol 1996; 20: 815–822
17. Hasleton PS, Al-Saffar N. The histological spectrum of bronchial carcinoid tumours. Appl Pathol 1989; 7: 205–218
18. Hasleton PS. Immunocytochemistry in the diagnosis of pulmonary carcinoid tumours. Cancer J 1996; 9: 177–178
19. Loy TS, Darkow GVD, Quesenberry JT. Immunostaining in the diagnosis of pulmonary neuroendocrine carcinomas: an immunocytochemical study with ultrastructural correlations. Am J Surg Pathol 1995; 19: 173–182
20. Travis WD, Linnoila RI, Tsokous MJ et al. Neuroendocrine tumors of the lung with proposed criteria for large cell neuroendocrine carcinoma: an ultrastructural, immunohistochemical and flow cytometric study of 35 cases. Am J Surg Pathol 1991; 15: 529–553
21. Arrigoni MG, Woolner LB, Bernatz PE. Atypical carcinoid tumors of the lung. J Thorac Cardiovasc Surg. 1972; 64: 413–421
22. Smolle-Juttner S-M, Popper H, Klemen H et al. Clinical features and therapy of 'typical' and 'atypical' bronchial carcinoid tumors (Grade I and II neuroendocrine carcinoma). Eur J Cardiothorac Surg 1993; 7: 121–125
23. Valli M, Fabris GA, Dewar A, Hornall D, Sheppard MN. Atypical carcinoid tumour of the lung: a study of 33 cases with prognostic features. Histopathology 1994; 24: 363–369
24. Hammond ME, Souse WT. Large cell neuroendocrine tumors of the lung: clinical significance and histopathologic definition. Cancer 1985; 56: 1624–1629
25. Miller RR. Bronchioloalveolar adenoma. Am J Surg Pathol 1990; 14: 904–912
26. Kitamura H, Kameda Y, Nakamura N et al. Atypical adenomatous hyperplasia and bronchoalveolar lung carcinoma: analysis by morphometry and the expressions of p53 and carcinoembryonic antigen. Am J Surg Pathol 1996; 20: 553–562
27. Miller RR, Nelem S, Evans KG, Muller LL, Ostrow DN. Glandular neoplasia of the lung: a proposed analogy of two colonic tumours. Cancer 1988; 61: 1009–1014
28. Kerr KM, Carey FA, King G, Lamb D. Atypical alveolar hyperplasia: relationship with pulmonary adenocarcinoma, p53 and *c-erb* B2 expression. J Pathol 1994; 174: 249–256
29. Logan PM, Miller RR, Evans K, Muller NL. Bronchogenic carcinoma and coexistent bronchioloalveolar cell adenomas: assessment of radiologic detection and follow-up in 28 patients. Chest 1996; 109: 713–717
30. Noguchi M, Morikawa A, Kawasaki M et al. Small adenocarcinoma of the lungs: histologic characteristics and prognosis. Cancer 1995; 75: 2844–2852
31. Hasleton PS, Hammar SP. Malignant mesothelioma. Curr Diag Pathol 1996; 3: 153–164
32. Doglioni C, Deitos AP, Laurino L et al. Calretinin: a novel immunocytochemical marker for mesothelioma. Am J Surg Pathol 1996; 20: 1037–1046
33. Peraltasoler A, Knusden KA, Jaurand M-C et al. The differential expression of N-cadherin and E-cadherin distinguishes pleural mesothelioma from lung adenocarcinomas. Hum Pathol 1995; 26: 1363–1369
34. Pepper C, Jasani B, Navabi H, Wynford-Thomas D, Gibbs AR. Simian virus 40 large T antigen (SV40 LT Ag) primer specific DNA amplification in human pleural mesothelioma tissue. Thorax 1996; 51: 1074–1076
35. Carbone M, Pass H, Rizzo P et al. Simian virus 40-like DNA sequences in human pleural mesothelioma. Oncogene 1994; 9: 1781–1790
36. Cicala C, Pompetti F, Carbone M. SV 40 induces mesotheliomas in hamsters. Am J Pathol 1993; 142: 1524–1533
37. Peto J, Hodgson JT, Matthews PE, Jones JR. Continuing increase in mesothelioma mortality in Britain. Lancet 1995; 345: 535–539
38. Strickler HD, Goedert JJ, Fleming M et al.Simian virus 40 and pleural mesothelioma in humans. Cancer Epidemiology, Biomakers and Prevention. 1996; 5: 473–475.

9

Epithelial lesions of the endocervix

Terence P. Rollason

This chapter selectively covers recent changes in opinion on lesions of the endocervical epithelium, both neoplastic and non-neoplastic. The non-neoplastic conditions described are significant because of their potential either to confuse the diagnosis of other clinically important lesions or because they may be misdiagnosed as malignant tumours.

NON-NEOPLASTIC LESIONS

Unusually deep crypts and cysts

The 'normal' maximum crypt depth is generally stated to be 5–7 mm but cystic crypts up to 9 mm deep are, in fact, not rare. Recently, it has been recognised that simple, cystic endocervical crypts may be present throughout the endocervical stroma[1,2] leading to possible misdiagnosis as minimal deviation adenocarcinoma of the cervix (MDA, adenoma malignum). In most cases, such deep crypts are clearly lined by benign endocervical cells without mitotic activity. No stromal reaction is seen and the crypts do not have the branching, complex pattern of the glands in MDA. Occasionally, however, the crypts are small and round or oval with some crowding, causing more serious diagnostic difficulty.[2] The lack of pleomorphism and stromal reaction are most important in correct diagnosis. In this diffuse, non-cystic type, typically, no CEA reactivity is seen. CEA is typically present in MDA but staining may be variable and focal and normal epithelium may occasionally stain, limiting its usefulness in the individual case. Endocervical crypts, particularly when cystic, may be associated with mucin spillage and stromal reactive changes, including a foreign body giant cell or histiocytic reaction. Such changes, particularly when seen deep within the cervical wall, may cause diagnostic difficulties if this occurrence is not borne in mind.

Dr T.P. Rollason, Department of Pathology, Birmingham Women's Hospital, Edgbaston, Birmingham B15 2TJ, UK

Atypical forms of microglandular endocervical hyperplasia (MEH)

MEH is a very common finding in normal cervices, being present in perhaps a quarter. It is associated with progestogen therapy, including combined-type oral contraceptive pill usage, and may be particularly florid in pregnancy, but is often seen with no stimulating cause. Occasionally, MEH may produce a polypoid mass that clinically may be mistaken for carcinoma. The typical

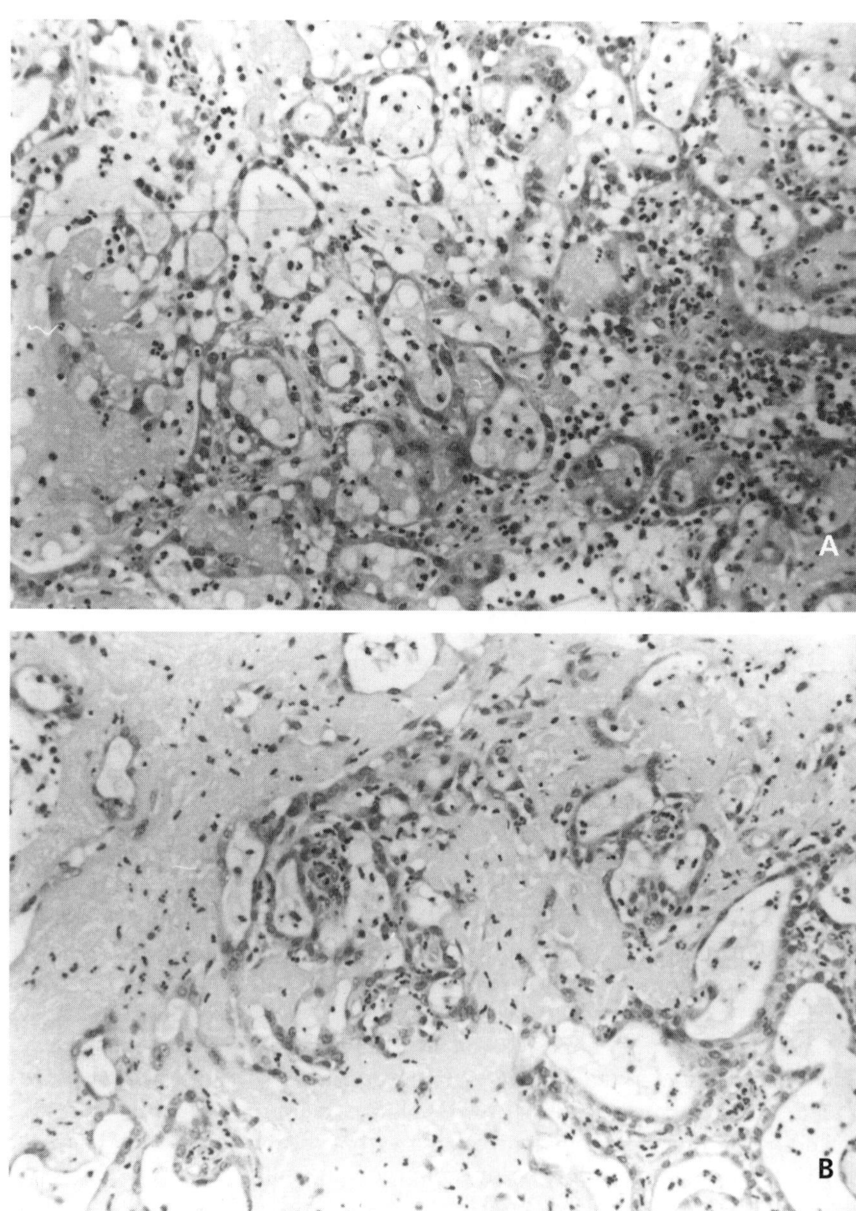

Fig. 1 (**A**) Atypical microglandular endocervical hyperplasia. Closely packed glands are seen with vacuolated cytoplasm and some nuclear pleomorphism. There is an acute inflammatory cell infiltrate present. (**B**) This field from the same case as (A) shows a pseudoinfiltrative pattern related to stromal hyalinization.

appearances of MEH, with closely packed glands lined by vacuolated cells, often with an acute inflammatory cell infiltrate, must be familiar to all pathologists, but it is not generally recognised that atypical forms of MEH may lead to considerable difficulties in differential diagnosis, in particular from clear cell carcinoma. The reasons for this difficulty are that MEH may show extensive hyalinization of the stroma, producing a 'pseudoinfiltrative' pattern (Fig. 1A,B); it may also show solid sheets of cells and cells with abundant eosinophilic cytoplasm or even hobnail cells, all features that may be present in clear cell carcinomas.[3] Signet ring cells also may occur adding to the difficulties in differentiation from adenocarcinoma. The degree of nuclear atypia and higher mitotic rate in clear cell carcinoma, together with the absence of intracellular mucin and presence of glycogen, help in differential diagnosis, but the differentiation may be extremely difficult. Lack of CEA staining in MEH may be useful in some cases[4,5] but the literature on this is confusing with some authors suggesting clear cell carcinomas are also commonly negative.[5] MIB1 staining has recently been suggested as useful in differentiation of MEH and endocervical adenocarcinoma and may be of help in this type of case.[6]

It should also be borne in mind that some adenocarcinomas can mimic, at least focally, the appearances of MEH.[7] For this reason, MEH should be diagnosed with circumspection in the postmenopausal woman though the use of hormone replacement therapy has made its occurrence in this age group not unusual. It has been known for some years that MEH may lead to problems in cytological diagnosis due to overcalling the MEH-derived cells as atypical endocervical cells. Recently, it has been shown that it may also result in overcall of squamous intra-epithelial neoplasia.[8]

Mesonephric hyperplasia

Mesonephric remnants are common in the cervix, being present in at least 10% of cervices and typically found laterally. Hyperplastic forms of such remnants are also quite common and have recently been divided into lobular, diffuse and pure ductal types.[10] The commonest type is a proliferation of small acini in poorly defined lobular aggregates surrounding the main duct or proliferated ducts (Fig. 2). Such acini are lined by cuboidal, regular cells and contain a dense central eosinophilic secretion which is weakly PAS positive and diastase resistant. The site, overall pattern and lack of pleomorphism are usually so typical that diagnosis is simple. Occasionally, however, the degree of proliferation may suggest mesonephric adenocarcinoma. This is a very rare tumour and is usually associated with hyperplasia. It shows destructive and extensive invasion, often with a clear stromal reaction. Mitoses may be frequent and pleomorphism evident, but these features are not always seen.[9]

Mesonephric hyperplasia may extend close to the endocervical surface and this is seen particularly after previous conization, diathermy loop excision of the transformation zone or laser destruction. The intermingling of the hyperplastic mesonephric glands with the endocervical crypts may lead to overdiagnosis as cervical intra-epithelial glandular neoplasia (CIGN) unless care is taken to assess the nuclear characteristics. CIN may also extend into mesonephric remnants leading to potential overdiagnosis as invasive squamous carcinoma due to their

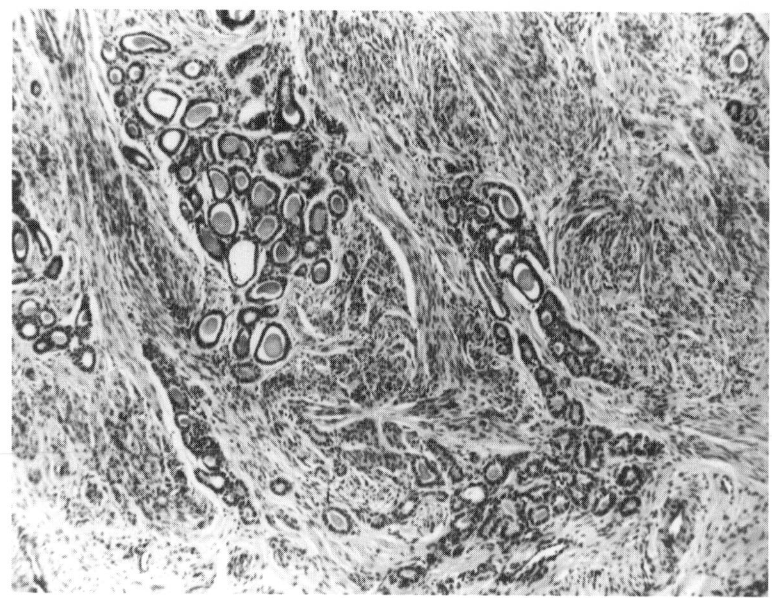

Fig. 2 Simple mesonephric duct hyperplasia. The proliferated ducts have a lobular pattern and show eosinophilic central secretion. No nuclear pleomorphism is evident.

deep site and varied architecture.[11] Confusion of mesonephric remnants with MDA and clear cell carcinoma may be avoided by attention to the columnar cell lining of the irregular branched glands in MDA and to the conspicuous clear cytoplasm, nuclear atypia and hobnail cells of clear cell carcinoma. Metastatic carcinomas to the cervix may also produce confusion, perhaps breast carcinoma metastases would be the likeliest to cause difficulty but, in the author's experience, breast carcinoma deposits usually show the typical diffusely infiltrative pattern seen in the primary tumour and the major problem is in overlooking the pale tumour cells on low power observation and disregarding them as a simple stromal hypercellularity.

Tubal and endometrial (endometrioid) metaplasia and endometriosis

Pure endometrial metaplasia of the endocervical epithelium is rare; in most cases the epithelium shows either pure tubal metaplasia (columnar ciliated, non-ciliated and peg cells) or admixed tubal and endometrial-type epithelium, hence the use of the term tubo-endometrial (or tubo-endometrioid) metaplasia. This change is common and is closely associated with previous cervical trauma, usually cone biopsy, loop excision or similar procedure. It is seen most commonly in the deeper crypts of the endocervix but not infrequently occurs in the surface epithelium or superficial crypts.[12,13]

Tubo-endometrial metaplasia may cause considerable diagnostic confusion with CIGN in cervical smears[14] and difficulties in histological differentiation from CIGN may also occur, particularly if there is co-existent reactive change related to inflammation or regeneration. The lack of significant pleomorphism, mixture of cell types, lack of mitotic activity and lack of stromal response are normally sufficient to allow histological differentiation. Some atypical cases of tubo-endometrial metaplasia may show deep involvement of the cervical wall, glandular crowding and stromal hypercellularity, suggesting malignancy.[15] In such cases, lack of diffuse cytoplasmic CEA immunoreactivity, low levels of Ki-67 and MIB1 staining,[16] amylase reactivity and lack of diffuse staining with HMFG1 and similar antibodies[17,18] may help in differentiation. AgNOR counts have also been suggested as helpful (*vide infra*).

Cervical endometriosis may be divided into two types – superficial and deep. Deep endometriosis is usually seen on the deep margin of the cervix, particularly posteriorly, and is associated with endometriosis elsewhere in the pelvis. Superficial endometriosis is most commonly seen at or near the squamo-columnar junction and has clear similarities to tubo-endometrial metaplasia, being closely and commonly associated with previous trauma.[12] It may be confused with glandular neoplasia, particularly in cases where proliferative or even hyperplastic changes are evident, related to hormonal state.

Other hyperplasias and metaplasias

Tunnel clusters

These are a very common finding, seen in perhaps 10% of normal cervices, and appear particularly common during and after pregnancy. They consist of well demarcated, usually rounded or lobulated, aggregates of either small (Type A) or cystic (Type B) tubular glands with inspissated mucin and pale cytoplasm. Mild nuclear atypia and occasional mitoses may be seen. The posterior lip appears to be the commoner site of occurrence and some distortion of the cervix may occur as the clusters may be multiple. The important differential diagnosis is MDA but the often superficial site of the clusters, lobularity, lack of atypia and lack of stromal response usually serves to differentiate the two conditions. The cystic variant of tunnel clusters particularly may be seen deep in the cervical wall and morphological overlap with mucus retention cysts (deep Nabothian follicles) is obvious. On rare occasions, Type A tunnel clusters show florid overgrowth and irregular borders to the aggregates may suggest invasion. The changes may be associated with nuclear atypia, cellular crowding and nuclear pseudostratification occasionally causing considerable diagnostic problems.[19] Mitotic activity in such atypical cases is usually absent, however, and they appear to behave in a benign fashion.

Diffuse laminar endocervical hyperplasia

In some cervices there appears to be a diffuse overgrowth of simple endocervical crypts with a clear demarcation from the deep cervical stroma;[20] this condition may be associated with non-specific inflammatory changes but does not appear to be associated with CIGN or invasive carcinoma. Only one case appears to have been associated with clinical symptoms[21] and the specificity of the diagnosis must at this stage be in some doubt, as overlap is evident with other types of non-specific simple overgrowth of endocervical crypts. Such examples of 'non specific simple glandular hyperplasia' may cause considerable diagnostic problems, particularly when the crypts are branched and crowded or when the hyperplasia is complicated by the co-existence of reserve cell hyperplasia or tubo-endometrial metaplasia.

Changes secondary to viral infections

Multinucleate endocervical cells are seen quite commonly in loop excision specimens and it has been suggested that human papillomavirus (HPV) or herpes virus infection may be their cause. This is still unproven. Epstein-Barr virus may be detected in the cervix and has been suggested in the past as a possible cause of cervical cancer; whilst recently overshadowed by HPV as a potential causative agent, the occasional co-existence of nasopharyngeal carcinoma in some patients with cervical cancer is of particular interest.[22]

Herpes simplex virus infection is common in the lower genital tract and must be considerably underdiagnosed histologically. The ground glass intranuclear inclusions are characteristic in the squamous epithelium but inflammation and reactive changes can also be severe and cause difficulties in diagnosis in the adjacent endocervix.

Cytomegalovirus produces classical basophilic 'owl's eye' inclusions in the endocervical epithelium and occasionally in endothelial cells. These cells may be stained by immunohistochemical agents against CMV but their isolation within an otherwise normal epithelium usually allows easy diagnosis.

Arias-Stella reaction

Most pathologists are aware of the common occurrence of decidualization of the cervix in pregnancy and occasionally in the non-gravid patient, particularly with exogenous progestogen usage, and recognise the risks both colposcopically and histologically of overdiagnosing squamous carcinoma in such cases. The fact that the Arias-Stella reaction may be seen, not only in cervical endometriosis but in normal endocervical epithelium, is often not realised. This occurs in approximately 10% of cervices during pregnancy[23] but is usually very focal. The appearances are similar to those in endometrial glands, with enlarged, pleomorphic nuclei, abundant, pale, vacuolated cytoplasm and a 'hobnail' appearance to the cells with displacement of the nuclei towards the lumen. Mitoses are uncommon. The changes may be misinterpreted as CIGN or clear cell carcinoma but the focal nature of the changes and close attention to cellular detail are the keys to diagnosis, together with the clinical history. Arias-Stella reaction may also involve endocervical polyps.

Goblet cell (intestinal) metaplasia

Goblet cells of hindgut type with or without associated argentaffin cells are a rare finding in the cervix except as a differentiation pattern in CIGN, when they are common (Type II CIGN), or in occasional adenocarcinomas.[24] For this reason the diagnosis of simple intestinal metaplasia should only be made after careful exclusion of CIGN, particularly as goblet cells in CIGN may appear deceptively benign.

'Unusual endocervical lesions with endocrine cells'

Recently a small series of cases of a proliferation of 'hypermucinous' endocervical glands with abnormal branched glandular architecture and proliferated smooth muscle has been described.[25] The lesions also showed numerous neuroendocrine cells. Whilst showing some similarity to MDA, they were non-infiltrative, small and well localized. The nature of these lesions is, as yet, uncertain.

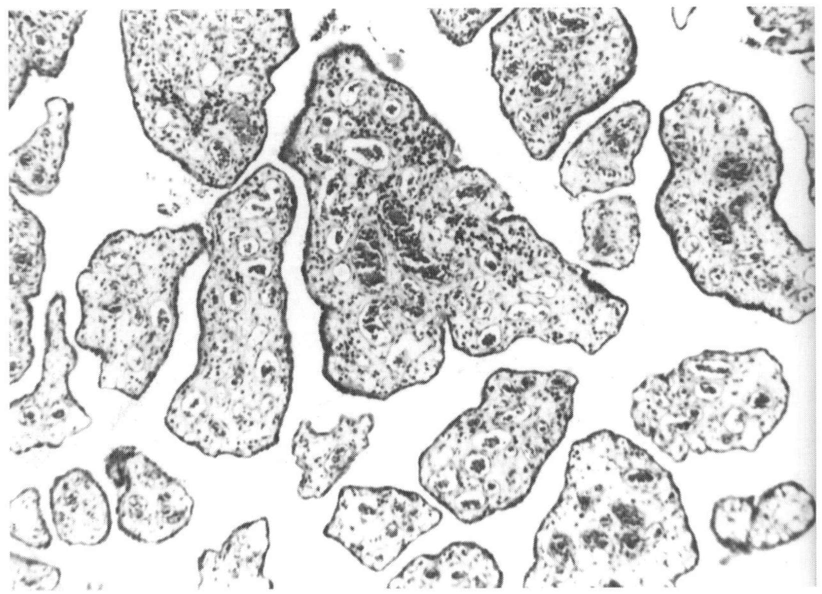

Fig. 3 Benign Müllerian papilloma. The papillae are of varying size and covered by cuboidal cells. The cores of the papillae are vascular but not highly cellular.

BENIGN ENDOCERVICAL TUMOURS

Müllerian (mesonephric) papilloma

This rare, benign tumour was originally thought to be of mesonephric origin but is now generally felt to be Müllerian in derivation. Although composed of glandular epithelium it usually presents on the ectocervix.[26] Classically, it occurs in children between the ages of 2 and 5 years and presents with vaginal bleeding or discharge. No clear association with DES or other exposure to hormones *in utero* has been reported but the author has recently seen a case occurring in a child exposed to maternal Tamoxifen in pregnancy.

The tumour is typically small (up to 2.0 cm diameter) and papillary. Histologically, it shows fine branching papillae covered by benign looking cuboidal to columnar cells (Fig. 3), sometimes with foci of squamous epithelium seen. The cores of the papillae tend to be oedematous and contain inflammatory cells. None of these tumours appear to have behaved in a malignant fashion.

Villous, tubulovillous and villoglandular adenomas

These rare lesions have an architecture similar to villoglandular papillary adenocarcinoma of the cervix (*vide infra*) but consist of uniformly benign cells.[27,28] Some of them may be associated with underlying invasive carcinoma, however, and the differentiation from invasive true villoglandular carcinoma in such cases appears arbitrary. Villous and tubulovillous adenomas have also been described showing enteric rather than endocervical Müllerian differentiation and again associated underlying adenocarcinomas may be present.[29,30]

IN SITU GLANDULAR NEOPLASIA

The past decade has seen a marked increase in interest in *in situ* glandular neoplasia of the cervix (CIGN, CGIN, glandular atypia, adenocarcinoma-in-situ). Whilst early attempts were made to divide such pre-invasive endocervical lesions into three grades in line with CIN, this is very difficult to do with any consistency and probably the best that can be achieved is to divide the cases into low and high grade, with high grade being essentially synonymous with adenocarcinoma-in-situ (AIS).

Pre invasive glandular lesions of low grade appear, despite some early suggestions that they might be common,[31] to be diagnosed less frequently by most pathologists than high grade and considerable debate continues on their clinical significance. Some studies suggest that they occur perhaps 5 years earlier than high grade lesions, suggesting progression over time, and some immunohistochemical studies, notably using markers for HMFG-1 and amylase, tend to support a continuum from low to high grade disease. Others hold that low grade cervical intra-epithelial glandular neoplasia (CIGN) should be separated from adenocarcinoma-in-situ and termed endocervical glandular dysplasia (EGD) to stress the lack of evidence of progression to adenocarcinoma[32] and some recent work suggests that the two diseases are unrelated topographically and morphologically and that only AIS has clear clinical relevance.[33]

The line separating low grade CIGN from high is subjective, as is that separating low grade from simple reactive hyperchromasia. Jaworski has suggested that for the diagnosis of EGD (low grade CIGN) the minimum requirements should be nuclear atypia and evidence of increased cell turnover, specifically apoptotic bodies and mitotic figures. Brown and Wells put emphasis on a spectrum of changes from minimal abnormalities to changes similar to, but less severe than, high grade CIGN, including nuclear enlargement, elongation and stratification limited to the lower two-thirds of the epithelial height, hyperchromasia and abnormal glandular profiles with decreased epithelial mucin.

High grade CIGN, in contrast to low grade, appears to be a robust diagnosis, though it is still underdiagnosed because of its often very focal nature. Studies utilizing retrospective review of biopsies and smears, together with evidence from the site of occurrence, continuity with invasive tumours, etc, provide strong evidence for high grade CIGN being the precursor lesion of invasive adenocarcinoma. The fact, however, that high grade CIGN has been diagnosed considerably less frequently than invasive adenocarcinoma in several centres where relative frequencies have been studied, suggests either that it has usually progressed to invasion before detection and is cytologically often missed or that it is not the precursor in a significant proportion of cases. Data on sensitivity of cytological diagnosis are highly conflicting with some claiming almost 100% success, but 50–60% is probably a more realistic figure (for review, see Young et al[33]). The lack of specific colposcopic appearances to allow biopsy diagnosis may also have played a part in underdiagnosis of

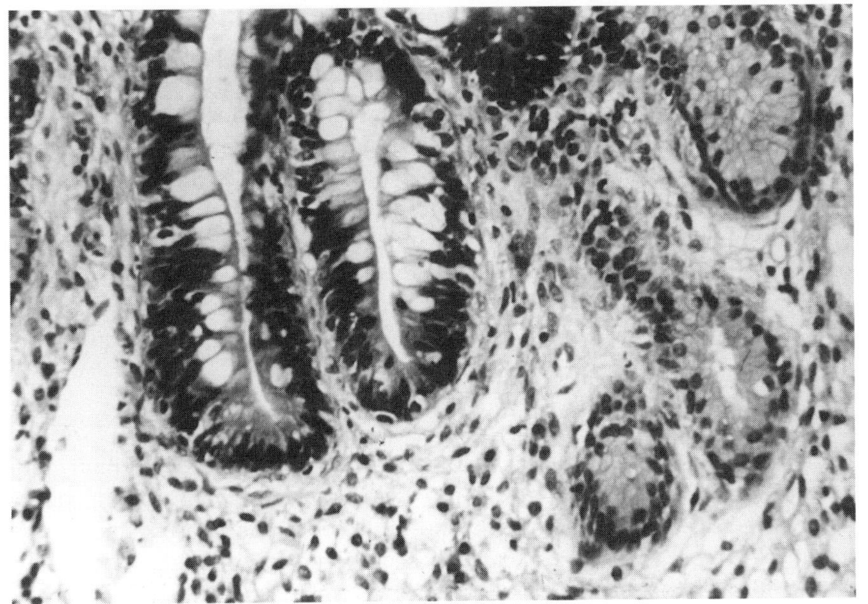

Fig. 4 Intestinal-type, high grade cervical intra-epithelial glandular neoplasia. The two larger crypts to the left of the field show goblet cells with nuclear hyperchromasia and enlargement evident.

CIGN prior to the widespread introduction of loop excision and previous studies on incidence are now likely to be outdated.

Whilst some studies suggest that low grade CIGN may be randomly distributed in the cervix, almost all agree that high grade typically occurs at or near the SCJ, with extension into the canal from this site, rather than by multifocal disease developing unconnected with the transformation zone.[33] 'Skip lesions' high in the canal probably occur in less than 10% of cases. Mean extension along the canal has been documented at 7.0 mm but a wide range is seen up to around 3.0 cm and the disease may vary from a single crypt to the majority of the crypt field. Usually both surface epithelium and crypts are involved. It appears uncommon for deep crypts to be involved in the absence of superficial.[34] Typically, a sharp demarcation is seen between normal crypt epithelium and high grade CIGN with no transitional zone of low grade disease. Perhaps 15% of cases are truly multifocal. Even disease confined to an endocervical polyp has been described on a few occasions.[35] CIN is very commonly seen in association with high grade CIGN (approximately 50% of cases); on what evidence exists its presence does not appear to affect the outcome of the disease.[36] Such co-existence argues for a common cell of origin, purportedly the subcolumnar reserve cell, and possibly a common aetiology.

The areas of crypt involvement by high grade CIGN are usually evident on low power microscopic examination because of the intense hyperchromasia of the epithelium; this is due to nuclear hyperchromasia, enlargement and atypia, which are usually prominent. Mitoses are often frequent and apoptosis common. A range of types of adenocarcinoma-in-situ have been described. The commonest is the endocervical cell type with mucin in the supranuclear cytoplasm, though this can be very difficult to differentiate from the endometrioid type as mucin reduction is a typical feature of CIGN. The second commonest type is the intestinal pattern with prominent goblet cells (Fig. 4) but this is almost always seen in association with the endocervical cell type, as is the endometrioid.[34] Rarer variants include adenosquamous,[35] signet ring, glassy cell, serous papillary and clear cell.[33] Of these the adenosquamous type is the least rare but should only be diagnosed in a multilayered CIN-like epithelium with extensive intracellular mucin secretion, to avoid misdiagnosis of CIN with simple mucin uptake from the crypt lumen.

Argyrophilic cells are common in intestinal and endocervical-type CIGN.[36] Differential diagnosis in CIGN is discussed under tumour-like conditions.

Therapy in CIGN

Until relatively recently the only therapy recommended for CIGN of high grade was hysterectomy. Over the past 5–10 years, more conservative treatment has become increasingly common with cold knife conization to a minimum canal length of 2.5 cm being recommended, based upon the morphological studies of CIGN alluded to earlier. Some workers now perform loop excision of the transformation zone. If the resection margins are clear, cytological follow-up by combined endocervical brush and spatula sampling is then recommended.[37] Results, in general, with these conservative techniques appear encouraging,[37,38] but further long-term studies are needed as the literature is still confused. One recent paper[39] has shown a 33% risk of residual high grade CIGN in repeat conization or hysterectomy specimens with **negative** original cone margins. This study is atypical, however, as some others have shown no invasive adenocarcinomas on follow-up for 3–5 years[37,38] and a less than 10% risk of residual high grade CIGN in repeat conization or hysterectomy specimens with previously clear margins. What does appear clear from most studies is that the major difficulty is not primary therapy but follow-up, as cytological surveillance, particularly after deep conization, is fraught with problems. It is also clear that if the conization specimen margins are involved then there is a high risk of finding residual high grade CIGN or invasive adenocarcinoma in a further specimen (40–70%). There is also early and unconfirmed evidence that loop excision may result in higher rates of disease recurrence than cold knife conization, even with negative margins.[40] No studies exist specifically dealing with therapy for low grade CIGN. In general, management at present is as for high grade disease.

EARLY INVASIVE ADENOCARCINOMA

There is, at present, no adequate definition of 'microinvasive' adenocarcinoma of the cervix, though the FIGO staging system for cervical carcinoma does not exclude adenocarcinoma specifically. The literature on outcome in early invasive adenocarcinoma is sparse and no consistent size and depth limits have been applied across series, some using 3, others 5, 2 or even 7 mm depth to define microinvasion. Most have used 5 mm (for review, see Young et al[33]). Tumour volume may be a better predictor of outcome, with 500 mm^3 being the cut off point for a group with very low risk of metastasis.[40,41] All of these studies, however, are small. On the available evidence, 2–3 mm would seem the likely maximum for an excellent prognosis group, if depth of invasion alone is the criterion used, but further data are needed.[42,43]

Most of the above studies fail to adequately address one major problem and that is the actual diagnosis of early invasion in the presence of high grade CIGN. The most common problem is that CIGN extends to involve the majority of the crypt field, with steadily increasing glandular complexity and crowding. It is then a highly subjective matter defining when early invasion is present. In such a case, even when early invasion can be confidently diagnosed, its specific point of origin may be impossible to define. One is then left with the problem that all that can be measured is really the full depth of the abnormal crypts from the surface epithelial base and as the 'normal' crypt depth may be 5–7 mm the 'microinvasive' limit may already be exceeded.

Despite the above problem there are a number of features which help in the differentiation of *in situ* from invasive adenocarcinoma at this site. The early invasive foci may be associated with an inflammatory and desmoplastic stromal response. The invasive glands may appear as small, irregular buds from a larger gland or solid cell nest and in some cases there may be distinct cytoplasmic eosinophilia in cells showing enlarged, rounded nuclei and prominent nucleoli, mimicking the pattern seen in squamous early stromal invasion.[44] Alternatively, the glands may become extremely crowded with cribriform foci seen and virtual or complete stromal exclusion between adjacent glands. Extension of glands beyond the limits of the normal crypt field is sometimes helpful, as is an abnormal relationship of glands to vessels, nerves etc. In perhaps 10–15% of cases of CIGN, major difficulty remains in confirming or excluding invasion.

There have been a number of studies attempting to apply special techniques to the differential diagnosis of *in situ* and invasive adenocarcinoma. AgNOR counts seem only of use in differentiating normal from neoplastic glands.[45] It has been claimed that laminin and type IV collagen staining is useful,[46] with basement membrane breaks being a specific feature of early invasion, but it is difficult to see why this should be the case as invasive tumours may produce new basement membranes and other studies fail to confirm its usefulness.[47]

INVASIVE ADENOCARCINOMA

The incidence of cervical adenocarcinoma appears to have increased over the past 20–30 years, perhaps from around 5 to around 15–20% of cervical carcinomas. Much of this increase may be due to the effect of screening on the incidence of invasive squamous carcinoma, together with changes in methods of early diagnosis and histological classification of adenocarcinoma. Considerable debate surrounds the question of how much, if any, of the increase is real. On balance, most opinion favours a real increase in incidence in women below 35–40 years of age,[48–50], though tumours in this age range are still uncommon.

The aetiological agents in adenocarcinoma are still ill-defined. HPV types 16 and 18 (particularly 18) appear implicated, but their prevalence in adenocarcinoma is less than in squamous.[51] Smoking also seems to increase risk and a role has been suggested for factors important in endometrial adenocarcinoma, in particular obesity, though less marked in the case of the cervix.[52] Associations with age at first intercourse and number of partners, particularly before the age of 20 years, exist. Earlier fears of a positive association with oral contraceptive usage have not been confirmed by some more recent studies,[53] but one supports an effect and shows a barrier contraceptive method to reduce incidence.[54]

There is still controversy over whether adenocarcinoma of the cervix has a poorer prognosis than squamous but the balance of opinion lies with adenocarcinoma being a more aggressive tumour,.[55] probably due in part to an increased risk of distant metastasis in large Stage IB tumours. Outcome does not appear to differ greatly in the common subtypes though endometrioid tumours may have a better prognosis than endocervical.

Considerable difficulty may be experienced in differentiating an endometrial from a cervical primary site of origin particularly in the case of endocervical and endometrioid types of carcinoma. Endometrial carcinomas may produce abundant mucin and may extend to produce *in situ* cervical adenocarcinoma, but the finding of co-existent complex hyperplasia in a curettage specimen of the endometrium is useful in differentiation as is very extensive cervical high grade CIGN. Squamous metaplasia tends to favour an endometrial primary tumour as does the presence of an endometrial-type tumour stroma and lipid laden stromal cells. CEA does not appear to be useful in the individual case but a recently described antibody, IC5, may be helpful,[56] as may some mucin-specific antigen stains,[57] but these findings are unconfirmed. A novel and particularly useful approach to the problem relates to the use of *in situ* hybridisation, or PCR, to detect HPV 16 or 18; positivity being taken as evidence in support of an endocervical primary site.[58] Caution is needed in interpretation of such results, however, as isthmic adenocarcinomas may contain HPV.

Histological typing

A classification of cervical adenocarcinoma and related tumours is given in the Table. This chapter will confine itself to those tumours where recent interest has focused or where new information is available, i.e. MDA, villoglandular carcinoma, adenosquamous carcinoma, adenoid cystic carcinoma and a few other recently described tumour variants.

Adenosquamous carcinoma

The frequency of diagnosis of adenosquamous carcinoma depends to a major extent on the criteria used for its diagnosis. If this term is applied to any cervical carcinoma with squamous differentiation and mucin production then perhaps 35% would be adenosquamous.[59] Many pathologists, however, require the presence also of unequivocal acinus formation and some demand tumour in which both glandular and squamous differentiation are clearly present in more than isolated foci. Certainly in cervical tumours adenosquamous carcinomas are usually dominated by the squamous component, though those with a balance of squamous and glandular or predominantly glandular

Table Classification of primary cervical glandular malignancy and related tumours

In situ		
	Low grade	
	High grade	Endocervical
		Endometrioid
		Intestinal (goblet cell)
		Adenosquamous (including glassy cell)
		Signet ring
		Serous
		Clear cell
Invasive		
	Adenocarcinoma	Endocervical
		Endometrioid
		Minimal deviation (including endometrioid and clear cell variant)
		Villoglandular (including endometrioid, endocervical and intestinal types)
		Clear cell
		Serous
		Mesonephric
		Non-Müllerian mucinous (intestinal and signet ring)
	Adenosquamous carcinoma (including glassy cell variant)	
	Adenoid basal carcinoma	
	Adenoid cystic carcinoma	

differentiation ('mucoepidermoid carcinoma') are by no means rare. It is very important not to mistakenly diagnose the aggressive small cell carcinoma of the cervix as adenosquamous; it commonly occurs in association with areas of adeno- or squamous carcinoma (50% or more of cases) but has a much poorer prognosis. The solid cell nests alongside adjacent glands may be mistaken for adenosquamous differentiation. Tumours in women below the age of 45 years appear to be more likely to produce mucin and some workers have shown an increased risk of nodal metastases in this subgroup; others, however, have been unable to confirm this finding.[60] It remains possible that adenosquamous carcinomas in younger women may contain or constitute a group of particularly aggressive tumours and some evidence exists that this group may show other poor prognostic markers,[61] but again this remains to be confirmed.

There is some evidence that HPV containing tumours are more likely to be mucin producing and that some oncogene products (e.g. C-erb B-2) may have more prognostic significance in adeno- than squamous carcinoma (*vide infra*).

So-called glassy cell carcinoma appears to be a very poorly differentiated variant of adenosquamous carcinoma composed of large polyhedral cells with ground glass cytoplasm, prominent nucleoli and well defined cell borders. Inflammatory cells tend to be numerous in the stroma leading to potential difficulties in differentiation from 'lymphoepithelioma-like carcinoma'. Occasional cases may show mucin droplets and/or squamous pearls. Outcome seems very similar to other very poorly differentiated adenosquamous carcinomas.

Minimal deviation adenocarcinoma (adenoma malignum)

Classically, MDA shows extremely well differentiated endocervical-type glands of irregular 'finger-in-glove' outline with only subtle differences in terms of nuclear pleomorphism to normal endocervical crypts. The key to the diagnosis is the abnormal glandular architecture on large biopsies, when the glandular outlines and deep infiltration of the tumour can be recognised and vessel invasion or a desmoplastic response may be seen focally. Increased mitoses are usually also seen compared to the very few seen in normal endocervical epithelium. A proportion of these tumours occur in association with Peutz-Jegher's syndrome.[62]

Diffuse cytoplasmic CEA staining has been suggested as a key feature in differentiating MDA from non-neoplastic endocervical conditions but such staining may be very focal and variable in intensity and thus of limited use in biopsy material, particularly as some normal glands may show staining.[63] The tumour also commonly shows argyrophil cells but these are also seen in other adenocarcinomas at this site. Immunoreactivity for transferrin receptor and HMFG 1, increased staining for neutral and sialomucins and inappropriate blood group antigen expression have also all been described. Recently, DNA cytometry on 3 cases suggested that the tumour has a hypodiploid stem cell population and is an aneuploid tumour.[64]).

The prognosis of adenoma malignum appears worse overall than adenocarcinoma generally (for review, see Young et al[65]). Around 50% of Stage I tumours appear to lead to death from disease. The spectrum of tumours placed in the MDA category has widened with endometrioid and clear cell types described, whose relationship to the more usual type is not clear;[66] some workers are also willing to include a tumour with small foci of otherwise unremarkable endocervical or endometrioid type adenocarcinoma in the MDA category. These varying diagnostic criteria probably account for the highly variable incidence rates quoted for MDA of 1–10% of cervical adenocarcinomas. An *in situ* phase in the development of MDA has been described. Even in the absence of Peutz-Jegher's syndrome associated ovarian tumours may be seen.[62,63]

Villoglandular adenocarcinoma

This recently described variant of adenocarcinoma appears to have a considerably better prognosis than adenocarcinoma overall[67] and to occur in a younger age group. The diagnosis should only be made in tumours exhibiting a papillary architecture with only mild cellular pleomorphism and with papillae covered by endometrioid, endocervical or intestinal-type cells, but not serous. The papillary cores are composed of normal cervical stroma and the infiltrating portion of the tumour underlying the exophytic papillary component is often inconspicuous and composed of irregular branching glands with little stromal desmoplastic response. Vessel invasion is rare. An inflammatory response to the tumour is common. Occasional cases do show deep stromal invasion and the prognosis in these is still not entirely clear.[65] In the larger published series to date, no recurrences or metastases have occurred, even in patients treated by cone biopsy alone, but recurrence has been noted in other series and anecdotal reports. A villous adenoma may be seen occasionally adjacent to the adenocarcinoma and adjacent adenocarcinoma-in-situ is common.

Whilst papillary adenofibromas, Müllerian papillomas and even simple 'papillary endocervicitis' may come into the differential diagnosis of villoglandular carcinoma the most important problem is differentiation from serous papillary adenocarcinoma of the cervix. Relative outcome for this rare primary tumour of the cervix is not known. The major points of difference from villoglandular adenocarcinoma are more pronounced nuclear atypia, the finer papillary pattern with prominent cellular budding and presence of psammoma bodies.[68]

Adenoid cystic and adenoid basal carcinoma

Both of these tumours appear to be more common in blacks than whites, at least in the US. Both predominantly occur in postmenopausal women and have some common histological features, i.e. uniform basaloid cells with little atypia arranged in solid nests and cords. Squamous differentiation can also be seen in both.[69] Adenoid basal carcinoma does not, however, have the characteristic hyaline intraluminal material seen in adenoid cystic carcinoma, which imparts the typical sieve-like pattern to the tumour, and nuclei are smaller with fewer mitoses and less or no necrosis. A stromal response is also usually inconspicuous. Both tumours may be associated with adjacent CIN or CIGN. Adenoid cystic carcinoma of the cervix may be a rather different tumour to that at other sites as it contains few immunohistochemically demonstrable myoepithelial cells. Solid variants are described.[70]

Despite their rather similar histological pattern, clinical outcome appears very different, with adenoid cystic tumours behaving aggressively and having a high rate of local recurrence and distant spread, whereas adenoid basal tumours are slow growing and often detected as an incidental finding during investigation for squamous dysplasia in smears.

Recently, a few cases of adenoid cystic carcinoma with malignant stromal change have been reported.[71] Their true nature is as yet unclear but they appear to be variants of carcinosarcoma and their included epithelial elements were not of purely adenoid cystic type.

'Stump adenocarcinoma'

Subtotal hysterectomy (leaving the cervix *in situ*) is becoming an increasingly popular operation. Its disadvantage is the need for continued cytological surveillance of the cervix due to the persisting low risk of cervical malignancy. There is little knowledge of the magnitude of the risk at present. One presumes that the risk of occurrence of cervical adenocarcinoma and squamous carcinoma will be similar to untreated patients but there may be additional risk related to any residual isthmic endometrial tissue, in the presence of continued oestrogenic stimulation. Older studies suggested a risk of 1–2% for development of invasive carcinoma, but most were squamous. A recent study looking at endocervical adenocarcinoma in the cervical stump showed a poorer prognosis than for either squamous carcinoma of the stump or adenocarcinoma of the cervix with an intact uterus.[72]

Adenocarcinoma with abundant mucin secretion

This variant of endocervical adenocarcinoma was recently described in a series of 14 cases. It is apparently distinguished only by the presence of abundant mucin production and may be either of MDA or other endocervical type.[73] The massive mucin production leads to considerable cervical enlargement of rubbery consistency and no surface ulceration occurs despite the large tumour size. Cytological diagnosis of malignancy in such tumours was said to be very difficult as was biopsy diagnosis in some. Outcome appeared to be poor despite the fact that the tumours were well differentiated.

Another recent paper on a related topic has suggested that cervical adenocarcinomas with mucin leakage into connective tissues and/or lymphatics are associated with a higher risk of lymph node metastasis than tumours not showing this feature.[74] This finding remains to be confirmed by further studies.

PROGNOSTIC FACTORS IN CERVICAL ADENOCARCINOMA

Apart from the established prognostic factors of tumour depth, volume, diameter, type, stage, vessel involvement and grade, a number of other potential prognostic factors have been recently investigated. Some are described below:

Ploidy

This appears to correlate with histological grade in both older and recent studies[75] and both ploidy and S-phase fraction appear to be independent prognostic factors.

Levels of apoptosis

In large (> 4 cm), Stage IB, cervical adenocarcinomas treated by radiation therapy, those with high levels of apoptosis had better overall survival than those with low,[76] but not a significantly better disease free survival. Further studies are needed to validate these findings.

Hormone receptors

Evidence as to the value of oestrogen and progesterone receptors as prognostic markers is at this stage unclear. Some have found them useful;[77] others, looking at both squamous and adenocarcinomas, have found them to have only weak predictive value. Endocervical-type carcinomas appear to show the highest proportion of receptor positive tumours. Progesterone may be more useful than oestrogen.

Oncogene studies

There is evidence that reduced expression of nm23-H1 protein with co-existent overexpression of C-erb B-2 may be associated with increased risk of lymph node metastasis and reduced survival in adenocarcinoma of the cervix,[78,79] but this has not been universally accepted, others arguing that overexpression of C-erb B-2 occurs late in the disease, being seen in high stage cases.[80]. p53 mutations have been suggested as a marker of biologically aggressive tumours with the same study suggesting that HPV containing tumours were a less aggressive subgroup.[81]

KEY POINTS FOR CLINICAL PRACTICE

- Non-neoplastic, cystic endocervical crypts may extend deep into the cervical stroma.
- Microglandular endocervical hyperplasia may mimic carcinomas of the endocervix and vice versa.
- Tubo-endometrial metaplasia and superficial endometriosis are closely related to cervical trauma. Deep endometriosis is not.
- CIGN can only be separated diagnostically into two grades, high and low, and the importance of low grade disease as a precursor of invasive carcinoma or high grade CIGN is unclear.
- No adequate definition of microinvasive adenocarcinoma exists and the term should be avoided.
- The relative frequency of diagnosis of adenosquamous carcinoma is increasing, particularly in relatively young women. This variant may include a poor prognosis group but the evidence for this at present is inconclusive.
- Villoglandular adenocarcinoma of the cervix appears to have a very good prognosis and specific histological features.

REFERENCES

1. Clement PB, Young RH. Deep Nabothian cysts of the endocervix. A possible source of confusion with minimal deviation adenocarcinoma (adenoma malignum). Int J Gynecol Pathol 1989; 8: 340–348
2. Daya D, Young RH. Florid deep glands of the uterine cervix. Another mimic of adenoma malignum. Am J Clin Pathol 1995; 103: 614–617
3. Young RH, Scully RE. Atypical forms of microglandular hyperplasia of the cervix simulating carcinoma: a report of five cases and review of the literature. Am J Surg Pathol 1989; 13: 50–56
4. Steeper TA, Wick MR. Minimal deviation adenocarcinoma of the uterine cervix ('adenoma malignum'). An immunohistochemical comparison with microglandular endocervical hyperplasia and conventional endocervical adenocarcinoma. Cancer 1986; 58: 1131–1138

5. Wahlstrom T, Lindgren J, Korhonen M, Seppala M. Distinction between endocervical and endometrial adenocarcinoma with immuno-peroxidase staining of carcinoembryonic antigen in routine histological tissue specimens. Lancet 1979; ii: 1159–1160
6. Van Hoeven KH, Ramondetta L, Kovatich AJ et al. Orientation image analysis of MIB1 reactivity in inflammatory hyperplastic and neoplastic endocervical lesions. Int J Gynecol Pathol 1997; 16: 15–21
7. Young RH, Scully RE. Uterine carcinomas simulating microglandular hyperplasia. A report of six cases. Am J Surg Pathol 1992; 16: 1092–1097
8. Valente PT, Schantz HD, Schultz M. Cytologic atypia associated with microglandular hyperplasia. Diagn Cytopathol 1994; 10: 326–331
9. Ferry JA, Scully RE. Mesonephric remnants, hyperplasia & neoplasia in the uterine cervix: a study of 49 cases. Am J Surg Pathol 1990; 14: 1100–1111
10. Seidman JD, Tavassoli FA. Mesonephric hyperplasia of the uterine cervix: a clinicopathologic study of 51 cases. Int J Gynecol Pathol 1995; 14: 293–299
11. Samaratunga H, Beresford A, Davison A. Squamous cell carcinoma *in-situ* involving mesonephric remnants. A potential diagnostic pitfall. Am J Surg Pathol 1994; 18: 1265–1269
12. Ismail SM. Cone biopsy causes cervical endometriosis and tubo-endometrioid metaplasia. Histopathology 1991; 18: 107–114
13. Jonasson JG, Wang HH, Antonioli DA, Ducatman BS. Tubal metaplasia of the uterine cervix: a prevalence study in patients with gynecologic pathologic findings. Int J Gynecol Pathol 1992; 11: 89–95
14. Novotny DB, Maygarden JJ, Johnson DE, Frable WY. Tubal metaplasia. A frequent potential pitfall in the cytologic diagnosis of endocervical glandular dysplasia on cervical smears. Acta Cytol 1992; 36: 1–10
15. Oliva E, Clement PB, Young RH. Tubal and tubo-endometrioid metaplasia of the uterine cervix. Unemphasized features that may cause problems in differential diagnosis: a report of 25 cases. Am J Clin Pathol 1995; 103: 618–623
16. McCluggage MG, Maxwell P, McBride HA, Hamilton PW, Bharucha H. Monoclonal antibodies Ki-67 and MIB1 in the distinction of tubo-endometrial metaplasia from endocervical adenocarcinoma and adenocarcinoma-in-situ in formalin-fixed material. Int J Gynecol Pathol 1995; 14: 209–216
17. Brown LJR, Griffin NR, Wells M. Cytoplasmic reactivity with the monoclonal antibody HMFG1 as a marker of cervical glandular atypia. J Pathol 1987; 151: 203–208
18. Rollason TP, Byrne P, Williams A, Brown G. Expression of epithelial membrane and 3 fucosyl-N-acetyllactosamine antigens in cervix uteri with particular reference to adenocarcinoma-in-situ. J Clin Pathol 1988; 41: 547–552
19. Jones MA, Young RH. Endocervical type A (non-cystic) tunnel clusters with cytologic atypia. A report of 14 cases. Am J Surg Pathol 1996; 20: 1312–1318
20. Jones MA, Young RH, Scully RE. Diffuse laminar endocervical glandular hyperplasia: a report of 7 cases. Am J Surg Pathol 1991; 15: 1113–1120
21. Maruyama R, Nagaoka S, Terao K et al. Diffuse laminar endocervical hyperplasia. Pathol Int 1995; 45: 283–286
22. Singh P, Ilancheran A, Ratnan SS et al. Cervical adenocarcinoma in women with nasopharyngeal carcinoma. Cancer 1989; 64: 1152–1155
23. Schneider V. Arias-Stella reaction of the endocervix. Frequency and location. Acta Cytol 1981; 25: 224
24. Trowell JE. Intestinal metaplasia with argentaffin cells in the uterine cervix. Histopathology 1985; 9: 551–559
25. Fetissof F, Heitzman A, Machet MC, Lausac J. Unusual endocervical lesions with endocrine cells. Pathol Res Pract 1993; 189: 928–939
26. Andrews CF, Jourdain L, Damjanov I. Benign cervical mesonephric papilloma of childhood. Report of a case studied by light and electron microscopy. Diagn Gynecol Obstet 1981; 3: 39–43
27. Young RH, Scully RE. Villiglandular papillary adenocarcinoma of the uterine cervix. A clinicopathological analysis of 13 cases. Cancer 1989; 63: 1773–1779
28. Young RH, Scully RE. Invasive adenocarcinoma and related tumors of the uterine cervix. Semin Diagn Pathol 1990; 7: 205–227

29. Michael H, Sutton G, Hull MT, Roth LM. Villous adenoma of the uterine cervix associated with invasive adenocarcinoma: a histologic, ultrastructural, and immunohistochemical study. Int J Gynecol Pathol 1986; 5: 163–169
30. Fox H, Wells M, Harris M, McWilliam LJ, Andersson GS. Enteric tumours of the lower female genital tract: a report of three cases. Histopathology 1988; 12: 167–176
31. Brown LJR, Wells M. Cervical glandular atypia associated with squamous intraepithelial neoplasia: a premalignant lesion? J Clin Pathol 1987; 39: 22–28
32. Jaworski RC. Endocervical glandular dysplasia, adenocarcinoma *in situ*, and early invasive (microinvasive) adenocarcinoma of the uterine cervix. Semin Diagn Pathol 1990; 7: 190–204
33. Young RH, Clement PB, Scully RE. Premalignant and malignant glandular lesions of the uterine cervix. In: Clement PB, Young RH, eds. Tumors and Tumorlike Lesions of the Uterine Corpus and Cervix. New York: Churchill Livingstone, 1993; 86–136
34. Jaworski RC, Pacey NF, Greenberg ML, Osborn RA. The histologic diagnosis of adenocarcinoma *in situ* and related lesions of the cervix uteri. Adenocarcinoma *in situ*. Cancer 1988; 61: 1171–1181
35. Steiner G, Friedell GH. Adenosquamous carcinoma *in situ* of the cervix. Cancer 1965; 18: 807
36. Lee SJ, Rollason T. Argyrophilic cells in cervical intraepithelial glandular neoplasia. Int J Gynecol Pathol 1994; 13: 131–132
37. Cullimore JE, Luesley DM, Rollason TP et al. A prospective study of conization of the cervix in the management of adenocarcinoma-in-situ and glandular atypia of the cervix – a preliminary report. Br J Obstet Gynaecol 1992; 99: 314–318
38. Muntz HG, Bell DA, Lage JM et al. Adenocarcinoma in situ of the uterine cervix. Obstet Gynecol 1992; 80: 935–939
39. Wolf JK, Leverback C, Malpica A et al. Adenocarcinoma in situ of the cervix: significance of cone biopsy margins. Obstet Gynecol 1996; 88: 82–86
40. Widrich T, Kennedy AW, Myers TM et al. Adenocarcinoma *in situ* of the uterine cervix: management and outcome. Gynecol Oncol 1996: 61: 304–308
41. Kaspar HG, Dinn TV, Doherty MG et al. Clinical implications of tumor volume measurement in Stage I adenocarcinoma of the cervix. Obstet Gynecol 1993; 81: 291–300
42. Teshima S, Shimosata Y, Kishi K et al. Early stage adenocarcinoma of the uterine cervix. Histopathologic analysis with consideration of histogenesis. Cancer 1985; 56: 167–172
43. Berek JS, Hacker NF, Fu Y-S et al. Adenocarcinoma of the uterine cervix: histologic variables associated with lymph node metastasis and survival. Obstet Gynecol 1985; 65: 46–52
44. Rollason TP, Cullimore J, Bradgate M. A suggested columnar cell equivalent of squamous carcinoma-in-situ with early stromal invasion. Int J Gynecol Pathol 1989; 8: 230–236
45. Darne JF, Polacarz SV, Sheridan E et al. Nucleolar organiser regions in adenocarcinoma *in situ* and invasive adenocarcinoma of the cervix. J Clin Pathol 1990; 43: 657–660
46. Yavner DL, Dwyer IM, Hancock WW, Ehrmann RL. Basement membrane of cervical adenocarcinoma: an immunoperoxidase study of laminin and type IV collagen. Obstet Gynecol 1990; 76: 1014–1019
47. Toki N, Kaku T, Tsukamoto N et al. Distribution of basement membrane antigens in uterine cervical adenocarcinomas: an immunohistological study. Gynecol Oncol 1990; 38: 17–21
48. Brand E, Berek JS, Hacker NF. Controversies in the management of cervical adenocarcinoma. Obstet Gynecol 1988; 71: 261–269
49. Vesterinen E, Forss M, Nieminen U. Increase of cervical adenocarcinoma: a report of 520 cases of cervical carcinoma including 112 tumors with glandular elements. Gynecol Oncol 1989; 33: 49–53
50. Nieminen P, Kallio M, Hakara M. The effect of mass screening on incidence and mortality of squamous and adenocarcinoma of cervix uteri. Obstet Gynecol 1995; 85: 1017–1021
51. Cooper K, Herrington CS, Lo ES et al. Integration of human papillomavirus types 16 and 18 in cervical adenocarcinoma. J Clin Pathol 1992; 45: 382–384
52. Parazzini F, La Vecchia C, Negin E et al. Risk factors for adenocarcinoma of the cervix: a case-control study. Br J Cancer 1988; 57: 2101–2104

53. Honore LH, Koch M, Brown LB. Comparison of oral contraceptive use in women with adenocarcinoma and squamous cell carcinoma of the uterine cervix. Gynecol Obstet Invest 1991; 32: 98–101
54. Ursin G, Pike MC, Preston-Martin S et al. Sexual, reproductive and other risk factors for adenocarcinoma of the cervix: results from a population-based case-control study. Cancer Causes Control 1995; 7: 391–410
55. Eifel PJ, Burke TW, Morris M, Smith TL. Adenocarcinoma as an independent risk factor for disease recurrence in patients with Stage IB cervical carcinoma. Gynecol Oncol 1995; 59: 38–44
56. Kudo R, Sasano H, Koizumi M et al. Immunohistochemical comparison of a new monoclonal antibody IC5 and carcinoembryonic antigen in the differential diagnosis of adenocarcinoma of the uterine cervix. Int J Gynecol Pathol 1990; 9: 325–336
57. Maes G, Flewen GJ, Bara J et al. The distribution of mucins, carcinoembryonic antigen, and mucus associated antigens in endocervical and endometrial adenocarcinomas. Int J Gynecol Pathol 1988; 7: 112–122
58. Johnson TL, Kim W, Plieth DA Sarkar FH. Detection of HPV 16/18 DNA in cervical adenocarcinoma using polymerase chain reaction (PCR) methodology. Mod Pathol 1992; 5: 35–40
59. Ireland D, Cole S, Kelly P, Monaghan JM. Mucin production in cervical intraepithelial neoplasia and in stage IB carcinoma of cervix with lymph node metastases. Br J Obstet Gynaecol 1987; 94: 467–472
60. Yazigi R, Sandstad J, Munoz AK et al. Adenosquamous carcinoma of the cervix: prognosis in stage IB. Obstet Gynecol 1990; 75: 1012–1015
61. Hale RJ, Buckley CH, Fox H, William J. Prognostic value of C-erb B-2 expression in uterine cervical carcinoma. J Clin Pathol 1992; 45: 594–596
62. Young RH, Welch WR, Dickersin GR, Scully RE. Ovarian sex cord tumor with annular tubules. Review of 74 cases including 27 with Peutz-Jegher's syndrome and four with adenoma malignum of the cervix. Cancer 1982; 50: 1384–1402
63. Gilks CB, Young RH, Aguirre P et al. Adenoma malignum (minimal deviation adenocarcinoma) of the uterine cervix. A clinicopathological and immunohistochemical analysis of 26 cases. Am J Surg Pathol 1989; 13: 717–729
64. Agorastos T, Vakiani A, Papaloucas A. Minimal deviation adenocarcinoma of the cervix: a hypodiploid tumour? Int J Gynecol Pathol 1994; 13: 211–219
65. Young RH, Clement PB, Scully RE. Premalignant and malignant glandular lesions of the uterine cervix. In: Clement PB Young RH eds. Tumors and Tumorlike Lesions of the Uterine Corpus and Cervix. New York: Churchill Livingstone 1993; 85–136
66. Young RH, Scully RE. Minimal deviation endometrioid adenocarcinoma of the uterine cervix. A report of five cases of a distinctive neoplasm that may be misinterpreted as benign. Am J Surg Pathol 1993; 17: 660–665
67. Jones MW, Silverberg SG, Kurman RJ. Well differentiated villoglandular adenocarcinoma of uterine cervix: a clinicopathological study of 24 cases. Int J Gynecol Pathol 1993; 12: 1–7
68. Gilks CB, Clement PB. Papillary serous adenocarcinoma of the uterine cervix. A report of three cases. Mod Pathol 1992; 5: 426–431
69. Ferry JA, Scully RE. 'Adenoid cystic' carcinoma and adenoid basal carcinoma of the uterine cervix. A study of 28 cases. Am J Surg Pathol 1988; 12: 134–144
70. Albores-Saavedra J, Manivel C, Mora A et al. The solid variant of adenoid cystic carcinoma of the cervix. Int J Gynecol Pathol 1992; 11: 2–10
71. Mentoff DT, Schiffman R, Haupt HM. Adenoid cystic carcinoma of the uterine cervix with malignant stroma. An unusual variant of carcinosarcoma? Am J Surg Pathol 1995; 19: 229–233
72. Goodman HM, Nilott JM, Buttlar CA et al. Adenocarcinoma of the cervical stump. Gynecol Oncol 1989; 35: 188–192
73. Ueki M, Ueda M, Okamura S, Yameda T. Clinicopathological features of well differentiated cervical adenocarcinoma with abundant mucin secretion. J Med 1995; 26: 17–30
74. Konishi I, Fujii S, Nanbu Y, Norogaki H, Mori T. Mucin leakage into the cervical stroma may increase lymph node metastasis in mucin producing cervical adenocarcinomas. Cancer 1990; 65: 229–237

75. Leminen A, Paavonen J, Vesterinen E et al. Deoxyribonucleic acid flow cytometric analysis of cervical adenocarcinoma: prognostic significance of deoxyribonucleic acid ploidy and S-phase fraction. Am J Obstet Gynecol 1990; 162: 848–853
76. Wheeler JA, Stephens LC, Tornos C et al. ASTRO Research Fellowship: apoptosis as a predictor of tumour response to radiation in stage IB cervical carcinoma. Int J Rad Oncol Biol Phys 1995; 32: 1487–1493
77. Masood S, Rhatigan RM, Wilkinson EW, Barwick KW, Wilson WJ. Expression and prognostic significance of oestrogen and progesterone receptors in adenocarcinoma of the uterine cervix. An immunocytolochemical study. Cancer 1993; 72: 511–518
78. Mandai M, Konishi I, Koshiyama T et al. Altered expression of nm23-H1 and C-erb B-2 proteins have prognostic significance in adenocarcinoma but not in squamous cell carcinoma of the uterine cervix. Cancer 1995; 75: 2523–2529
79. Kihana T, Tsuda H, Toshima J et al. Prognostic significance of the overexpression of C-erb-B-2 protein in adenocarcinoma of the uterine cervix. Cancer 1994; 73: 348–353
80. Costa MJ, Walls J, Trelford JD. C-erb B-2 protein overexpression in uterine cervix carcinoma with glandular differentiation. A frequent event but not an independent prognostic marker because it occurs late in the disease. Am J Clin Pathol 1995; 104: 634–642
81. Jiko K, Tsuda H, Sato S, Hirohashi S. Pathogenetic significance of *p53* and *C-Ki-ras* gene mutations and human papillomavirus DNA integration in adenocarcinoma of the uterine cervix and uterine isthmus. Int J Cancer 1994; 59: 601–606

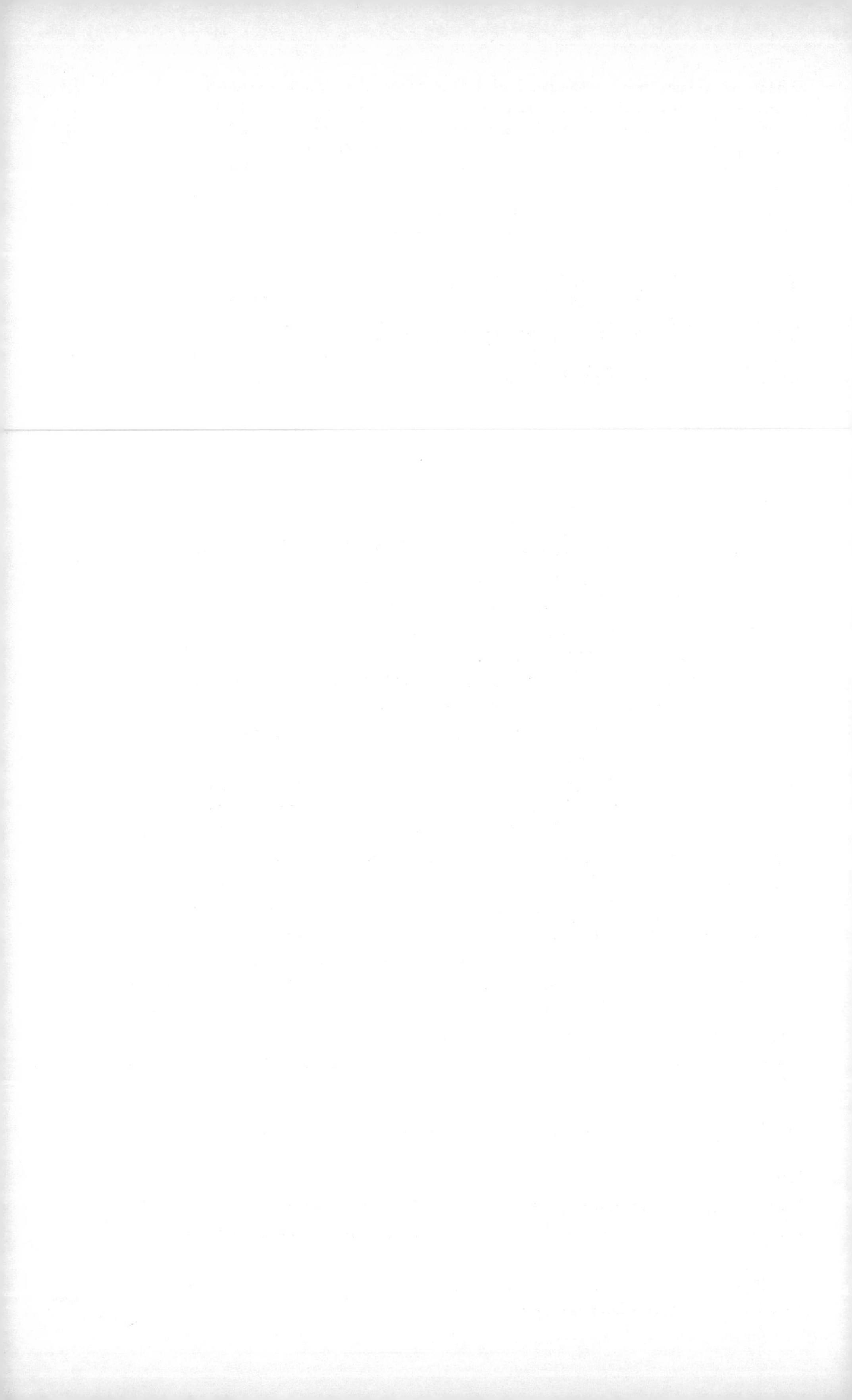

10

The pathologist, the surgeon and colorectal cancer – get it right because it matters

Philip Quirke

VITAL PARTNERSHIP OF PATHOLOGIST AND SURGEON

Cuthbert Dukes and subsequently Basil Morson at St Mark's Hospital created and publicised the vital partnership between the surgeon and the pathologist. The importance of this relationship is even greater today than it was then because of changes in the management of colorectal cancer. The relationship has been lost in many centres for a range of reasons but probably most importantly because of the increased workloads in surgical histopathology and the demands of other clinicians such as the gynaecologists, endoscopists and breast surgeons directing the way we practice histopathology. It is necessary to re-establish the close working relationship between the surgeon and the pathologist and to include the oncologists and radiologists. Surgeons are having to sub-specialise and, with development in the UK of specialised Calman Cancer Units, each District General Hospital will have a lead colorectal cancer surgeon. Each Calman Cancer Unit will also have to have a pathologist who leads in colorectal cancer and is responsible for the quality of reporting. Thus we are being forced to re-establish the links between the colorectal surgeon and the pathologist. We should not see this as a threat but as a recognition of the vital role of the pathologist in the clinical team. We must embrace it, for not only is it good for the patient but here lies the salvation of the histopathologist from being relegated to the realms of a privatised support service. Why has the quality of pathology and the efforts of the pathologist become so important? This is addressed in the next section.

VITAL ROLE OF THE PATHOLOGIST IN COLORECTAL CANCER

Quality

Many pathologists believe that colorectal cancer reporting is relatively unimportant compared to the other specimens that appear beneath their

Professor Philip Quirke, Professor and Honorary Consultant, Division of Clinical Sciences, School of Medicine, University of Leeds, Leeds LS2 9JT, UK

microscope. They delegate the dissection of the specimen to the senior house officer or specialist registrar, believe that 10–15 min is adequate to assess a cancer resection specimen and that a brief report with a Dukes stage is more than enough to keep the surgeon happy. That a problem exists was shown by Blenkinsop et al[1] in 1981 who audited the reports from the Large Bowel Cancer Project and showed marked variation in the frequency not only of different Dukes stages (e.g. the frequency of Dukes A's varying from 5–30%) and the mean lymph node yield (1–11.2 per centre) but of grade and many other parameters. One might expect that 16 years on things would be different. After all, audit is now an accepted part of modern practice and guidelines are sprouting from every angle. Bull et al[2] in a regional audit in Wales, together with unpublished data from Trent and Wessex, show that little has changed in 1997. The standard quality of colorectal cancer reporting is poor especially with respect to lymph node yields and circumferential margin (CRM) involvement. In Wales, only 11.3% of colonic cancer reports and 4% of rectal cancer reports met the minimum standards. When the criteria were relaxed, only 78% of colonic reports and 46.6% of rectal cancer reports met the absolute minimum standards. Only 51.6% of laboratories reported the status of the CRM in rectal cancer in spite of good evidence for its importance.[3–6] It is probable that it is not just the pathology of colorectal cancer that is poorly understood, but also the anatomy. How many pathologists could recite the names of the arteries of the colorectum which form the important high tie of the specimen? How many could identify the insertion of the levator muscles? How many understand the importance of the anatomy of the non-peritonealised surface of the rectum which forms the CRM in the rectum to the development of local recurrence? It is not just the DGH pathologist who may have difficulty answering these questions. How many pathologists were asked these questions in their Part 1 or Part 2 MRCPath?

Why is it that the same pathologist who reports colorectal cancer badly will spend hours looking at a difficult lymph node or an early screen detected atypical hyperplasia/*in situ* breast cancer and will easily pass their quality assurance tests in cervical cytology? It is probably because they have not been kept up to date with the changes in the management of colorectal cancer and colorectal surgeons have tolerated poor reporting, unlike haematologists, breast surgeons and gynaecologists. There is now no excuse for poor reporting of colorectal cancer as histopathology is central to the management of colorectal cancer patients. After all, one patient with a colorectal cancer is equivalent to one patient with a lymphoma or any other tumour and colorectal cancer is a common disease. Furthermore, the quality of the diagnosis may have more effect on the management of the patient!

IMPORTANCE OF PATHOLOGY TO THE MANAGEMENT OF COLORECTAL CANCER

In colonic cancer, adjuvant chemotherapy is now accepted as reducing the risk of relapse by 30% and the 5 year mortality by 5–10% in lymph node positive patients undergoing a curative resection. Whilst there is still some debate, especially in the light of the ongoing Dutch and Swedish adjuvant studies, there is now no doubt that the majority of patients in the UK classified as Dukes stage C should get adjuvant chemotherapy for 6 months. In the future, the 17-1A antibody Panorex may also be used for adjuvant therapy in Dukes C colorectal cancer.[7] These regimens have a significant morbidity and cost. The decision to treat is directly related to the pathological stage. Failure of the pathologist to correctly stage a patient as a Dukes C reduces that patient's life expectancy.

In rectal cancer, the situation is less clear, but nearly all Dukes C's will receive adjuvant chemotherapy. It is, however, in rectal cancer that the greatest improvement is required. If a patient with rectal cancer develops local recurrence, then the prognosis is poor with a 90% chance of death. Frequently, this can be the only manifestation of the disease and it may be amenable to therapy if predicted from the resection specimen. In a recent MRC trial, 33% of patients with operable rectal cancer treated by surgery alone developed local recurrence.[8] These patients had frequently had sub-optimal or poor surgery. This can be recognised by the pathologist who may gently feed this back to the surgeon who can then change his or her surgical technique or obtain further surgical experience at a centre known for excellence in rectal surgery. The pathologist should also be auditing the abdomino-perineal excision rate. In many centres this is above 40%, whereas in specialist centres it can be as low as 15%. Pathologists are afraid to audit surgeons but we perform this duty everyday in the *post mortem* room. Do we cover up the transected bile duct which lead to death? – no, because our duty is to the patient. Likewise, the poor rectal resection and the frequency of involved circumferential margins should be constructively reported so that the management of patients is improved. In a review of published papers on rectal cancer surgery, McCall et al[9] showed marked variation in local recurrence rates and survival depending on whether the surgeons had felt they had performed a total mesorectal excision. There is growing evidence that an improvement in the quality of surgery, e.g. the ability to remove the mesorectum intact without violation, can lead to a 20% improvement in 4 year survival.[10] Early evidence is accruing in other Scandinavian hospitals (Lund and Ulleskelf) which have been visited and the surgeons trained by Mr Heald, an acknowledged expert in rectal surgery with a low local recurrence rate, of a dramatic reduction in local recurrence (Mr Heald, personal communication).

To improve the value of pathology reports, we need to concentrate on what is important. There are many prognostic factors in colorectal cancer but most of them are not independent, add little information or may be subject to a large degree of interobserver variation. A group of UK gastrointestinal pathologists have now created a minimum data set which we believe records the essential features for reporting colorectal cancer. This is shown in Figure 1.

It is important that British patients should benefit from knowledge acquired in European and North American trials of adjuvant therapy and from advances in imaging which may allow the identification of patients amenable for local surgery. To enable these data to be easily translated into British practice requires common staging methods on both Continents. We have, therefore, recommended the use of both Dukes and TNM,[11–17] since the latter is commonly used in Europe and North America. TNM has the advantages of better description of the extent of invasion, the inclusion of peritoneal and direct spread into other organs and the use of the R0, R1 and R2 stages.[17] Dukes' staging is simple and well understood all over the world. Astler-Coller[18] and its modifications do not help if TNM has been adopted and TNM encompasses the Australian classification,[19–21] albeit in many more groups.

DEVELOPING THE MINIMUM DATA SET

The poor quality of examination of the specimen and the recording of data has lead to the development of a minimum data set by Professor G.T. Williams, Dr I.C. Talbot, Dr N. Shepherd and myself with valuable input from many other colleagues, especially within Yorkshire. This is shown in Figure 1 and has been accepted by the Royal College of Pathologists, the Royal College of Surgeons of England, the United Kingdom Co-ordinating Committee for Cancer Research Colorectal Cancer Subcommittee, the Association of Coloproctology of Great Britain and Ireland, The Association of Clinical Pathologists and the Pathology section of the British Society of Gastroenterology. It is also identical to the Scottish recommendations drawn up by Professor Levison. This data set has been arrived at by extensive discussion between gastrointestinal pathologists, District General Hospital pathologists and surgeons. An early version has been tested in the old Yorkshire region in all the DGHs and teaching hospitals with good to excellent compliance and the final proforma has been discussed in the South-West and Wessex Regions. It has been presented to the British Society of Gastroenterology Gastrointestinal Pathology Group and to the pathologists participating in the MRC/ICRF Flexible Endoscopy Screening Trial. Many pathologists have had an input into the form and we believe that we have arrived at a reasonable minimum data set. Why use a proforma? A proforma is necessary because we forget to report important features.[1,2] The introduction of a proforma appears to have rapidly improved the data going into the Yorkshire Cancer Registry. We now routinely obtain information on Dukes and TNM stage, the number of lymph nodes found together with involvement of the circumferential margin in rectal cancer. The pathologists have been excellent in submitting their data and soon it will be possible to obtain an accurate assessment of these important features in the Yorkshire population. The introduction of a national proforma should do the same for the rest of the country and allow the development of a comparable set of pathological data across the country.

THE PROFORMA

The clinical information allows 3 points of identification, the surgeon, hospital and histology accession number. Under the gross description is included the site of the tumour as this is important for prognosis and the type of failure (e.g. rectal cancer has a worse prognosis than colonic cancer and a higher local recurrence rate), for epidemiological studies, and an assessment of the ease of clinical diagnosis and likelihood of being picked up in a screening trial.

The distance to the nearest distal or proximal margin is only important if the margin is very close, i.e. < 3 cm[22] or if the tumour is very poorly differentiated or very invasive where spread up to 5 cm from the primary may occur.[23–26] In these situations, the nearer margin should be sampled histologically.

The presence of perforation of the tumour is an adverse prognostic feature[27,28] and will classify the tumour as stage pT4.

Joint National Guidelines Minimum Data Set
Colorectal Cancer Histopathology Report

Patient Name:... Date of Birth:...

Hospital: .... Hospital No: ....

Histology No:... Surgeon: ....

Gross Description

Site of Tumour...

Maximum tumour diameter ....cm

Distance of tumour to nearer margin (cut end) ....cm

	Yes	No
Presence of tumour perforation (pT4)	☐	☐

For rectal tumours

Tumour is: Above ☐ At ☐ Below ☐ the peritoneal reflection

Distance from pectinate line.....................................cm

Histology

Type

	Yes	No
Adenocarcinoma (to include mucinous and signet ring adenocarcinomas)	☐	☐

If No, Other...

Differentiation by predominant area

Poor ☐ Other ☐

Local Invasion

Submucosa (pT1) ☐

Muscularis propria (pT2) ☐

Beyond Muscularis propria (pT3) ☐

Tumour cells have breached the peritoneal surface or invaded adjacent organs (pT4) ☐

Margins

Tumour involvement	N/A	Yes	No
doughnut	☐	☐	☐
margin (cut end)	☐	☐	☐
circumferential margin	☐	☐	☐

Histological measurement

from tumour to circumferential margin .... mm

Metastatic Spread

No of lymph nodes examined...

No of positive lymph nodes ....

(pN1 1-3 nodes, pN2 4+ nodes involved)

	Yes	No
pN3 nodes positive along named artery	☐	☐
Apical node positive (Dukes C2 and pN3)	☐	☐
Extramural vascular invasion	☐	☐

Background Abnormalities

	Yes	No
Adenoma(s)	☐	☐
Synchronous carcinoma(s)	☐	☐
Complete a separate form for each cancer		
Ulcerative colitis	☐	☐
Crohn's	☐	☐
Familial adenomatous polyposis	☐	☐

Other Comments...

....

Pathological Staging

	Yes	No
Complete resection at all margins	☐	☐

TNM

T ☐ N ☐ M ☐

Dukes

Dukes A ☐ (Growth limited to wall, nodes negative)

Dukes B ☐ (Growth beyond M. propria, nodes negative)

Dukes C1 ☐ (Nodes positive and apical node negative)

Dukes C2 ☐ (Apical node positive)

	Yes	No
Histologically confirmed liver metastases	☐	☐

Signature...

Date...

Approved by the Royal Colleges of Pathologists and Surgeons (England), Associations of Coloproctology and Clinical Pathologists, the Pathology Section of the British Society of Gastroenterology, SIGN/SCTN and CROPS

Fig. 1 Joint national guidelines minimum data set: colorectal cancer histopathology report.

The relationship of the tumour to the anterior peritoneal reflection is important, as tumours below the peritoneal reflection have a higher rate of local recurrence. The distance from the pectinate line is important as this identifies the height of the tumour and signifies the patient has undergone an abdomino-perineal excision and lost their anal sphincter. The frequency of abdomino-perineal excision varies substantially between surgeons and is data of interest to surgical audit.

The histological features of the tumour have been confined to the minimum information to give the TNM classification. The presence of invasive adenocarcinoma is noted (invasion of the submucosa) and if there is not an adenocarcinoma present the type of tumour is recorded, e.g. squamous cell carcinoma, lymphoma, etc.

The histopathological assessment of differentiation in colorectal cancer is fraught with interobserver variation and problems with methodology. It appears important to recognise poorly differentiated cancers, but less important to subclassify well and moderately differentiated adenocarcinoma. We recommend the use of the method of Halvorsen et al[29] of grading a tumour by its predominant area rather than the area of worst differentiation.

The level of invasion of the primary tumour is recorded because of its importance to the possibility of local resection and for audit of the quality of preoperative imaging by endorectal ultrasound, computed tomography or magnetic resonance. Invasion into the sub-mucosa (pT1), into muscularis propria (pT2), beyond muscularis propria (pT3), if tumour cells are present on the serosal surface or have ulcerated the serosal surface (pT4), or if there is involvement of adjacent organs (pT4). Serosal involvement should be stated to be present when tumour cells have broken through the peritoneal surface or are on the surface.[30]

For rectal tumours, the circumferential margin (CRM) should be assessed as stated below for the MRC CR07 rectal cancer study. The distance of the CRM from the tumour should be measured. Tumours with a clearance of 1 mm or less had the same level of local recurrence as tumours with no clearance and should be reported as involved. Tumours with clearance of more than 1 mm had a much lower rate of local recurrence.

In assessing metastatic spread, the number of lymph nodes found should be noted, as this is an indicator of the quality of the pathological examination. The number of positive lymph nodes should be recorded. If 1–3 nodes contain tumour it should be staged as pN1 and if 4 or more nodes are positive, as pN2. If the C2 node is found to be involved this should be recorded. If the tumour is colonic, it may lie between two of the major arteries and there may be two high ties. In this situation nodes should be submitted from both high ties for examination as C2 nodes. The assessment of pN3 lymph nodes is more difficult. pN3 nodes are nodes which lie above the bifurcation of the major arteries supplying the colon and rectum. These are the ileo-colic, right colic, middle colic, left colic, sigmoid and superior rectal arteries. If the C2 node is involved by tumour then the case should also be classified as pN3. In the new 1997 TNM classification pN3 has been dropped as it adds no further data to pN2.

The presence of venous invasion has been reported to be an adverse predictive factor in many series (e.g. Talbot et al[31]) yet, in others, it has failed to predict prognosis, the balance of evidence would support its retention, especially as it may predict the future development of liver metastases and, as such, may emerge as an important predictor of patients in need of adjuvant therapy.

The presence of background abnormalities such as adenomas, synchronous carcinomas, ulcerative colitis, Crohn's disease or familial adenomatous polyposis should be noted and any other significant abnormality recorded in the space provided.

The final TNM stage should be derived from the form and the Dukes stage given. If there is a record of liver metastases, or if a positive liver biopsy was received, this should be recorded. The R0, R1 and R2 stage has not been included but this information can easily be derived from the form. An R0 resection is when the tumour has been completely excised. An R1 resection is when there is microscopic involvement of margins and an R2 resection when there is macroscopic residual disease.[17] The form should be signed by the pathologist responsible for the case. A free text report can also be issued if the pathologist wishes. The above information should allow very good reporting of colonic cancer but a description of the dissection of rectal cancer has been included to help pathologists as this area generates more confusion.

PATHOLOGICAL ASSESSMENT OF A RECTAL CANCER SPECIMEN

This is the current method in routine NHS use in Leeds and will form the basis of the new CR07 rectal cancer study. The pathological assessment of a rectal cancer specimen has been described previously,[32,33] but minor modifications are presented here. Where possible, specimens should be received fresh and then opened by the pathologist. If this is not possible, then the surgeon should open the bowel in the way described below and pin it out on a cork board for fixation. If neither of these are possible, then the specimen should be placed in an adequate volume of formalin, usually 20 times the volume of the specimen.

The rectum is opened anteriorly apart from the area 2 cm above and below the tumour where the anterior part of the rectum is left intact. This change is because of the importance of the anterior quadrant with respect to local spread. Below the peritoneal reflection the surgeon can usually only remove between 0.5 and 1.0 cm anteriorly, thus tumours involving this area are at greater risk of CRM involvement because of the small amount of tissue that can be removed. In tumours above the peritoneal reflection, involvement of the peritoneal surface can occur and it is best to avoid destroying this area and the pathologist's ability to sample it by avoiding opening the site of the tumour. If possible, a macroscopic photograph of the posterior and anterior aspects of the specimen is valuable as an audit record of the quality of surgery.

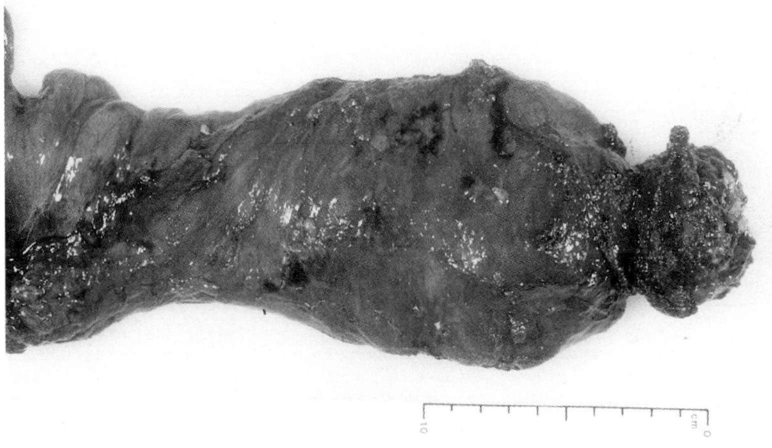

Fig. 2 Good quality abdomino-perineal excision of the rectum. Note the smooth surface of the mesorectum with no irregularity and the very small waist on the specimen at the insertion of the levator muscles.

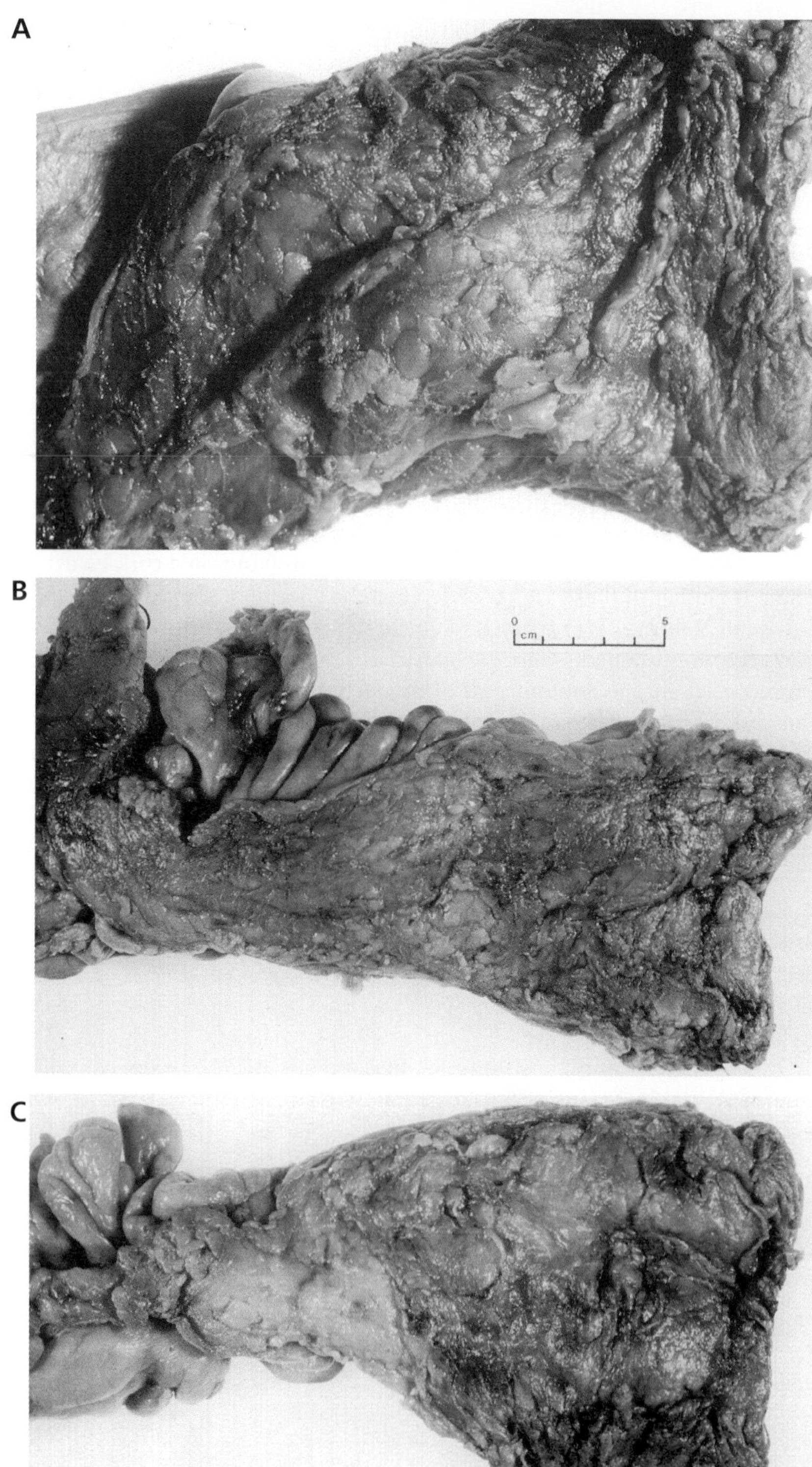

Fig. 3

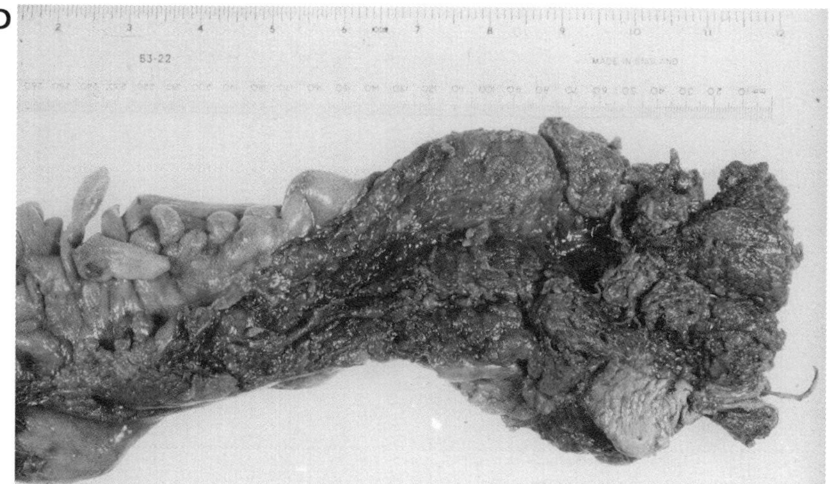

Fig. 3 Resections of vasrying quality. A,B and C are sub-optimal and D is poor. (**A**) Surgical incisions into the mesorectum. These can be as deep as the muscularis propria on occasion and involve the tumour. (**B,C**) Mid-way through the mesorectum the surgeon has lost the mesorectal plane and there is irregularity of the mesorectum towards the distal margin. This is the commonest type of problem seen. (**D**) This is a poor mesorectal excision. The upper and lower mesorectum are irregular and there are defects extending to the muscularis propria.

The opened specimen should be pinned to a cork board and fixed for 48–72 h. Lengthy fixation is valuable as it allows easier dissection. After fixation, the specimen should be removed from the board and the non-peritonealised surfaces painted with ink by the method in use locally. The macroscopic description of the specimen is then performed. Failing to open the specimen does cause a problem with recording the tumour characteristics, but the length, width and area of the tumour are not prognostic, whereas CRM and peritoneal involvement are. The best possible estimate of size should be made after slicing the tumour. The segment of the rectum containing the tumour that has been left intact should now be sectioned transversely as thinly as possible.

The fixed slices should be laid out under good light, photographed, if possible, to form an audit record, and then inspected macroscopically. The maximum depth of extension of the tumour from the muscularis propria should be measured and the distance from the CRM to the tumour. If the tumour is between 0–1 mm on histological sections then CRM involvement is said to have occurred. This distance was chosen by analysis of previous studies.[3,5] If any lymph nodes abut the CRM, then these should be taken in continuity with the CRM so that involvement by this route can be identified, similarly if there is any evidence of isolated deposits or thickening/fibrosis in this area it should be sampled. Again, if tumour is less than 1 mm from the CRM, the CRM is said to be involved. Any peritumoral lymph nodes will be collected at this time. If the tumour approaches the peritoneal surface, this must also be sampled to exclude malignant cells on the surface or ulceration of the serosa by tumour.[30] Four blocks of the primary tumour must be taken to assess the status of the peritoneum and the tumour characteristics. These may be the same blocks as those used for assessment of the CRM or peritoneal involvement, if there is adequate tumour represented.

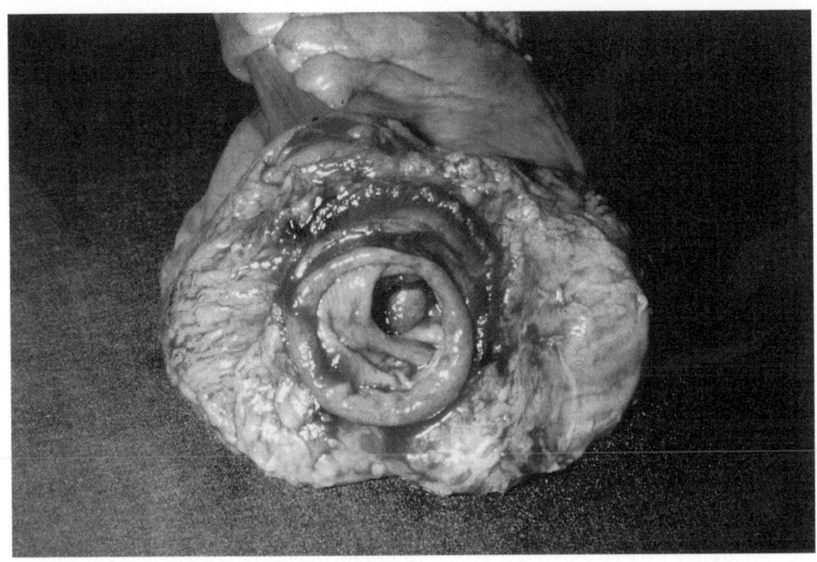

Fig. 4 The correct distal margin with the mesorectal transection occurring at 90°. (Photograph courtesy of Mr R.J. Heald)

After assessing the primary tumour, attention should be turned to the lymph nodes. Starting at the high vascular resection margin, the high tie lymph nodes should be visualised by cross cutting the vessels and mesorectum. Vessels along the inferior mesenteric or superior rectal artery should be identified and embedded separately (pN3) as should the highest lymph node (Dukes C2). All other lymph nodes should be identified and embedded. If any lymph nodes lie against the circumferential margin, then they should be taken in continuity with the margin to exclude CRM involvement. Again, if tumour is < 1 mm, CRM involvement is said to occur. The distal margin and doughnuts (if present) should then be sampled. The proximal margin does not need to be examined unless within 5 cm of the tumour. Any mucosal lesions seen should be sampled. The status of the background mucosa can be obtained from the distal margin.

Standard histological examination of the haematoxylin and eosin sections should then be performed. If tumour is within 1 mm of the CRM, then it should be deemed to be involved. This measurement should be made on the glass slide using the Vernier scale on the microscope stage. If tumour is close to the margin but greater then 1 mm, then deeper levels should be cut to exclude involvement. If fibrosis has led to a mistaken impression of the depth of invasion from the muscularis propria, then this measurement should be corrected from the slide.

AUDITING THE QUALITY OF RECTAL SURGERY

In Figures 2–4, examples are shown of good quality, sub-optimal and poor surgery. A total mesorectal excision should have a bulky mesorectum with a smooth surface covered in mesorectal fascia (Fig. 2). Surgeons commonly make three types of mistake: firstly, incising the mesorectum (Fig. .3A) sometimes

Table 1 The quality of rectal surgery assessed on a three point scale (MRC CLASICC study)

One (poor)	Irregular mesorectum with defects > 1 cm^2 or incision down to muscularis propria. Irregular CRM with little bulk and little clearance anteriorly.
Two (sub-optimal)	Moderate bulk of mesorectum but some irregularity. Moderate coning distally may be present.
Three (optimal)	Good bulk of mesorectum, smooth surface, good clearance anteriorly, no defects in mesorectum.

down to the muscularis propria; secondly, creating a new plane of excision which approaches close to the tumour (Fig. 3B,C); and, thirdly, fail to transect the rectum at 90 degrees so there is coning of the mesorectum leading to an inadequate circumferential margin distal to the tumour. The correct distal margin is shown in Figure 4. The old style method of removing the rectum was by blunt digital dissection where the rectum was quite literally ripped from the pelvis. The effect of this is to leave substantial amounts of mesorectal tissue behind and denuding areas of muscularis propria such that any Dukes B/T3 tumour would involve the CRM, an example of which is shown in Figure3D.

In the MRC CLASICC study of laparoscopic assisted versus open resection for colorectal cancer, the quality of rectal surgery is being assessed on a three point scale as shown in Table 1. The value of the addition of this assessment to the frequency of CRM involvement is currently unknown but will emerge from the trial. The aim being to identify sub-optimal surgery at the earliest opportunity to allow further surgical training.

CONCLUSIONS

Good pathology reporting is essential for the management of colorectal cancer. Audit evidence suggests that many pathology reports are sub-optimal and a major effort is required to improve the quality of pathology. It is very important for the pathologist to concentrate on the macroscopic dissection of the specimen. The pathologist influences postoperative adjuvant chemotherapy as well as the decision for postoperative radiotherapy in rectal cancer and, as such, must provide the required information. Standard free text pathology reporting leads to the omission of important information and the use of proformas ensures that all the relevant information is included and is easy to find by the clinicians. Pathologists can audit the quality of surgery and play a role in helping the surgeon improve. New trials in rectal cancer surgery are planned and pathologists will play a major role in quality control of rectal cancer surgery.

ACKNOWLEDGEMENTS

Our colorectal cancer research is supported by grants from the Yorkshire Cancer Research Campaign, Medical Research Council, Northern & Yorkshire NHS R&D and Special Trustees of Leeds General Infirmary. The manuscript has been prepared by Mrs J. Fearnley and the photographs by Mr S. Toms.

REFERENCES

1. Blenkinsopp WK, Stewart-Brown S, Blesovsky L, Kearney G, Fielding LP. Histopathology reporting in large bowel cancer. J Clin Pathol 1981; 34: 598–613
2. Bull AD, Biffin AHB, Mella J et al. Colorectal cancer pathology reporting: a regional audit. J Clin Pathol 1997; 50: 138–142
3. Quirke P, Durdey P, Dixon MF, Williams NS. The prediction of local recurrence of rectal adenocarcinoma due to inadequate surgical resection. Histopathological study of lateral tumour spread and surgical excision. Lancet 1986; 2: 996–999
4. Ng IOL, Luk ISC, Yuen ST et al. Surgical lateral clearance in resected rectal carcinomas. A multivariate analysis of clinicopathological features. Cancer 1993; 71: 1972–1976
5. Adam JJ, Mohamdee MO, Martin IG et al. Role of circumferential margin involvement in the local recurrence of rectal cancer.Lancet 1994; 344: 707–711
6. de Haas-Kock DF, Baeten CG, Jager JJ et al. Prognostic significance of radial margins of clearance in rectal cancer. Br J Surg 1996; 83: 781–785
7. Riethmuller G, Schneider-Gadicke E, Schlimok G et al and the German Cancer Aid 17-1A Study Group. Randomised trial of monoclonal antibody for adjuvant therapy of resected Dukes' C colorectal carcinoma. Lancet 1994; 343: 1177–1183
8. Medical Research Council Rectal Cancer Working Party. Randomised trial of surgery alone versus surgery followed by radiotherapy for mobile cancer of the rectum. Lancet 1996; 348: 1610–1614
9. McCall JL, Cox MR, Wattchow A. Analysis of local recurrence rates after surgery alone for rectal cancer. Int J Colorect Dis 1995; 10: 126–132
10. Arbman G, Nilsson E, Hallbook O, Sjodahl R. Local recurrence following total mesorectal excision for rectal cancer. Br J Surg 1996; 83: 375–379
11. Denoix PF. French Ministry of Public Health. Paris: National Institute of Hygiene monograph No. 4, 1954
12. Beahrs OH, Myers MD. American Joint Committee on Cancer. Manual for staging cancer, 2nd Edn. Philadelphia: Lippincott, 1983
13. Hermanek P. Problems of pTNM classification of carcinoma of the stomach, colorectum and anal margin. Pathol Res Pract 1986; 181: 296–300
14. Hermanek P, Giedl J, Dworak O. Two programmes for examination of regional lymph nodes in colorectal carcinoma with regard to the new pN classification. Pathol Res Pract 1989; 185: 867–873
15. UICC. In: Hermanek P, Sobin LH (eds). TNM classification of malignant tumours, 4th Edn, 2nd revision. Berlin: Springer, 1992
16. UICC. In: Hermanek P, Henson DE, Hunter RVP, Sobin L. (eds). TNM supplement 1993. A commentary on uniform use. Berlin: Springer, 1993
17. Hermanek P, Wittekind Ch. The pathologist and the residual tumour (R) classification. Pathol Res Pract 1994; 190: 115–123
18. Astler VB, Coller FA. The prognostic significance of direct extension of carcinoma of the colon and rectum. Ann Surg 1954; 139: 846–852
19. Davis NC, Newland RC. The reporting of colorectal cancer. The Australian clinico-pathological staging system. Aust N Z J Surg 1982; 53: 211–221
20. Chapuis PH, Dent OF, Fisher R et al. A multivariate analysis of clinical and pathological variables in prognosis after resection of large bowel cancer. Br J Surg 1985; 72: 698–702
21. Newland RC, Chapuis PH, Smyth EJ. The prognostic value of substaging colorectal carcinoma: a prospective study of 1117 cases with standardised pathology. Cancer 1987; 60: 852–857
22. Cross SS, Bull AD, Smith JH. Is there any justification for the routine examination of bowel resection margins in colorectal adenocarcinoma? J Clin Pathol 1989; 42: 1040–1042
23. Sidoni A, Bufalari A, Alberti PF. Distal intramural spread in colorectal cancer: a reappraisal of the extent of distal clearance in fifty cases. Tumori 1991; 77; 514–517
24. Shirouza K, Isomoto H, Kakegawa T. Distal spread of rectal cancer and optimal distal margin of resection for sphincter-preserving surgery. Cancer 1995; 76: 388–392
25. Williams NS, Dixon MF, Johnston D. Reappraisal of the 5 centimetre rule of distal excision for carcinoma of the rectum: a study of distal intramural spread and of patients' survival. Br J Surg 1983; 70: 150–154

26. Scott N, Jackson P, Al-Jaberi T, Dixon MF, Quirke P, Finan PJ. Total mesorectal excision and local recurrence: a study of tumour spread in the mesorectum distal to rectal cancer. Br J Surg 1995; 82: 1031–1033
27. Griffin MR, Bergstralh EJ, Coffey RJ, Beart Jr RW, Melton 3rd LD. Predictors of survival after curative resection of carcinoma of the colon and rectum. Cancer 1987; 60: 2318–2324
28. Abulafi AM, Williams NS. Local recurrence of colorectal cancer: the problem, mechanisms, management and adjuvant therapy. Br J Surg 1994; 81: 7–19
29. Halvorsen TB, Seim E. Association between invasiveness, inflammatory reaction, desmoplasia and survival in colorectal cancer. J Clin Pathol 1989; 42: 162–166
30. Shepherd NA, Baxter KJ, Love SB. Influence of local peritoneal involvement on pelvic recurrence and prognosis in rectal cancer. J Clin Pathol 1995; 48: 849–855
31. Talbot IC, Ritchie S, Leighton MH, Hughes AO, Bussey HJR, Morson BC. The clinical significance of invasion of veins by rectal cancer. Br J Surg 1980; 67: 439–442
32. Quirke P, Dixon MF. How I do it: the prediction of local recurrence in rectal adenocarcinoma by histopathological examination. Int J Colorect Dis 1988; 3: 127–131
33. Quirke P, Scott N. The pathologists role in the assessment of local recurrence in rectal carcinoma. Surg Oncol Clin North Am 1992; 1: 1–17

11

Growth factor receptor gene mutations and human pathology

K. E. Leverton W. J. Gullick

INTRODUCTION

Many extracellular signals, such as growth factors and hormones, are involved in the regulation of cell proliferation, differentiation and survival. Growth factors mediate their effects through high affinity receptors, which, in turn, interact with downstream signalling systems and ultimately regulate the expression and activity of genes involved in cellular control systems. Aberrant signalling by growth factor receptors may lead to developmental abnormalities or, in the case of overexpressed or constitutively activated receptors, excessive cell proliferation and oncogenesis. Many growth factors are ligands for receptor tyrosine kinases (RTKs), a group of proteins comprising several families which share common structural features, including an extracellular ligand-binding domain, short membrane-spanning region and intracellular tyrosine kinase catalytic domain.

Activation of RTKs is initiated by ligand binding,[1,2] inducing receptor dimerisation, tyrosine kinase activation and autophosphorylation of intracellular tyrosine residues.[3] Receptor phosphotyrosine residues act as docking sites for proteins (e.g. GAP, Grb2, Shc, PI 3-kinase, PLC-γ) containing phosphotyrosine binding domains such as SH2 or PTB[4,5] or, alternatively, the activated tyrosine kinase may also directly phosphorylate intracellular proteins, ultimately leading to the activation of a cascade of intracellular signalling pathways. A model for the involvement of receptor oligomerisation in RTK transmembrane signalling was initially established for the epidermal

Dr K. E. Leverton BSc PhD, ICRF Molecular Oncology Unit, Imperial College School of Medicine, Hammersmith Campus, London W12 0NN, UK

Professor W. J. Gullick BSc PhD FRCPath, ICRF Molecular Oncology Unit, Imperial College School of Medicine, Hammersmith Campus, London W12 0NN, UK

growth factor receptor[6] and has since been confirmed for many other RTKs. This proposes that inactive receptor monomers are in equilibrium with active dimers and that ligand binding stabilises the active, dimeric form. An exception is the insulin receptor family, in which receptors are naturally dimeric and activation is assumed to occur through a ligand-induced conformational change. Conventionally, it has been viewed that ligand-induced dimerisation of naturally monomeric receptors causes activation via allosteric changes in the receptor. More recently, however, models involving bivalent ligand binding stabilising dimers[7] have received experimental support.[8] Dimerisation may occur between identical receptors (homodimerisation) or between different members of the same receptor family (heterodimerisation). Overexpression of RTKs is often involved in malignancy and, according to the dimerisation model, increased receptor expression, even in the absence of ligand, would increase the level of receptor dimers on the cell surface, resulting in increased stimulation of signalling pathways involved in cellular proliferation. An increase in cell surface receptor dimers would be predicted both due to the increase in the absolute number of receptors expressed on the cell surface and also, perhaps, because the increased density may shift the equilibrium towards the dimeric form. Ligand expression with receptor overexpression also commonly occurs, which has been termed autocrine signalling.

Enhanced signalling can also occur through mutations which cause constitutive receptor activation, for example by the induction or stabilisation of ligand-independent dimerisation, as well as by mutations which directly enhance tyrosine kinase activity, alter substrate specificity or extent of receptor downregulation. Mutational activation of RTKs in general has recently been reviewed.[9] In this review we will, therefore, focus in more detail on activating mutations in the type I family of RTKs, with particular emphasis on the role of mutations which may cause constitutive activation of receptors by the induction of ligand-independent dimerisation.

The type I growth factor receptor family in humans comprises the epidermal growth factor receptor (EGFR/c-erbB-1), c-erbB-2, c-erbB-3 and c-erbB-4 (also known as HER1–4). These are encoded by separate genes but are highly related in sequence and overall layout. The extracellular domain of the receptors comprise two regions involved in ligand-binding (sub-domains I and III, or L1 and L2) and two cysteine-rich regions (II and IV, or S1 and S2). Studies of EGFR have suggested that domain III is directly involved in binding EGF, although domain I is also implicated.[10–14] The cysteine-rich regions are assumed to be involved in maintaining the structure of the extracellular domain via the formation of intramolecular disulphide bonds and it has been suggested that conserved cysteine residues form a pattern resembling that found in the tumour necrosis factor receptor and other proteins.[15] The membrane-spanning domain is composed of a single, short α-helical region. The intracellular domain of the receptor consists of a short juxtamembrane region followed by an intracellular tyrosine kinase domain and C-terminal tail. The highest level of homology between members of the family occurs in the tyrosine kinase domain, whilst the greatest sequence divergence occurs in the C-terminal tail and it is thought that this region, which contains all of the mapped sites of phosphorylation on tyrosine, may be involved in the determination of substrate specificity of the activated receptor.

EGFR, c-erbB-2 and c-erbB-3 are widely expressed in normal epithelial, mesenchymal and neuronal tissues[16] and a recent study in our laboratory has shown c-erbB-4 expression in many adult and fetal tissues.[17] Overexpression of EGFR and c-erbB-2 occurs widely in carcinomas, either as a consequence of increased transcription or of gene amplification, or both.[18] As a generalisation, EGFR overexpression is more common in squamous cell carcinomas (such as of the head and neck and lung) whereas c-erbB-2 is more often increased in adenocarcinomas (such as breast or ovary), although many exceptions occur. EGFR is also notably overexpressed in gliomas (see below). To date, fewer studies have been performed on c-erbB-3. Overexpression without amplification is not uncommon, but it is not clear if this has an oncogenic influence.[19] Studies on c-erbB-4 have only just begun but it has been found to be overexpressed in meduloblastomas,[20] but is absent in malignant prostate and present in normal prostatic epithelium.[21] Our own preliminary studies suggest that reduced expression in cancers relative to normal tissues is the more common presentation,[17] but whether this is a driving force for transformation or whether it is merely characteristic of the state of differentiation of the tumour cells is currently unknown. Since several extensive reviews are available on receptor overexpression (see, for instance, Salomon et al[18]), this chapter will concentrate instead on activating mutations which have been reported more frequently in the literature over the last few years.

MUTATIONS IN *EGFR*

EXTRACELLULAR DOMAIN DELETIONS

The *EGFR* gene,[3] which encodes a 1210 amino acid sequence that is post-translationally glycosylated to produce a protein with a molecular weight of 170 kDa, is the cellular homologue of the *v-erbB* oncogene originally identified in avian erythroblastosis viruses.[22] The chicken *c-erbB* gene can be converted into an oncogene in two ways (Fig. 1). Avian leukosis virus induces erythroblastosis by insertional mutagenesis within the *c-erbB* gene of the chicken genome, removing most of the extracellular ligand-binding domain and encoding a protein containing the erbB sequence beginning at residue 556 compared with the full length protein, fused to the gag sequence of the viral gene. The mutant receptor does not bind ligand, but has constitutive tyrosine kinase activity[23,24] and can transform erythroblasts.[25] Alternatively, the truncated receptor sequence can be acquired by avian erythroblastosis virus, an infectious retrovirus. When contained within the virus, subsequent mutations occur in the cytoplasmic domain of the truncated receptor which enable transformation of other cell types, such as fibroblasts and endothelial cells and several highly tumourigenic viral mutants have been isolated and characterised as reviewed by Carter & Kung[26] (Fig. 1). It has been suggested that deletion of the ligand binding domain of the receptor permits receptor packing, resulting in constitutively active receptors. Indeed, constitutive dimerisation of receptors present at the cell surface of fibroblasts, erythroblasts and endothelial cells has been demonstrated by analysis of various v-erbB products with or without additional C-terminal deletions.[27]

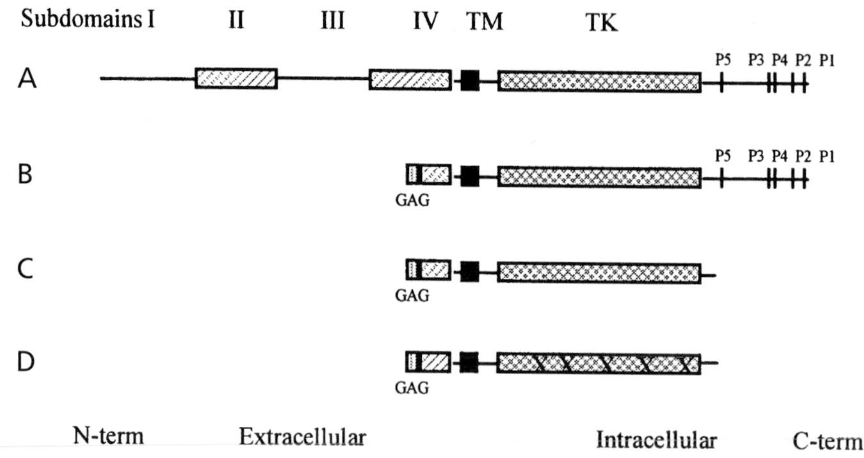

Fig. 1 Activation of the chicken c-erbB receptor. (**A**) Wild-type receptor. (**B**) Insertional mutagenesis of avian leukosis virus (ALV) within the genome interrupts the *c-erbB* gene encoding receptors lacking most of the extracellular domain, with a 5′ fusion to the viral *gag* sequence. Following acquisition of the truncated receptor sequence by avian erythroblastosis virus (AEV), C-terminal deletions (**C**) and subsequent point mutations occur (**D**). I, II, III, IV – extracellular sub-domains; TM – transmembrane region; TK – tyrosine kinase domain; P1–P5 – cytoplasmic autophosphorylation sites.

As described above, activation of the *EGFR* gene by overexpression has been seen in many human tumours and experiments have shown that overexpression of EGFR leads to ligand-dependent transformation of mammalian fibroblasts.[28–30] Some tumours also show amplification of altered *EGFR* genes. At the genomic level, re-arrangements are not uniformly found at specific sequences, but generally occur between exons leading to a limited number of possible transcripts obtained by aberrant splicing.[31] Amplification of altered genes generally co-exists with amplification of wild type sequences, suggesting, perhaps, that amplification of the wild type gene is followed by re-arrangement and then subsequent amplification of the altered gene. Furthermore, it is notable that re-arrangements are rarely, if ever, detected without amplification, suggesting that the encoded changes are not sufficient *per se* to induce transformation and that it is the combination of overexpression with deletion of specific regions of the receptor which confers tumourigenicity.

Deletions of the extracellular domain are the most common structural mutations affecting the EGFR. To date, three truncated forms of EGFR have been reported (Fig. 2). In the type I deletion, identified in a single human malignant glioma,[32] most of the extracellular domain is absent. The predicted protein sequence begins at amino acid 543 of the wild type sequence, encoding a protein very similar (8 amino acids longer at the amino-terminus) to the c-erbB-derived region of the many avian v-erbB products, which is also unable to bind ligand but is catalytically active.[33] Sucrose gradient centrifugation analysis of preparations of this receptor suggested that it is dimeric in the absence of the ligand-binding domain.[34] Expression of human EGF receptors with artificial deletions including most of the extracellular domain has shown that these deletions do appear to activate the receptors in vitro. Analysis of N-terminal *v-erbB*-type

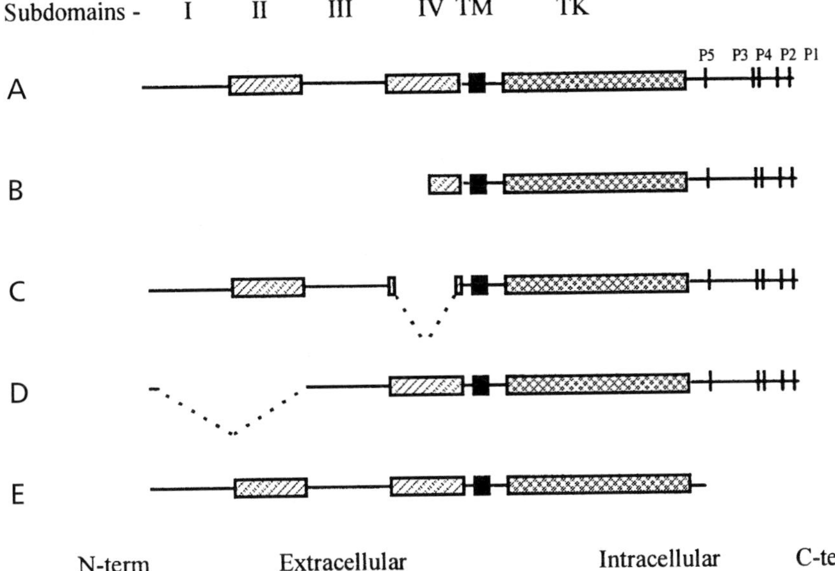

Fig. 2 Structural mutations of the EGFR in human tumours. (**A**) Wild-type receptor. (**B**) In the type I deletion, identified in a glioma,[32] most of the extracellular domain is absent. (**C**) The type II mutant, identified in 2 gliomas[33,34] has a deletion in extracellular sub-domain IV of the receptor. (**D**) The type III mutant[31,32,38] has a deletion within the extracellular domain of the receptor spanning sub-domains I and II, and is the most commonly observed alteration. (**E**) Deletions in the cytoplasmic domain have also been observed,[38] with or without the type III extracellular domain deletion. I, II, III, IV – extracellular sub-domains; TM – transmembrane region; TK – tyrosine kinase domain; P1–P5 – cytoplasmic autophosphorylation sites.

mutations in human *EGFR* inserted into avian retroviral vectors[35] showed that the expression of mutant receptors, in the absence of ligand, was weakly transforming in avian fibroblasts and erythroblasts (an effect which was enhanced by deletion of C-terminal sequences), whereas expression of wild-type receptors was only transforming in the presence of EGF. Haley et al[36] mutated the human *EGFR* gene, removing a region encoding amino acids 18–589 in the extracellular domain of the protein. In the absence of ligand, mutant receptors showed ligand-independent tyrosine kinase activity and transformation of immortalised rodent fibroblasts, although again the effects were enhanced by deletion of C-terminal sequences.

The type II mutant, identified as an amplified gene in 2 malignant human gliomas, has an in-frame deletion of 83 amino acids in sub-domain IV of the extracellular domain, removing amino acids 520–603 of the receptor.[32,37] One tumour, D-298, was established as a xenograft which allowed the properties of the receptor to be examined.[37] Both EGF and TGFα retained high affinity binding and could stimulate tyrosine kinase activity. The mutant receptor, however, displayed an elevated catalytic rate in the absence of ligand relative to wild-type receptor. Tumour growth was still EGF-dependent, but was 3-fold enhanced relative to cells expressing wild-type receptor and the cells were more invasive in co-culture experiments. To date, the types I and II deletions have only been observed in a very small number of gliomas.

By far the most commonly observed rearrangement is the type III deletion, also known as *EGFRvIII* or *ΔEGFR*), which comprises genomic rearrangements leading to the deletion of exons 2–7 of the gene and causing an in-frame deletion of 801 bp of the coding sequence in the extracellular domain of the receptor.[31,32,38] This results in the expression of receptors of 140–155 kDa, lacking 267 amino acids (6–273) spanning the first and second extracellular sub-domains (Fig. 2). *EGFRvIII* was first isolated in the highly malignant CNS neoplasm, glioblastoma multiforme, in which *EGFR* gene amplification occurs in 40–50% of tumours.[33,39,40] Of these tumours exhibiting *EGFR* amplification, around 50% also contain the amplified *EGFRvIII* gene.[40–43] Clinical studies have shown that overexpression of EGFRvIII is related to a shorter interval to relapse and decreased survival, suggesting that this mutation plays a prominent role in progression of the malignancy.[44,45]

Amplification of *EGFR* in gliomas has been shown to be associated with increased expression of EGFR mRNA,[46] which is assumed to stimulate growth by increased levels of membrane receptor expression. Studies of the overexpressed EGFRvIII have shown that the mutant receptor has features which may further contribute to stimulation of cellular proliferation pathways and the frequent amplification and recurrent identical structural alteration strongly implicates the mutant EGFR in tumour formation. In vitro analysis of the amplified, re-arranged gene has been difficult because it is usually lost during the growth of tumour cells in tissue culture.[47] However, transfection experiments have shown that EGFRvIII mediates the formation of tumours in nude mice.[48,49]

Investigation of the mechanism by which expression of *EGFRvIII*-transfected glioblastoma cells caused enhanced tumourigenicity in an in vivo model of glioma formation in mouse brain showed that cells proliferated via clonal expansion rather than exerting a field effect on surrounding cells.[50] Cells expressing EGFRvIII showed increased proliferation and also a decreased rate of apoptosis and, therefore, a selective growth and survival advantage. Further analysis of the molecular mechanisms of enhanced tumourigenicity by EGFRvIII[51] has shown that constitutively autophosphorylated mutant receptors are expressed on the cell surface, although the level of phosphorylation is much lower than that seen in ligand-stimulated wild type receptors. Introduction of a tyrosine kinase-negative mutation into EGFRvIII abolished these effects, as did mutation of any of the major intracellular autophosphorylation sites, suggesting that both the intrinsic tyrosine kinase activity and each of the autophosphorylation sites located in the regulatory C-terminus are essential for the enhanced tumourigenesis characteristic of EGFRvIII. Studies of the signalling pathways activated by the mutant receptor showed that Shc, Grb2 and Ras are involved in the enhanced mitogenesis and tumour forming potential of cells expressing the EGFRvIII receptor.[52] It is also likely that the effect of enhanced signalling by the constitutively phosphorylated receptor is amplified by a lack of signal attenuation by receptor downregulation[51,53] and a combination of these factors may contribute to enhanced tumourigenicity.

EGFRvIII receptors have a constitutive tyrosine kinase activity at a level of approximately 10% compared with the fully-activated wild-type receptor,[49] but are unable to bind ligand[49,54] and thus cannot be further activated. Higher levels of activation must then be achieved by an alternative mechanism, namely overexpression of the mutant receptor and this would perhaps explain why tumours in which EGFRvIII is detected always show amplification of the rearranged gene – presumably a low level of constitutive receptor activation is not sufficient to induce cellular transformation. This further leads to an assumption that intrinsic levels of EGFR activation in normal brain cells are low and that the levels achieved by a combination of low-level constitutive activation together with overexpression provide a selective advantage for the proliferation of cells expressing the mutant receptor. Overexpressed EGFRvIII has recently been reported to occur in many other human malignant tumours, including carcinomas of the breast, lung, kidney, ovary and cervix.[55–57] Studies have used various methods to identify and quantify the EGFRvIII gene and/or protein levels. However, individual studies have not used multiple approaches to the analysis, which would perhaps give a more complete picture of the actual involvement of amplified and/or rearranged *EGFR* in these tumours. Some evidence suggests that EGFR is not commonly overexpressed in breast tumours.[58] Of 189 tumours analysed, only 4 showed amplification of the *EGFR* gene and, of these, only one showed genomic re-arrangement. It is currently unclear, therefore, what mechanism is responsible for the reported expression of mutant receptors in such a high proportion of these tumours.

It has been reported by some authors that EGFRvIII receptors are constitutively dimeric,[53] although others have suggested that the mutant receptor is unable to dimerise.[59] If dimerisation is responsible, it could be due to disruption of the cysteine-rich sub-domain II causing abnormal folding of the extracellular domain, and producing a structure that is unable to bind ligand and yet is similar to the conformational change induced by ligand, resulting in activation via ligand-independent dimerisation. This is reminiscent of results obtained through deletion studies of the human αPDGF receptor although it is not clear that the mechanism is identical. PDGF receptors have an extracellular region which comprises 5 immunoglobulin (Ig)-like loops, and exist in α or β isoforms which can homo- or heterodimerise depending on the inducing ligand. Analysis of mutant αPDGF receptors with deletions of individual extracellular domain loops[60] showed that deletion of loop 3, which is required for PDGF binding, causes ligand-independent transformation of NIH3T3 cells and also constitutive receptor autophosphorylation in vitro and in vivo, mediated by ligand-independent receptor dimerisation. It is postulated that extracellular domain 3 of the receptor acts as a negative regulator of receptor dimerisation and that ligand-binding induces an altered conformation that releases this negative regulation, so that in αPDGFR mutants lacking loop 3 the oncogenic potential of the RTK is activated by constitutive receptor dimerisation. Alternatively, it is possible that deletion of loop 3 creates an unpaired cysteine residue causing constitutive dimerisation via the formation of covalent sulphydryl bonds between receptors, as discussed in detail below. Studies of artificially mutagenised human EGFR containing inserted regions of 20–40 hydrophilic amino acids in the extracellular and/or intracellular juxtamembrane regions[61] showed that insertion into the extracellular region results in the formation of receptors which are constitutively dimeric, phosphorylated and transforming in vitro and it is postulated that this occurs via a mechanism which allows activation through constitutive dimerisation, again either by conformational changes

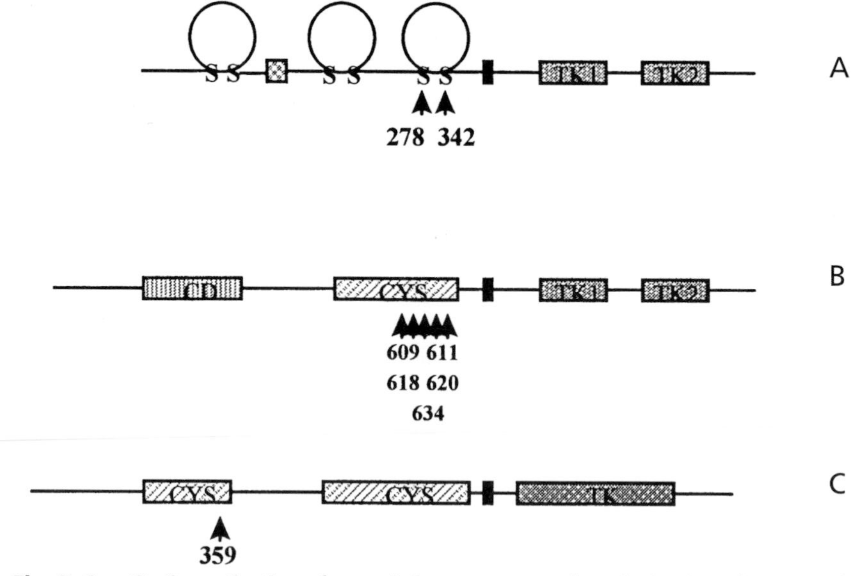

Fig. 3 Constitutive activation of growth factor receptors by substitution of conserved cysteine residues. (**A**) Crouzon, Pfeiffer and Jackson Weiss syndromes are commonly caused by mutation of one of two conserved cysteine residues in loop III of the human FGFR2 extracellular domain.[63–65] (**B**) MEN2A and FMTC syndromes commonly involve the mutation of one of 5 conserved cysteine residues close to the transmembrane region in the extracellular cysteine-rich domain of the human Ret receptor.[69–71] (**C**) An activating mutation in the *C. elegans EGFR* gene homologue, *let-23*, involves the substitution of a conserved cysteine residue in the extracellular (S1) cysteine-rich region of the receptor.[81] I, II, III – extracellular Ig-like loops in human FGFR2; CD – cadherin-like domain in human Ret receptor; CYS – cysteine-rich region; TM – transmembrane domain; TK – tyrosine kinase domain.

which result in the loss of an inhibitory effect on receptor dimerisation, or through the gain of interactions which stabilise receptor dimers.

EXTRACELLULAR DOMAIN MUTATIONS

Other types of growth factor receptors can be activated by extracellular mutations (Fig. 3). FGFR2 is a RTK with an extracellular domain containing three Ig-like loops, which has been implicated in the negative regulation of bone development.[62] Many cases of autosomal dominant Crouzon and Pfeiffer syndromes and a few reported cases of Jackson Weiss syndrome (craniosynostosis syndromes) are caused by missense point mutations in *FGFR2*, leading to the loss of one of two conserved cysteine residues (Cys278 and Cys342) which are thought to be involved in a disulphide bond that stabilises the IgIII loop structure (reviewed elsewhere[63–65]). Such mutations create an unpaired cysteine residue that is available to form an intermolecular disulphide bond (Fig. 4). Experiments have shown that mutation of either of the two equivalent cysteine residues in *Xenopus* FGFR2[66,67] results in (abnormal) ligand-independent induction of mesoderm and analysis of the mutant receptors revealed covalent homodimers which showed increased tyrosine phosphorylation and were unable to bind ligand. It would appear that

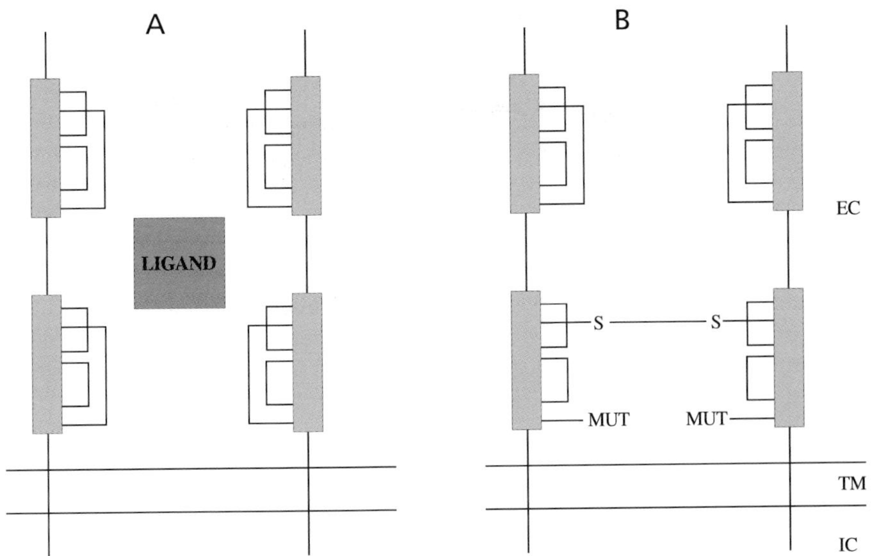

Fig. 4 Activation of growth factor receptors by induction of constitutive dimerisation due to extracellular domain mutations. (**A**) Dimerisation of wild-type receptors is induced by ligand-binding. (**B**) Loss or gain of a conserved extracellular domain cysteine residue may lead to the disruption of intramolecular disulphide bonding, leaving an unpaired cysteine residue which may be involved in aberrant disulphide bonding with other mutant receptors. MUT – mutation; EC – extracellular domain; TM – transmembrane region; IC – intracellular domain;] indicates intradomain disulphide bond.

these mutations imitate ligand binding by inducing constitutive dimerisation of the receptor. Simultaneous mutation of these two cysteine residues, however, did not result in the production of covalent dimers or in greatly enhanced mesoderm induction, which further supports the supposition that the receptors are activated by the formation of covalent dimers due to the presence of a free sulphydryl group. Crouzon and Pfeiffer syndromes may, however, also be caused by mutations or deletions involving conserved amino acid residues other than cysteine within the IgIII loop of FGFR2[63,64] and, although the mechanism has not been determined, it is possible that this causes constitutive dimerisation solely by disruption of the normal structure of the loop or due to conformational changes resulting in the creation of an unpaired cysteine residue.

Induction of constitutive dimerisation has also been suggested as the mechanism by which extracellular domain mutations activate the human Ret receptor in the multiple endocrine neoplasia type 2A (MEN2A) syndrome. The *RET* proto-oncogene encodes a membrane-spanning RTK which is involved in the differentiation and proliferation of neurectoderm-derived cells (reviewed by Pasini et al[68]). Mutations in the extracellular domain of the receptor are associated with the inherited autosomal dominant cancer syndromes MEN2A and the less severe familial medullary thyroid carcinoma (FMTC).[69,70] The vast majority of mutations identified involve substitution of one of five conserved cysteine residues (609, 611, 618, 620, 624) in the cysteine-rich extracellular domain of the protein, with the most commonly observed mutations at Cys620 and Cys634.[71] These alleles have been shown to have transforming potential due to constitutive activation of the RTK caused by the generation of disulphide bridge-stabilised Ret dimers.[72,73] This is in contrast to the transforming Ret intracellular domain mutant, (Met918Thr, seen in MEN2B) which shows constitutive activity, although receptors are monomeric. Again it is postulated that the cysteine residues, disrupted by the MEN2A mutations, are normally involved in intramolecular disulphide bonds and that mutations render the partner cysteine available for aberrant disulphide bonding with other mutant Ret molecules, creating active homodimers.[73] Further work[74] has suggested that different cysteine substitutions induce varying levels of Ret activation (mutation of Cys634 is more activating and transforming than Cys620) both in vitro and in vivo and that this correlates with a higher level of constitutive dimerisation in receptors containing the Cys634 mutation. Cys634 is most frequently affected in families with MEN2A (approximately 80% of reported cases) whilst Cys620 and Cys618 mutations are rarely associated with MEN2A, but account for approximately 60% of FMTC, and it is postulated that the increased activating capacity of Cys634 mutations accounts for their involvement in the more severe clinical phenotype, due to threshold levels of activation required to transform different cell-types. A few sporadic medullary thyroid carcinomas (MTCs) have also shown alterations in the extracellular juxtamembrane region of Ret. In-frame deletions of 6 bp and 9 bp in exon 11 of the gene have been detected, in each case encoding proteins in which Cys634 is deleted.[75–77] Two other deletions in this region did not directly involve the removal of a cysteine residue, but involved amino acids in the immediate vicinity.[78] Indeed one of these deletions encoded the removal of amino acids 632 and 633, immediately prior to Cys634 and analysis of this mutant in vitro showed a transforming capacity almost 5 times greater than that of the Cys634Arg mutant seen in many cases of MEN2A,[78] correlating with the clinical severity of the corresponding tumour. A mutation encoding Cys634Tyr has also been observed in a sporadic MTC.[75]

It is feasible that amino acid substitutions which create a functional free cysteine may be involved in activation of other human growth factor receptors and this has been supported by mutagenesis studies. Artificial mutation of the erythropoietin receptor, a member of the non-tyrosine kinase cytokine receptor family, introducing an amino acid substitution (Arg129Cys) in the extracellular domain of the receptor, caused constitutive activation through the formation of disulphide linked-dimers.[79] Activation of receptors by the stabilisation of dimers has also been described for in vitro mutagenised EGFR,[80] in which the insertion of a cysteine residue in the extracellular juxtamembrane region (between residues 618 and 619) resulted in ligand-induced covalently bonded receptor dimers which showed a significantly higher level of activity than monomers. Furthermore, an activating point mutation has been described in the *Caenorhabditis elegans EGFR* homologue, *let-23*, encoding the substitution of a conserved cysteine residue (Cys359Tyr) in extracellular domain II of the receptor[81] and resulting in development of the multivulval phenotype associated with increased stimulation of the *let-23* pathway. In vivo analysis of this mutant demonstrated activation via a ligand-independent mechanism, although expression of the equivalently mutated human *EGFR* gene in vitro showed enhanced levels of EGF-dependent tyrosine phosphorylation, but no ligand-independent dimerisation. There have been no reports, as yet, of such mutations in human *EGFR* occurring naturally, although it is likely that screening methods, which to date have focussed on the detection of amplification or gross re-arrangements of coding sequences, would not have identified them. Studies in our laboratory have, however, identified a variant human EGFR cDNA in which a single base change encodes substitution of tyrosine for a conserved cysteine residue in extracellular domain IV and in vitro studies of the encoded receptors have shown that they are unable to bind ligand and appear to be constitutively dimeric and phosphorylated (Tuzi & Gullick, unpublished observations). It is notable that, where pathological mutations encoding cysteine substitutions in other RTKs occur, the position of the altered cysteine residue appears to be important. For instance, in the case of the Ret receptor, the extracellular domain of the protein contains 28 cysteine residues, but mutations are only seen in 5 of these residues, all of which are close to the membrane-spanning region of the receptor. Likewise activating mutations in FGFR2 only seem to occur in the third Ig-like loop, which again is close to the transmembrane domain. In contrast, the activating mutation seen in the *C. elegans* let-23 receptor is in extracellular domain II (S1), although it may be that in the folded structure this region is close to the transmembrane domain. It would appear that the occurrence of mutations in a position close to the membrane allows for the productive dimerisation of receptors and, thus, by inference, the region encoding extracellular domain IV of human *EGFR* is a particular candidate for mutation screening.

TRANSMEMBRANE DOMAIN MUTATIONS

Although a highly transforming mutation (Val664Glu) has been identified in the transmembrane domain of rat erbB2 (neu) (see below), transmembrane mutations have not been observed in human EGFR. Initial reports suggested that the equivalently mutated EGFR (Val627Glu substitution, corresponding to Val664Glu in neu) is not activated or transforming at all.[82,83] However, a subsequent, more detailed, analysis[84] suggested that this mutant is partially activated, showing low levels of ligand-independent transformation and autophosphorylation, constitutive phosphorylation of SHC and MAP kinase (but not PLC-γ) and constitutive association with GRB-2. It has been suggested that the equivalent neu* mutation is not seen in human c-erbB-2 because conversion of valine to glutamic acid requires a 2 bp mutation (GTT to GAA or GAG), as discussed later. However, this is not the situation for human EGFR, where Val627 is encoded by the triplet GTG, which requires only a T to A substitution to encode glutamic acid. Furthermore, if there was a polymorphism in the wild-type sequence at this codon (GTG to GTA), this would still encode valine but would also represent a sequence that only required a further single base change to encode glutamic acid. It is not clear whether many cancers have been examined for such mutations but, if they did occur, they would potentially provide a selective advantage.

CYTOPLASMIC DOMAIN MUTATIONS

Although deletions of regions of the extracellular domain of EGFR, particularly the EGFRvIII deletion, are the most common alterations seen in human tumours, alterations of the cytoplasmic domain of the receptor have also been reported (Fig. 2). Analysis of 70 grade IV glioblastomas for amplification of *EGFR*[38] revealed that 32 (46%) contained more than 10 times the normal number of gene copies per cell. Of these, 16 also showed co-amplification of *EGFRvIII* and 8 had in-frame deletions of a 3′ region of the transcript, with 3 of the 8 cases displaying both a 3′ and 5′ alteration. The alterations in the cytoplasmic region of the receptor have a consensus region of deletion from bases 3133–3387 in the 3′ regulatory region. This deletion encompasses a region of the protein (between amino acid residues 991–1022) which is thought to be important for receptor internalisation and degradation,[85,86] thus overexpression of this mutant in glioblastomas may be functionally significant in the development of the malignancy through impaired downregulation of the receptor.

As discussed above, dual truncation of N-terminal and C-terminal sequences in v-erbB and artificially engineered into human EGFR are more transforming than deletion of the extracellular domain alone. It has been reported[38] that in a single glioma patient the first tumour biopsy showed a 3′ truncation but that at relapse the tumour now contained an amplified *EGFR* deleted at both the 3′ and 5′ ends. Presumably, this represents an original event occurring in a single cell in one copy of the 3′ deleted gene which was then amplified in that cell. Clonal expansion must then have occurred during tumour growth so that this became dominant in the population.

MUTATIONS IN *c-erbB-2*

The *c-erbB-2* proto-oncogene[87,88] encodes a 1255 amino acid transmembrane RTK with significant homology to other members of the EGFR family,[89] which is expressed as a post-translationally glycosylated 185 kDa protein. To date, no ligand has been identified for c-erbB-2, although the receptor has been shown to be very active in heterodimers with other members of the type I receptor family.[90–92] Overexpression of c-erbB-2, via a mechanism of gene amplification, has been implicated in many human tumours[18] and the significance of overexpression of the receptor in tumourigenesis has been supported by the demonstration that very high levels of expression of wild type c-erbB-2 cause transformation in vitro and tumour formation in transgenic mice.[93–96] The mechanism by which activation occurs is still uncertain although, as for EGFR, it is suggested that either overexpression alters the equilibrium towards active, dimeric forms of the receptor or it enhances the response to ligands presented by other type I receptors (or both).

Unlike *EGFR*, there have been very few, if any, reports of activating point mutations or deletions occurring in the extracellular domain of *c-erbB-2*. It is not clear why this is, but it may be that a mechanism of aberrant splicing following exon deletion, as seems likely for the *EGFR* extracellular domain deletions, produces transcripts that are in the wrong reading frame for the expression of a functional protein. It would be necessary to know the sequences surrounding each intron/exon boundary to know this, but these are not currently available. It has been shown that artificial deletions equivalent to *v-erbB*, i.e. removing almost all of the extracellular domain of *neu*[97] and *c-erbB-2*[98] are activating but it may be that similar *c-erbB-2* mutations are simply not transforming in glial cells. It would be interesting to create artificially such a deletion in *c-erbB-2* to ask if this is indeed capable of transformation.

TRANSMEMBRANE DOMAIN MUTATIONS

The highly transforming oncogene *neu**[99,100] was originally identified in a system in which treatment of pregnant rats with alkylating agents led to the development of tumours in the offspring[101–103] and the equivalent mutation has since been identified in the Syrian hamster gene[104]. *neu** differs from wild type *neu* by a single point mutation (T to A), encoding an activated form of the receptor with an amino acid substitution Val664Glu in the transmembrane domain. In parallel with activating mutations seen in EGFR, neu* resembles the ligand-stimulated receptor, showing constitutive tyrosine kinase activity, autophosphorylation and phosphorylation of cellular proteins, increased receptor dimerisation and increased receptor turnover.[105–108] It has been postulated that activation of neu* by a single amino acid change occurs by stabilisation of receptor dimerisation, due to a structural change of the transmembrane region. Studies have suggested that the specific amino acid substitution, its precise position within the primary structure of the protein and, also, the nature of the surrounding amino acids in the vicinity of Glu664, are important in activation. Various mutations at Val664 were examined[100] and both glutamic acid and glutamine were found to be equally activating, whilst aspartic acid and tyrosine were weakly activating. Substitution of glutamic acid at positions 663 or 665 did not activate the receptor, demonstrating that the location of the change is important. However, mutation of Val663 and Gly665 abolished transforming activity of the Glu664 mutant and thus the ValGluGly motif at residues 663–665 appears to be necessary for constitutive dimerisation and activation, although introduction of this motif into other regions of the transmembrane domain does not significantly enhance dimerisation or induce transformation.[109]

Two theories have been proposed as to how the structural changes caused by substitution of glutamic acid for valine may stabilise dimer formation. Sternberg and Gullick[110] suggested that a five residue sequence, Ala661–X–X–Glu664–Gly665 is involved in activation and, in this model, interhelical hydrogen bonds are formed either between pairs of protonated glutamic acid side chains or between the Glu664 carboxylic acid side chain and the peptide backbone carbonyl group of Ala661 in the second monomer (Fig. 5). The small side chains of Gly665 are required to allow close helix packing. Recent biophysical studies[111] and structural modelling[112] have provided support for this model. An alternative model[113] is based on minimum energy calculations for conformation of the wild-type and mutant transmembrane regions and suggests that the wild-type receptor shows a sharp bend at positions 664–665, whilst the corresponding region in neu* is straight, allowing packing of α-helices to occur. The structure of synthetic peptides determined by NMR representing the wild-type or mutant sequence did not, however, show any tendency for a distorted helix in this region.[114]

Theories of neu* activation centre on the stimulation of constitutive dimerisation as the first step in activation of the receptor and it has been shown

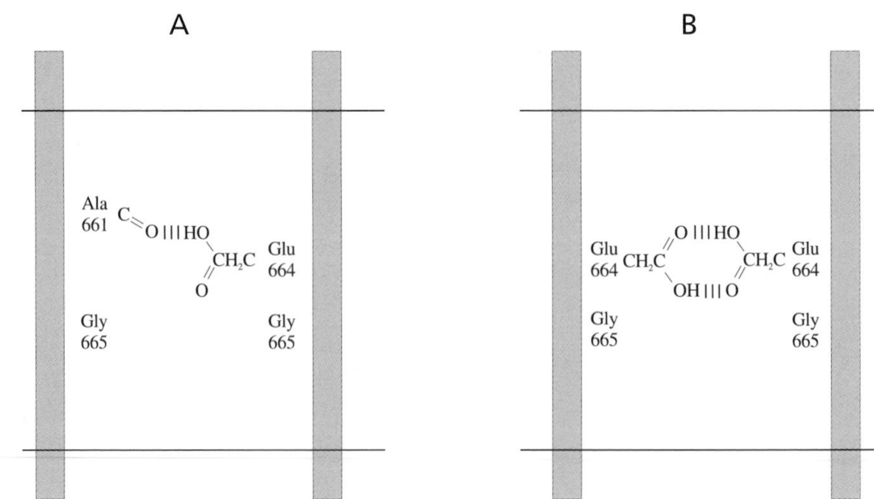

Fig. 5 Substitution of glutamic acid for valine at residue 664 of the rat neu receptor leads to constitutive dimerisation via the formation of inter-receptor hydrogen bonds in the transmembrane region.[110–112] **(A)** It is possible that interhelical hydrogen bonds are formed between a Glu664 side chain and the peptide backbone carbonyl group of Ala661, or **(B)** between pairs of Glu664 side chains. In either case the small side chains of Gly665 allow close helix packing to occur.

that activated receptors are constitutively dimeric.[108,109] However, other studies have suggested that dimerisation of receptors is necessary, but not sufficient, for activation *per se*. Introduction of a well-characterised dimerisation motif from the transmembrane region of glycophorin A into the transmembrane region of neu and neu* in both cases produced receptors which showed a high level of constitutive dimerisation, but only those with the Val664Glu mutation were transforming.[109] Thus, dimerisation of the receptor alone does not appear to be sufficient for transformation to occur. Interpretation of this evidence suggests that, as well as the formation of dimers, the geometry with which receptors pack is crucial to their ability to cross-phosphorylate and activate one another and for the binding of substrates and other interacting proteins.

Analysis of human tumours for the presence of activating point mutations in the *c-erbB-2* transmembrane-encoding region has proved negative[115–120] and it is likely that the lack of occurrence of the equivalent *neu** mutation in human *c-erbB-2* is due to the necessity for a 2 bp change (GTT to GAA or GAG).[116] However, artificial introduction of the equivalent mutation into human *c-erbB-2* (at codon 659) has been shown to cause cell transformation in vitro and tumourigenesis in vivo.[106] This observation is an example of the theoretical premise that a polymorphism (silent or specifying alternative amino acids) in an oncogene at a critical position might alter an individual's susceptibility to cancer. If each base change had a mutation frequency of (say) 10^{-6}, the risk in one individual where two changes are required would be a million-fold less than in a person with a different codon usage, where a single base change would result in a transforming amino acid substitution. This, of course, presumes that mutation rate is important in the incidence of cancer which is currently a matter of debate. In principle, this could be tested in animals by altering their codon usage and observing their cancer incidence in the chemical carcinogenesis model.

Activating transmembrane mutations have also been identified in other human growth factor receptors. Approximately 97% of cases of achondroplasia (dwarfism) in humans are caused by missense mutations encoding a single amino acid change (Gly380Arg) in the transmembrane region of FGFR3,[121,122] a RTK which is thought to act as a negative regulator of long-bone growth in chondrocytes.[123,124] This mutation is in an analogous position to the Val664Glu mutation in neu* and has also been shown to induce ligand-independent kinase activity of the receptor.[125,126] In addition, the Gly380Arg mutation causes activation of neu when the mutated transmembrane region of FGFR3 is substituted for the equivalent segment of neu.[126] A few cases of achondroplasia are caused by mutations encoding an amino acid substitution Gly375Cys in the TM region of FGFR3[127,128] and it has been suggested that both the Gly380Arg and this mutation result in the formation of hydrogen-bonded dimers between α-helices.[64] By contrast, mutations involving the gain of a cysteine residue at the extracellular/transmembrane domain junction of FGFR3 (amino acids 370, 371, 373) have been identified in the lethal thanatophoric dysplasia type I and it is suggested that the more severe phenotype caused by these mutations is due to the formation of stronger, disulphide-bonded dimers,[64] although it is also possible that the gain of a cysteine at position 375 leads to inter-receptor disulphide bond formation, but in a less productive configuration than at the transmembrane domain border.

EXTRACELLULAR DOMAIN MUTATIONS

Recent studies on the induction of mammary tumours in mice provide evidence that extracellular domain mutations which promote receptor dimerisation are likely to be involved in the activation of the rat *neu* proto-oncogene.[129,130] Transgenic mice expressing wild-type neu under the control of the MMTV promoter develop mammary tumours after a period of latency, which suggests that additional genetic events occur during this period. Analysis of the neu receptors expressed in these tumours showed increased tyrosine kinase activity and phosphorylation of several cellular proteins, without receptor overexpression. *neu* genes isolated from these tumours were analysed for the *neu** transmembrane mutation and although this was not observed, small deletions were identified in the extracellular, membrane-proximal region of the gene. Of 34 tumours analysed from 4 different transgenic lines, 22 (65%) showed in-frame deletions of 21–36 bp (7–12 amino acids). The majority of the deletions that were identified involved the loss of one of five conserved cysteine residues proximal to the transmembrane domain and it was hypothesised that this may leave an unpaired cysteine residue capable of forming a covalent interaction with another receptor. (Of the deletions that did not remove a conserved cysteine residue, one encoded a 3 amino acid insertion between 2 conserved cysteine residues and another the deletion of a conserved proline next to a conserved cysteine, both of which may well disrupt Cys-Cys pairing in the extracellular domain of the receptor). Expression of receptors containing such deletions in vitro showed enhanced catalytic activity, transformation levels of 18–56% compared with neu* in focus formation assays and levels of stable dimer formation which correlated with transforming activity. In order to test the significance of cysteine residue loss, point mutations encoding substitution of serine for 3 of the conserved cysteine residues involved (Cys 635, 639 and 647) were introduced separately into wild type *neu*. The Cys635 and 647 mutants were constitutively dimeric and these constructs also induced tumour formation in transgenic mice with a shorter latency period than wild type *neu*. However, the Cys639Ser mutant was only very weakly transforming and mostly monomeric, suggesting that disruption of amino acid spacing is also involved in the altered properties of deletion mutants which have lost this residue. It is interesting that the results obtained by analysis of this animal model and in subsequently engineered molecules are very reminiscent of the types of mutations discussed above which are characteristic of the MEN2A syndrome involving the Ret receptor.

To date, there is no evidence of activating point mutations or deletions in the extracellular domain of human *c-erbB-2*. Artificial introduction of a cysteine residue into the transmembrane-proximal extracellular region of human c-erbB-2[131] resulted in the formation of stable dimers, but mutants did not show increased transforming potential, further supporting evidence from studies of artificial transmembrane mutants that constitutively dimeric receptors must also have a particular geometry in order to be activated. Again, it is possible that were such mutations to occur in human *c-erbB-2* they may not be detected by screening methods which have been used to date.

MUTATIONS IN *c-erbB-3* AND *c-erbB-4*

The human *c-erbB-3* gene[132,133] encodes a 1342 amino acid sequence which is expressed as a 180 kDa, post-translationally glycosylated protein in human cells. Gene targeting studies have shown that homozygous *c-erbB-3*-deficient mice have defective development of the peripheral nervous system, and in particular in the growth and development of Schwann cells.[134] c-erbB-3 is unusual amongst tyrosine kinases in that two normally conserved amino acid residues are different (His740 and Asn815 instead of glutamate and aspartate, respectively). It has been shown that mutation of the equivalent aspartic acid residue in other tyrosine kinase receptors reduces or abolishes kinase activity[135,136] and analyses of c-erbB-3 have shown that it has a defective tyrosine kinase which has at most only 1% of 'normal' kinase activity.[137] Simple mutation of these two residues to the consensus sequence was not sufficient to restore kinase activity.[138] In contrast to EGFR and c-erbB-2, and perhaps as a consequence of negligible levels of receptor tyrosine kinase activity, overexpression of c-erbB-3 alone is not transforming in NIH3T3 cells,[139] although overexpression is transforming if moderate levels of c-erbB-2 are co-expressed indicating that c-erbB-3 has the potential for involvement in tumour formation.[140] Preliminary studies have identified variable levels of c-erbB-3 overexpression in a range of human tumours (reviewed by Gullick[19]), but gene amplification has not been detected and it would appear that increased expression occurs via a mechanism of increased gene transcription.[141] Indeed, in a recent major study of gene amplification in breast cancer, only one case in a series of 1365 tumours appeared to be amplified at the *c-erbB-3* locus.[142]

The human *c-erbB-4* gene encodes a protein of 1283 amino acids which is post-translationally glycosylated to give a product of molecular weight 180 kDa.[143] Although the cytoplasmic domain of the receptor shows almost 80% homology with EGFR and c-erbB-2, the extracellular domain is most similar to c-erbB-3. Studies of c-erbB-4 are in their infancy. It has been shown that ligand-mediated activation of the receptor in vitro induces autophosphorylation on tyrosine[144] and association with PI 3-kinase and cell chemotaxis.[145] However, in this study, activation did not lead to cellular proliferation whereas others have reported that it does, although it is possible that this was because the NIH3T3 cells employed in the latter study expressed low levels of EGF receptors in addition to c-erbB-4.[146] Studies of *c-erbB-4* knockout mice have shown that the protein is important in the development of cardiac muscle and in neural development.[147] Analysis of c-erbB-4 mRNA and protein expression in human tumours has shown loss of expression in most tumours,[17,21] although a few tumours show overexpression[17,148] and a combination of c-erbB-4 with c-erbB-2 appears to correlate with increased tumour aggressiveness and poor prognosis in some brain tumours.[20] To date the mechanisms of altered *c-erbB-4* expression have not been investigated and the occurrence of gene amplification or re-arrangement have not been examined. However, two splice variants of human c-erbB-4 have recently been described, which differ by the insertion of either 23 or 13 alternative amino acids in the extracellular juxtamembrane region and show tissue-specific differential expression.[149] This observation has been related to the report that the c-erbB-4 protein can be cleaved to release a soluble extracellular domain as a result of protein kinase C-mediated proteolysis.[150] The 23 amino acid form (termed JM-a) was sensitive to proteolysis whereas the 13 amino acid form (JM-b) was not.[149] In addition, although not yet published in full, it is apparent that another site of splicing occurs in the cytoplasmic domain alternatively including or not a 16 amino acid sequence containing the receptor's single site capable of interacting with PI 3-kinase. The presence of alternatively spliced transcripts should be taken into consideration when screening for mutant transcripts in tumours.

To date, activating mutations of *c-erbB-3* or *c-erbB-4* have not been described, although studies of these genes and the receptors which they express are very limited. However, as it is likely that the normal function of these receptors is in cellular differentiation, rather than proliferation, it is perhaps less likely that activating mutations of these two genes will be seen in human pathology.

CONCLUSIONS

Activation of a receptor may be achieved through a limited number of mechanisms, such as increased or constitutive dimerisation, direct activation of the tyrosine kinase catalytic function, alteration of regions involved in the determination of substrate specificity or in receptor internalisation and/or degradation. It is, however, possible to achieve these effects in a number of ways, which may involve overexpression of the normal protein product and/or structural alteration(s) creating an abnormal protein. Normal activation of receptors is postulated to be initiated by ligand-induced dimerisation, but activation may also be achieved by overexpression of receptors which, it is suggested, leads to an increase in the level of receptor dimers. Constitutive dimerisation also occurs via a number of structural alterations which increase the affinity of receptors for one another, for example major deletions of all or part of the extracellular domain, creation of covalently bonded receptor dimers through unpaired sulphydryl groups (*C. elegans* EGF receptor, human FGFR2 and Ret receptors), or stabilisation of dimers through non-covalent interactions (hydrogen bonding in rat neu* and human FGFR3). The pathological activation of type I growth factor receptors in human tumours has been studied in most detail for EGFR and c-erbB-2. It is interesting that, although in both cases activation appears to occur mainly through increased stimulation of receptor dimerisation, in the case of the EGFR this may be achieved by overexpression with or without structural mutation, whilst many tumours show c-erbB-2 overexpression but few structural mutations have been identified. The reasons for this are not known.

REFERENCES

1. Yarden Y, Schlessinger J. Epidermal growth factor induces rapid, reversible aggregation of the purified epidermal growth factor receptor. Biochemistry 1987; 26: 1443–1451
2. Yarden Y, Schlessinger J. Self-phosphorylation of epidermal growth factor receptor: evidence for a model of intermolecular allosteric activation. Biochemistry 1987; 26: 1434–1442
3. Ullrich A, Coussens L, Hayflick JS et al. Human epidermal growth factor receptor cDNA sequence and aberrant expression of the amplified gene in A431 epidermoid carcinoma cells. Nature 1984; 309: 418–425
4. Pawson T. Protein modules and signalling networks. Nature 1995; 373: 573–580
5. van der Geer P, Pawson T. The PTB domain: a new protein module implicated in signal transduction. Trends Biochem Sci 1995; 20: 277–280
6. Schlessinger J. Signal transduction by allosteric receptor oligomerization. Trends Biochem Sci 1988; 13: 443–447
7. Gullick WJ. A new model for the interaction of EGF-like ligands with their receptors: the new one-two. Eur J Cancer 1994; 30 (Suppl A): 2186
8. Tzahar E, Pinkas-Kramarski R, Moyer JD et al. Bivalence of EGF-like ligands drives the ErbB signaling network. EMBO J 1997; 16: 4938–4950
9. Lohermeyer M, Gullick WJ. Mutational activation of receptor tyrosine kinases. In: Dickson RB, Salomon DS. (eds). Hormones and Growth Factors in Development and Neoplasia. New York: Wiley-Liss, 1997; 289–309
10. Lax I, Bellot F, Howk R, Ullrich A, Givol D, Schlessinger J. Functional analysis of the ligand binding site of EGF-receptor utilizing chimeric chicken/human receptor molecules. EMBO J 1989; 8: 421–427
11. Wu DG, Wang LH, Sato GH et al. Human epidermal growth factor (EGF) receptor sequence recognized by EGF competitive monoclonal antibodies. Evidence for the localization of the EGF-binding site. J Biol Chem 1989; 264: 17469–17475
12. Lax I. Bellot F, Honegger AM et al. Domain deletion in the extracellular portion of the EGF-receptor reduces ligand binding and impairs cell surface expression. Cell Reg 1990; 1: 173–188
13. Lax I, Fischer R, Ng C et al. Noncontiguous regions in the extracellular domain of EGF receptor define ligand-binding specificity. Cell Reg 1991; 2: 337–345
14. Schlessinger J. Mutational analysis of the epidermal growth factor-receptor kinase. Biochem Soc Symp 1990; 56: 13–19

15. Ward CW, Hoyne PA, Flegg RH. Insulin and epidermal growth factor receptors contain the cysteine repeat motif found in the tumour necrosis factor receptor. Proteins 1995; 22: 141–153
16. Prigent SA, Lemoine NR, Hughes CM, Plowman GD, Selden C, Gullick WJ. Expression of the c-*erb*B-3 protein in normal human adult and fetal tissues. Oncogene 1992; 7: 1273–1278
17. Srinivasan R, Poulsom R, Hurst HC, Gullick WJ. Expression of the c-erbB-4/HER4 protein and mRNA in normal human foetal and adult tissues and in a sample survey of nine solid tumour types. J Pathol 1997; In press
18. Salomon DS, Brandt R, Ciardiello F, Normanno N. Epidermal growth factor-related peptides and their receptors in human malignancies. Crit Rev Oncol Hematol 1995; 19: 183–232
19. Gullick WJ. The c-erbB3/HER3 receptor in human cancer. Cancer Surveys 1997; 27: 339–349
20. Gilbertson RJ, Perry RH, Kelly PJ, Pearson ADJ, Lunec J. Prognostic significance of HER2 and HER4 coexpression in childhood medulloblastoma. Cancer Res 1997, 57, 3272–3280
21. Lyne JC, Melhem MF, Finley GG et al. Tissue expression of Neu differentiation factor/heregulin and its receptor complex in prostate cancer and its biologic effects on prostate cancer cells in vitro. Cancer J Sci Am 1997; 3: 21–30
22. Downward J, Yarden Y, Mayes E et al. Close similarity of epidermal growth factor receptor and v-erb-B oncogene protein sequences. Nature 1984; 307: 521–527
23. Gillmore T, DeClue JE, Martin GS. Protein phosphorylation at tyrosine is induced by the v-*erbB* gene product in vivo and in vitro. Cell 1985; 40: 609–618
24. Kris RM, Lax, I, Gullick W et al. Antibodies against a synthetic peptide as a probe for the kinase activity of the avian EGF receptor and v-erbB protein. Cell 1985; 40: 619–625
25. Pelley RJ, Moscovici C, Hughes S, Kung HJ. Proviral-activated *c-erbB* is leukemogenic but not sarcomagenic: characterization of a replication-competent retrovirus containing the activated *c-erbB*. J Virol 1988; 62: 1840–1844
26. Carter TH, Kung H-J. Tissue-specific transformation by oncogenic mutants of epidermal growth factor receptor. Crit Rev Oncog 1994; 5: 389–428
27. Adelsman MA, Huntley BK, Maihle NJ. Ligand-independent dimerization of oncogenic v-erbB products involves covalent interactions. J Virol 1996; 70: 2533–2544
28. Di Fiore PP, Pierce JH, Fleming TP et al. Overexpression of the human EGF receptor confers an EGF-dependent transformed phenotype to NIH-3T3 cells. Cell 1987; 15: 1063–1070
29. Velu TJ, Beguinot L, Vass WC et al. Epidermal growth factor-dependent transformation by a human EGF receptor proto-oncogene. Science 1987; 238: 1408–1410
30. Reidel H, Massoglia S, Schlessinger J, Ullrich A. Ligand activation of overexpressed EGF receptors transforms NIH-3T3 mouse fibroblasts. Proc Natl Acad Sci USA 1988; 85: 1477–1481
31. Sugawa N, Ekstrand AJ, James CD, Collins VP. Identical splicing of aberrant epidermal growth factor receptor transcripts from amplified rearranged genes in human glioblastomas. Proc Natl Acad Sci USA 1990; 87: 8602–8606
32. Wong AJ, Ruppert JM, Bigner SH et al. Structural alterations of the epidermal growth factor receptor gene in human gliomas. Proc Natl Acad Sci USA 1992; 89: 2965–2969
33. Humphrey PA, Wong AJ, Vogelstein B et al. Amplification and expression of the epidermal growth factor receptor gene in human glioma xenografts. Cancer Res 1988; 48: 2231–2238
34. Kwatra MM, Bigner DD, Cohn JA. The ligand binding domain of the epidermal growth factor receptor is not required for receptor dimerization. Biochim Biophys Acta 1992; 1134: 178–181
35. Khazaie K, Dull TJ, Graf T et al. Truncation of the human EGF receptor leads to differential transforming potentials in primary avian fibroblasts and erythroblasts. EMBO J 1988; 7: 3067–3071
36. Haley JD, Hsuan JJ, Waterfield MD. Analysis of mammalian fibroblast transformation by normal and mutated human EGF receptors. Oncogene 1989; 4: 273–283
37. Humphrey PA, Gangarosa LM, Wong AJ et al. Deletion-mutant epidermal growth factor receptor in human gliomas: effect of type II mutation on receptor function. Biochem Biophys Res Commun 1991; 178: 1413–1420

38. Ekstrand AJ, Sugawa N, James CD, Collins VP. Amplified and rearranged epidermal growth factor receptor genes in human glioblastomas reveal deletions of sequences encoding portions of the N- and/or C-terminal tails. Proc Natl Acad Sci USA 1992; 89 4309–4313
39. Libermann TA, Nusbaum HR, Razon N et al. Amplification, enhanced expression and possible rearrangement of EGF receptor gene in primary human brain tumours of glial origin. Nature 1985; 313: 144–147
40. Ekstrand AJ, James CD, Cavenee WK, Seliger B, Petterson RF, Collins VP. Genes for epidermal growth factor receptor, transforming growth factor (, and epidermal growth factor and their expression in human gliomas in vivo. Cancer Res 1991; 51: 2164–2172
41. Schlegel J, Stumm G, Brandle K et al. Amplification and differential expression of members of the *erbB*-gene family in human glioblastoma. J Neurooncol 1994; 22: 210–217
42. Olson JJ, Hames CD, Krisht A, Barnett D, Hunter S. Analysis of epidermal growth factor receptor gene amplification and alteration in sterotactic biopsies of brain tumours. Neurosurgery 1995; 36: 740–748
43. Schwechheimer K, Huang S, Cavenee WK. EGFR gene amplification-rearrangement in human glioblastomas. Int J Cancer 1995; 62: 145–148
44. Hurtt MR, Moossy J, Donovan PM, Locker J. Amplification of epidermal growth factor receptor gene in gliomas: histopathology and prognosis. J Neuropathol Exp Neurol 1992; 51: 84–90
45. Schlegel J, Merdes A, Stumm G et al. Amplification of the epidermal-growth-factor-receptor gene correlates with different growth behaviour in human glioblastoma. Int J Cancer 1994; 56: 72–77
46. Wong AJ, Bigner SH, Bigner DD, Kinzler KW, Hamilton SR, Vogelstein B. Increased expression of the epidermal growth factor receptor gene in malignant gliomas is invariably associated with gene amplification. Proc Natl Acad Sci USA 1987; 68: 6899–6903
47. Bigner SH, Humphrey PA, Wong AJ et al. Characterization of the epidermal growth factor receptor in human glioma cell lines and xenografts. Cancer Res 1990; 50: 8017–8122
48. Nishikawa R, Ji X-D, Harmon RC et al. A mutant epidermal growth factor receptor, common in human glioma, confers enhanced tumorigenicity. Proc Natl Acad Sci USA 1994; 91: 7727–7731
49. Hills D, Rowlinson-Busza G, Gullick WJ. Specific targeting of a mutant, activated EGF receptor found in glioblastoma using a monoclonal antibody. Int J Cancer 1995; 63: 537–543
50. Nagane M, Coufal F, Lin H, Bogler O, Cavenee WK, Huang H-JS. A common mutant epidermal growth factor receptor confers enhanced tumorigenicity on human glioblastoma cells by increasing proliferation and reducing apoptosis. Cancer Res 1996; 56: 5079–5086
51. Huang H-J Su Nagane M, Klingbeil CK et al. The enhanced tumourigenic activity of a mutant epidermal growth factor receptor common in human cancers is mediated by threshold levels of constitutive tyrosine phosphorylation and unattenuated signalling. J Biol Chem 1997; 272: 2927–2935
52. Prigent SA, Nagane M, Lin H et al. Enhanced tumorigenic behavior of glioblastoma cells expressing truncated epidermal growth factor receptor is mediated through the Ras-Shc-Grb2 pathway. J Biol Chem 1996; 271: 25639–25645
53. Moscatello DK, Montgomery RB, Sundareshan P, McDanel H, Wong MY, Wong AJ. Transformation and altered signal transduction by a naturally occurring mutant EGF receptor. Oncogene 1996; 13: 85–96
54. Ekstrand AJ, Longo N, Hamid ML et al. Functional characterization of an EGF receptor with a truncated extracellular domain expressed in glioblastomas with EGFR gene amplification. Oncogene 1994; 9: 2313–2320
55. Garcia de Palazzo IE, Adams GP, Sundareshan P et al. Expression of mutated epidermal growth factor receptor by non-small cell lung carcinomas. Cancer Res 1993; 53: 3217–3220
56. Moscatello DK, Holgado-Madruga M, Godwin AK et al. Frequent expression of a mutant epidermal growth factor receptor in multiple human tumors. Cancer Res 1995; 55: 5536–5539
57. Wikstrand CJ, Hale LP, Batra SK et al. Monoclonal antibodies against EGFRvIII are tumor specific and react with breast and lung carcinomas and malignant gliomas. Cancer Res 1995; 55: 3140–3148

58. Slamon DJ, Clark GM, Wong ST, Levin WJ, Ullrich A, McGuire WL. Human breast cancer: correlation of relapse and survival with amplification of the HER-2/*neu* oncogene. Science 1987; 235: 177–182
59. Chu CT, Everiss KD, Wikstrand CJ, Batras SK, Kung H-J, Bigner DD. Receptor dimerization is not a factor in the signalling activity of a transforming variant epidermal growth factor receptor (EGFRvIII). Biochem J 1997; 324: 855–861
60. Uren A, Yu JC, Karcaaltincaba M, Pierce JH, Heidaran MA. Oncogenic activation of the alphaPDGFR defines a domain that negatively regulates receptor dimerization. Oncogene 1997; 14: 157–162
61. Sorokin A. Activation of the EGF receptor by insertional mutations in its juxtamembrane regions. Oncogene 1995; 11: 1531–1540
62. Peters KG, Werner S, Chen G, Williams LT. Two FGF receptor genes are differentially expressed in epithelial and mesenchymal tissues during limb formation and organogenesis in the mouse. Development 1992; 114: 233–243
63. Lewanda AF, Meyers GA, Jabs EW. Craniosynostosis and skeletal dysplasias: fibroblast growth factor receptor defects. Proc Assoc Am Physicians 1996; 108: 19–24
64. Webster MK, Donoghue DJ. FGFR activation in skeletal disorders: too much of a good thing. Trends Genet 1997; 13: 178–182
65. Tartaglia M, Dirocco C, Lajeunie E, Valeri S, Velardi F, Battaglia P-A. Jackson-Weiss-syndrome – identification of 2 novel FGFR2 missense mutations shared with Crouzon and Pfeiffer craniosynostotic disorders. Hum Genet 1997; 101: 47–50
66. Neilson KM, Friesel RE. Constitutive activation of fibroblast growth factor receptor-2 by a point mutation associated with Crouzon syndrome. J Biol Chem 1995; 270: 26037–26040
67. Neilson KM, Friesel R. Ligand-independent activation of fibroblast growth factor receptors by point mutations in the extracellular, transmembrane and kinase domains. J Biol Chem 1996; 271: 25049–25057
68. Pasini B, Ceccherini I, Romeo G. *RET* mutations in human disease. Trends Genet 1996; 12: 138–145
69. Donis-Keller H, Dou S, Chi D et al. Mutations in the *RET* proto-oncogene are associated with MEN2A and FMTC. Hum Mol Genet 1993; 2: 851–856
70. Mulligan LM, Kwok JBJ, Healey CS et al. Germ-line mutations of the *RET* proto-oncogene in multiple endocrine neoplasia type 2A. Nature 1993; 363: 458–460
71. Ponder BA, Smith D. The MEN II syndromes and the role of the ret proto-oncogene. Adv Cancer Res 1996; 70: 179–222
72. Asai N, Iwashita T, Matsuyama M, Takahashi M. Mechanism of activation of the *ret* proto-oncogene by multiple endocrine neoplasia 2A mutations. Mol Cell Biol 1995; 15: 1613–1619
73. Santoro M, Carlomagno F, Romano A et al. Activation of *RET* as a dominant transforming gene by germline mutations of MEN2A and MEN 2B. Science 1995; 267: 381–383
74. Carlomagno F, Salvatore G, Cirafici AM et al. The different *RET*-activating capability of mutations of cysteine 620 or cysteine 634 correlates with the multiple endocrine neoplasia type 2 disease phenotype. Cancer Res 1997; 57: 391–395
75. Kimura T, Yoshimoto K, Yokogoshi Y, Saito S. Mutations in the cysteine-rich region of the *RET* proto-oncogene in patients diagnosed as having sporadic medullary thyroid carcinoma. Endocr J 1995; 42: 517–525
76. Alemi M, Lucad SD, Sallstrom JF, Akerstrom G, Wilander E. A novel deletion in the *RET* proto-oncogene found in sporadic medullary thyroid carcinoma. Anticancer Res 1996; 16: 2619–2622
77. Alemi M, Lucas SD, Sallstrom JF, Bergholm U, Akerstrom G, Wilander E. A complex nine base pair deletion in RET exon 11 common in sporadic medullary thyroid carcinoma. Oncogene 1997; 14: 2041–2045
78. Ceccherini I, Pasini B, Pacini F et al. Somatic in frame deletions not involving juxtamembranous cysteine residues strongly activate the *RET* proto-oncogene. Oncogene 1997; 14: 2609–2612
79. Watowich SS, Yoshimura A, Longmore GD, Hilton DJ, Yoshimura Y, Lodish HF. Homodimerization and constitutive activation of the erythropoietin receptor. Proc Natl Acad Sci USA 1992; 89: 2140–2144

80. Sorokin A, Lemmon MA, Ullrich A, Schlessinger J. Stabilization of an active dimeric form of the epidermal growth factor receptor by introduction of an inter-receptor disulphide bond. J Biol Chem 1994; 269: 9752–9759
81. Katz WS, Lesa GM, Yannoukakos D, Clandinin TR, Schlessinger J, Sternberg PW. A point mutation in the extracellular domain activates LET-23, the *Caenorhabditis elegans* epidermal growth factor receptor homolog. Mol Cell Biol 1996; 16: 529–537
82. Kashles O, Szapary D, Bellot F, Ullrich A, Schlessinger J, Schmidt A. Ligand-induced stimulation of epidermal growth factor receptor mutants with altered transmembrane regions. Proc Natl Acad Sci USA 1988; 85: 9567–9571
83. Carpenter CD, Ingraham HA, Cochet C et al. Structural analysis of the transmembrane domain of the epidermal growth factor receptor. J Biol Chem 1991; 266: 5750–5755
84. Miloso M, Mazzotti M, Vass WC, Beguinot L. SHC and GRB-2 are constitutively activated by an epidermal growth factor receptor with a point mutation in the transmembrane domain. J Biol Chem 1995; 270: 19557–19562
85. Chen WS, Lazar CS, Lund KA et al. Functional independence of the epidermal growth factor receptor from a domain required for ligand-induced internalization and calcium regulation. Cell 1989; 59: 33–43
86. Wells A, Welsh JB, Lazar CS, Wiley HS, Gill GM, Rosenfeld MG. Ligand-induced transformation by a noninternalizing epidermal growth factor receptor. Science 1990; 247: 962–964
87. King CR, Draus MH, Di Fiore PP, Paik S, Kasprzyk PG. Implications of *erbB-2* overexpression for basic science and clinical medicine. Semin Cancer Biol 1985; 1: 329–227
88. Coussens L, Yang-Feng TL, Liao YC et al. Tyrosine kinase receptor with extensive homology to EGF receptor shares chromosomal location with *neu* oncogene. Science 1985; 230: 1132–1139
89. Ullrich A, Schlessinger J. Signal transduction by receptors with tyrosine kinase activity. Cell 1990; 61: 203–212
90. Riese DJ, van Raaij TM, Plowman GD, Andrews GC, Stern DF. The cellular response to neuregulins is governed by complex interactions of the erbB receptor family. Mol Cell Biol 1995; 15: 5770–5776
91. Tzahar E, Waterman H, Chen X et al. A hierarchical network of interreceptor interactions determines signal transduction by *Neu* differentiation factor/neuregulin and epidermal growth factor. Mol Cell Biol 1996; 16: 5276–5287
92. Graus-Porta D, Beerli RR, Daly JM, Hynes NE. ErbB-2, the preferred heterodimerization partner of all ErbB receptors, is a mediator of lateral signaling. EMBO J 1997; 16: 1647–1655
93. Di Fiore PP, Pierce JH, Draus MH, Segatto O, King CR, Aaronson A. *erb*-B2 is a potent oncogene when overexpressed in NIH/3T3 cells. Science 1987; 237: 178–182
94. Hudziak RMJ, Schlessinger J, Ullrich A. Increased expression of the putative growth factor receptor p185 *HER2* causes transformation and tumorigenesis of NIH3T3 cells. Proc Natl Acad Sci USA 1987; 84: 7159–7163
95. Guy CT, Webster MA, Schaller M, Parsons TJ, Cardiff RD, Muller WJ. Expression of the *neu* protooncogene in the mammary epithelium of transgenic mice induces metastatic disease. Proc Natl Acad Sci USA 1992; 89: 10578–10582
96. Baasner S, von Melchner H, Klenner T, Hilgard P, Beckers T. Reversible tumorigenesis in mice by conditional expression of the HER2/c-*erb*B2 receptor tyrosine kinase. Oncogene 1996; 13: 901–911
97. Bargmann CI, Weinberg RA. Oncogenic activation of the *neu*-encoded receptor protein by point mutation and deletion. EMBO J 1988; 7: 2043–2052
98. Di Fiore PP, Segatto O, Taylor WG, Aaronson SA, Pierce JH. EGF receptor and *erb*B-2 tyrosine kinase domains confer cell specificity for mitogenic signaling. Science 1990; 248: 79–83
99. Bargmann CI, Hung MC, Weinberg RA. The *neu* oncogene encodes an epidermal growth factor receptor-related protein. Nature 1986; 319: 226–230
100. Bargmann CI, Hung MC, Weinberg RA. Multiple independent activations of the *neu* oncogene by a point mutation altering the transmembrane domain of p185. Cell 1986; 45: 649–657
101. Schubert D, Heinemann S, Carlisle W et al. Clonal cell lines from the rat central nervous system. Nature 1974; 249: 224–227

102. Rajewski MF, Augenlicht LH, Biessman H et al. Nervous system specific carcinogenesis by ethylnitrosourea in the rat: molecular and cellular aspects. In: Haitt H, Watson J, Winsten J. (eds). Origins of Human Cancer. New York: Cold Spring Haror Laboratory, 1977; 708–726
103. Shih C, Padhy LC, Murray M, Weinberg RA. Transforming genes of carcinomas and neuroblastomas introduced into mouse fibroblasts. Nature 1981; 290: 261–264
104. Nakamura T, Ushijima T, Ishizaka Y et al. Cloning and activation of the Syrian hamster *neu* proto-oncogene. Gene 1994; 140: 251–255
105. Bargmann CI, Weinberg RA. Increased tyrosine kinase activation associated with the protein encoded by the activated *neu* oncogene. Proc Natl Acad Sci USA 1988; 85: 5394–5398
106. Segatto O, King CR, Pierce JH, Di Fiore PP, Aaronson SA. Different structural alterations upregulate in vitro tyrosine kinase activity and transforming potency of the *erbB-2* gene. Mol Cell Biol 1988; 8: 5570–5574
107. Stern DF, Kamps MP, Cao H. Oncogenic activation of p185 stimulates tyrosine phosphorylation in vivo. Mol Cell Biol 1988; 8: 3969–3973
108. Weiner DB, Liu J, Cohen JA, Williams WV, Greene MI. A point mutation in the *neu* oncogene mimics ligand induction of receptor aggregation. Nature 1989; 229: 230–231
109. Burke CL, Lemmon MA, Coren BA, Engelman DM, Stern DF. Dimerization of the $p185^{neu}$ transmembrane domain is necessary but not sufficient for transformation. Oncogene 1997; 14: 687–696
110. Sternberg MJE, Gullick WJ. Neu receptor dimerization. Nature 1989; 339: 587
111. Smith SO, Smith CS, Bormann BJ. Strong hydrogen bonding interactions involving a buried glutamic acid in the transmembrane sequence of the neu/erbB-2 receptor. Nat Struct Biol 1996; 3: 252–258
112. Garnier N, Genest D, Duneau JP, Genest M. Molecular modeling of c-erbB2 receptor dimerization: coiled-coil structure of wild and oncogenic transmembrane domains – stabilization by interhelical hydrogen bonds in the oncogenic form. Biopolymers 1997; 42: 157–168
113. Brandt-Rauf PW, Rackovsky S, Pincus MR. Correlation of the structure of the transmembrane domain of the *neu* oncogene-encoded p185 protein with its function. Proc Natl Acad Sci USA 1990; 87: 8660–8664
114. Gullick WJ, Bottomley AC, Lofts FJ et al. Three dimensional structure of the transmembrane region of the proto-oncogenic and oncogenic forms of the *neu* protein. EMBO J 1992; 11: 43–48
115. Hall PA, Hughes CM, Staddon SL, Richman PI, Gullick WJ, Lemoine NR. The *c-erb B-2* proto-oncogene in human pancreatic cancer. J Pathol 1990; 161: 195–200
116. Lemoine NR, Staddon S, Dickson C, Barnes D, Gullick WJ. Absence of activating transmembrane mutations in the *c-erbB-2* proto-oncogene in human breast cancer. Oncogene 1990; 5: 237–239
117 Lemoine NR, Wyllie FS, Lillehaug JR et al. Absence of abnormalities of the c-*erbB*-1 and c-*erbB*-2 proto-oncogenes in human thyroid neoplasia. Eur J Cancer 1990; 26: 777–779
118. Lemoine NR, Jain S, Silvestre F et al. Amplification and overexpression of the EGF receptor and c-*erbB*-2 proto-oncogenes in human stomach cancer. Br J Cancer 1991; 64: 79–83
119. Tuzi NL, Venter DJ, Kumar S, Staddon SL, Lemoine NR, Gullick WJ. Expression of growth factor receptors in human brain tumours. Br J Cancer 1991; 63: 227–233
120. Sachse R, Murakami Y, Shiraishi M, Hayashi K, Sekiya T. Absence of activating mutations in the transmembrane domain of the *c-erbB-2* proto-oncogene in human lung cancer. Jpn J Cancer Res 1992; 83: 1299–1303
121. Rousseau F, Bonaventure J, Legeai-Mallet L et al. Mutations in the gene encoding fibroblast growth factor receptor-3 in achondroplasia. Nature 1994; 371: 252–254
122. Shiang R, Thompson LM, Zhu Y-Z et al. Mutations in the transmembrane domain of FGFR3 cause the most common genetic form of dwarfism, achondroplasia. Cell 1994; 78: 335–342
123. Colvin JS, Bohne BA, Harding GW, McEwen DG, Ornitz DM. Skeletal overgrowth and deafness in mice lacking fibroblast growth factor receptor 3. Nat Genet 1996; 12: 390–397
124. Deng, CA, Wynshaw-Boris, A, Zhou F, Kuo A, Leder P. Fibroblast growth factor receptor 3 is a negative regulator of bone growth. Cell 1996; 84: 911–921

125. Naski MC, Wang Q, Xu J, Ornitz DM. Graded activation of fibroblast growth factor receptor 3 by mutations causing achondroplasia and thanatophoric dysplasia. Nat Genet 1996; 13: 233–237
126. Webster MK, Donoghue DJ. Constitutive activation of fibroblast growth factor receptor 3 by the transmembrane domain point mutation found in achondroplasia. EMBO J 1996; 15: 520–527
127. Superti-Furga A, Eich G, Bucher HU et al. A glycine 375-to-cysteine substitution in the transmembrane domain of the fibroblast growth factor receptor-3 in a newborn with achondroplasia. Eur J Pediatr 1995; 154: 215–219
128. Ikegawa S, Fukushima Y, Isomura M, Takada F, Nakamura Y. Mutations of the fibroblast growth factor receptor-3 gene in one familial and six sporadic cases of achondroplasia in Japanese patients. Hum Genet 1995; 96: 309–311
129. Siegel PM, Dankort DL, Hardy WR, Muller WJ. Novel activating mutations in the *neu* proto-oncogene involved in induction of mammary tumors. Mol Cell Biol 1994; 14: 7068–7077
130. Siegel PM, Muller WJ. Mutations affecting conserved cysteine residues within the extracellular domain of Neu promote receptor dimerization and activation. Proc Natl Acad Sci USA 1996; 93: 8878–8883
131. Cao H, Bangalore L, Dompe C, Bormann B-J, Stern DF. An extra cysteine proximal to the transmembrane domain induces differences cross-linking of p185neu and p185neu*. J Biol Chem 1992; 267: 20489–20492
132. Kraus MH, Issing W, Miki T, Popescu NC, Aaronson SA. Isolation and characterization of ErbB3, a third member of the erbB/epidermal growth factor receptor family: evidence for overexpression in a subset of human mammary tumors. Proc Natl Acad Sci USA 1989; 86: 9193–9197
133. Plowman GD, Whitney GS, Neubauer MG et al. Molecular cloning and expression of an additional epidermal growth factor receptor-related gene. Proc Natl Acad Sci USA 1990; 87: 4905–4909
134. Riethmacher D, Sonnenberg-Riethmacher E, Brinkmann V, Yamaai T, Lewin GR, Birchmeier C. Severe neuropathies in mice with targeted mutations in the ErbB3 receptor. Nature 1997; 389: 725–730
135. Moran MF, Koch CA, Sadowski I, Pawson T. Mutational analysis of a phosphotransfer motif essential for v-fps tyrosine kinase activity. Oncogene 1988; 3: 665–672
136. Tan JC, Nocka K, Ray P, Traktman P, Besmer P. The dominant W^{42} spotting phenotype results from a missense mutation in the c-kit receptor kinase. Science 1990; 247: 209–212
137. Guy PM, Platko JV, Cantley LC, Cerione RA, Carraway KL. Insect cell-expressed p180erbB3 possesses an impaired tyrosine kinase activity. Proc Natl Acad Sci USA 1994; 91: 8132–8136
138. Prigent SA, Gullick WJ. Identification of c-erbB-3 binding sites for phosphatidylinositol 3'-kinase and SHC using an EGF receptor/c-erbB-3 chimera. EMBO J 1994; 13: 2831–2841
139. Kraus MH, Fedi P, Starks V, Muraro R, Aaronson SA. Demonstration of ligand-dependent signaling by the erbB-3 tyrosine kinase and its constitutive activation in human breast-tumor cells. Proc Natl Acad Sci USA 1993; 90: 2900–2904
140. Alimandi M, Romano A, Curia MC et al. Cooperative signaling of ErbB3 and ErbB2 in neoplastic transformation and human mammary carcinomas. Oncogene 1995; 10: 1813–1821
141. Skinner A, Hurst HC. Transcriptional regulation of the *c-erbB-3* gene in human breast carcinoma cell lines. Oncogene 1993; 8: 3393–3401
142. Courjal F, Cuny M, Simony-Lafontaine J et al. Mapping of DNA amplification at 15 chromosomal localizations in 1875 breast tumors: definition of phenotypic groups. Cancer Res 1997; 57: 4360–4367
143. Plowman GD, Culouscou JM, Whitney GS et al. Ligand-specific activation of HER4/p180erbB4, a fourth member of the epidermal growth factor receptor family. Proc Natl Acad Sci USA 1993; 90: 1746–1750
144. Culouscou J-M, Plowman GD, Carlton GW, Green JM, Shoyab M. Characterization of a breast cancer cell differentiation factor that specifically activates the HER4/p180^{erbB4} receptor. J Biol Chem 1993; 268: 18407–18410
145. Elenius K, Subroto P, Allison G, Sun J, Klagsbrun M. Activation of HER4 by heparin-binding EGF-like growth factor stimulates chemotaxis but not proliferation. EMBO J 1997; 16: 1268–1278

146. Baulida J, Kraus MH, Alimandi M, Di Fiore PP, Carpenter G. All ErbB receptors other than the epidermal growth factor receptor are endocytosis impaired. J Biol Chem 1996; 271: 5251–5257
147. Gassmann M, Casagranda F, Orioli D et al. Aberrant neural and cardiac development in mice lacking the ErbB4 neuregulin receptor. Nature 1995; 378: 390–394
148. Faksvag Haugen DR, Akslen LA, Varhaug JE, Lillehaug JR. Expression of c-erbB-3 and c-erbB-4 proteins in papillary thyroid carcinomas. Cancer Res 1996; 56: 1184–1188
149. Elenius K, Corfas G, Paul S et al. A novel juxtamembrane domain isoform of HER4/ErbB4: isoform-specific tissue distribution and differential processing in response to phorbol ester. J Biol Chem 1997; 272: 26761–26768
150. Vecchi M, Baulida J, Carpenter G. Selective cleavage of the heregulin receptor ErbB-4 by protein kinase C activation. J Biol Chem 1996; 271: 18989–18995

12

Malignant melanoma: progress in diagnosis and prognosis

Nigel Kirkham

INTRODUCTION

Malignant melanoma continues to cause problems to the pathologist. In diagnosis, in differential diagnosis and in prognosis there are developments and continuing uncertainties to consider. This chapter will discuss various of these matters with the aim of outlining a fail-safe approach to diagnosis. Further consideration will be given to the recommended content of the biopsy report. In recent years, many areas of diagnostic pathology have seen an increasing demand for more diagnostic and staging information in reports. Much of this demand has been prompted by the development of adjuvant therapies that may improve long term survival, but at a cost to cash limited health care systems.

At the present time there is no generally accepted effective adjuvant therapy for melanoma, so, to some extent, there is no justification for extra detail in biopsy reports. On the other hand, a great deal is already known about the likely behaviour of melanoma based on morphological variables easily identified in routine sections of biopsies. The effective adjuvant therapy may appear at any time, so we should be prepared for the inevitable demand for more detail that such a development will bring with it. All of the information that is known to have a bearing on prognosis is derived from haematoxylin and eosin stained sections, so we have no present need for any sophisticated or expensive technology. As with many other cancers, what is required is a greater level of uniformity in the information reported.[1,2]

THE BIOPSY

In the clinical diagnosis of melanoma, the form of biopsy procedure undertaken will depend on the clinical situation. In the majority of cases, the patient

Dr Nigel Kirkham MD FRCPath, Histopathology Laboratory, Royal Sussex County Hospital, Brighton BN2 5BE, UK

will present with a darkly pigmented lesion on some reasonably accessible part of the body. A history of recent change or darkening of pigmentation, enlargement of the lesion, or of bleeding will increase the level of clinical suspicion. In this typical situation, most patients will have an excision biopsy with a clinical margin of 2 mm of normal skin around the lesion. To the apparent surprise of many pathologists, the average dermatologist is perfectly capable of excising a darkly pigmented lesion in its totality in this way.

In some anatomically more sensitive sites, such as the face, the initial approach may be to undertake a punch biopsy from the area of the lesion that appears to be the thickest. This approach offers an opportunity to assess the lesion and, especially, whether it is intraepidermal or has an invasive dermal component. Occasionally, an incisional biopsy will be performed, but this approach does not play any substantial part in the investigation of melanoma.

Finally, there are occasions when the clinical diagnosis is not one of melanoma but of some other, and perhaps benign, condition such as a seborrhoeic keratosis. In these circumstances, the lesion may be removed by curettage, producing the familiar fragmented specimen that is difficult to orientate

TRIMMING THE BIOPSY

EXCISION BIOPSY

There are two possible approaches to an ellipse excision biopsy. One can either try to look at all of the margins of the specimen to see if the lesion is excised or, alternatively, sample the lesion completely and obtain less clear information about the margins. For primary excision biopsies of melanoma, the first approach is of no relevance. As mentioned above, it is a relatively straightforward matter to excise a darkly pigmented lesion arising in pale skin because the lesion is easily seen and easily excised. This is not the case for basal cell carcinomas which are usually not pigmented and may be difficult to delineate clinically. Furthermore, an excision biopsy of a basal cell carcinoma is an attempt at complete treatment. It is important in these circumstances to examine the excision margins to confirm the completeness of the excision. The tumour itself is usually easily identified as a basal cell carcinoma and there is little more to be said about it. In all but the smallest excision ellipses, it may be entirely reasonable to sample the tissue by taking 'cruciate blocks' transversely across the centre and longitudinally from the ends of the ellipse.

With melanoma there is an entirely different set of questions to be answered and most of these require a full examination of the tumour. Once the diagnosis of melanoma is confirmed, then, in almost all cases, a re-excision procedure will be undertaken to reduce the chances of local tumour recurrence.

It is, therefore, much more important to examine the whole tumour so that variations in tumour thickness and variations in mitotic activity, regression and so on can be identified. To achieve this end it is recommended that the tumour in its ellipse of skin should be sliced transversely at intervals of 1–2 mm. It may be worthwhile to ink the margins of the biopsy before slicing it, although this is not an absolute requirement because the biopsy will usually have a coating of blood on it, which acts as an alternative marker of the margins of the specimen.

It is also important to use a sharp blade to slice the biopsy. Especially with thinner lesions, a blunt knife will introduce artefacts, in particular slicing with a blunt knife will often lead to disruption of the dermal–epidermal interface, making interpretation of possible early dermal invasion even more difficult than usual.

Depending upon the size of the lesion, this slicing will produce something between 3 and 8 or 10 slices. These can be divided between more than one cassette for processing if necessary. It is usually not advisable to put more than three or four slices into one cassette.

Finally, it is important to examine each block of tissue at several levels. Typically, sections cut at three levels are examined. This additional precaution reduces the chances of missing variations in the tumour. By adopting this approach of slicing the whole tumour and examining each slice at multiple levels one can be a sure as it is possible to be that the worst aspects of the tumour will come to light.

PUNCH BIOPSY

A punch biopsy requires no further dissection before processing. However, it is important to examine the biopsy in multiple sections cut to at least three levels. It is such a common experience to find a feature in only a few of the sections cut from a punch biopsy that this examination of multiple sections must be taken as mandatory.

CURETTING BIOPSY

When the diagnosis of melanoma has not been apparent at the time of biopsy, a curettage may be performed. In these circumstances there may also be no suspicion of anything unusual when the curettings are put into a cassette for processing. When the diagnosis becomes evident at the time of microscopic examination of sections, further levels should be requested if they have not been already.

DIAGNOSIS

CLINICAL INFORMATION

It perhaps goes without saying, but is worth reiterating, that the clinical history is important when diagnosing melanoma. In a typical straightforward case, the diagnosis of melanoma will have been made clinically. The request form accompanying the biopsy will usually convey a high clinical suspicion of melanoma very clearly using terms such as 'clinically melanoma', 'enlarging and bleeding recently' and so on. The pathologist must pay attention to this sort of information. If a benign diagnosis is going to be offered on the biopsy report then the reporting pathologist must think several times before dismissing the possibility of melanoma.

The request form must, of course, give the name and other identifying details of the patient, including gender, and the doctor in charge of the case and address for delivery of the report. The age of the patient (or date of birth) will usually also be given. This is of some help. Most melanomas occur in middle-aged people. Young age does not, however, exclude the diagnosis. Young age alone cannot be taken as grounds for offering a benign diagnosis.

The site of the biopsy should also be given. This has no particular bearing on the diagnosis but may be a factor in determining prognosis.

Full recommendations on the reporting of melanomas have recently been published by the Association of Directors of Anatomic and Surgical Pathology.[3,4]

DYSPLASTIC NAEVUS OR MELANOMA?

The dysplastic naevus is a risk factor for melanoma and is now rarely excised unless there is clinical concern that transformation to a malignant melanoma may have taken place.[5–8] The criteria for diagnosis of a dysplastic naevus are:

1. A diameter of at least 4 mm
2. A host lymphocytic response around blood vessels in the underlying dermis
3. Nested and lentiginous melanocytic proliferation
4. The presence of random (variable) cytological atypia
5. Delicate elongation of rete ridges and fusion of adjacent rete
6. Narrow elongated spindle-shaped melanocytes orientated horizontally
7. Lamellar dermal fibroplasia around rete ridges.

There is clearly an overlap between a dysplastic naevus as defined and the earliest of melanomas. In the diagnosis of melanoma, it is likely that, by comparison with a dysplastic naevus, a melanoma would show a larger diameter, typically at least 6 or 7 mm. It would also show more marked and more uniformly non-random cytological atypia. The melanocytic proliferation is likely to be more marked a feature with pagetoid or 'buckshot' spread of melanocytes into the upper layers of the epidermis being likely to be found in a melanoma.

RADIAL GROWTH PHASE OR MELANOMA *IN SITU*?

The recognition that there does really seem to be a group of melanomas that lack the capacity to metastasise has led to the emergence of various terms to describe and attempt to define examples of such lesions.[9] All such descriptions are inevitably approximations in the absence of any true discriminators between tumours that can and tumours that cannot metastasise.

The best available definition is simple to apply and merely depends upon the ability to recognise two features: the presence of the largest nest of abnormal melanocytes in the lesion and the presence of mitoses.

If the largest nest of cells is in the epidermis and if there are no mitoses in any dermal component that may be present, then the lesion fulfils the criteria for classification as a radial growth phase melanoma. The absence of a dominant dermal component and of dermal mitoses is taken as evidence that the tumour is not proliferating in the dermis and so is unlikely to have the capacity to metastasise.

The term 'melanoma *in situ*' at first sight seems to be a good one in that it clearly conveys the information that the melanoma is intraepidermal with the implication that benign behaviour is guaranteed. Inevitably things are not so simple in practice. In routine haematoxylin and eosin stained sections, it may be extremely difficult to decide whether a melanoma is intraepidermal or is showing early dermal invasion. This difficulty is partly explained by the tendency of proliferating melanocytes to form large nests which tend to show expansile growth with consequent downward extension of the basal layer of the epidermis. We do not have a good marker of basement membrane to apply in paraffin sections.

The advantage of the radial growth phase definition is that it avoids the need to decide whether the melanoma is *in situ* or not. The distinction seems to be of little, although not of no, importance.

In studies of prognosis it is the thinnest tumours that usually have the best prognosis. The best prognosis is typically associated with tumours less than 0.75 mm thick. Melanomas with this degree of thinness are most likely to be *in situ* or to fulfil the criteria for classification as radial growth phase melanomas.

VERTICAL GROWTH PHASE

The description 'vertical growth phase' is used to describe those tumours that show clear evidence of growth in the dermis. This is defined morphologically by the presence in the dermis of either (i) the largest nest of cells in the tumour and/or (ii) mitoses. The presence of one or both of these features gives unequivocal evidence that the tumour has developed beyond the *in situ* phase. The fact that the tumour is growing in the dermis is taken as an indication that there is a finite possibility that the tumour may progress to the development of distant metastases. The presence of a vertical growth phase morphology in itself does not guarantee that metastases will develop. It is the possibility that they may that has led to attempts to develop prognostic models that might offer a greater degree of accuracy in defining that possibility.

VARIANT VERTICAL GROWTH PHASE

Melanocytes are unusual cells in that they are destined to migrate. In the development of benign moles or naevi, it is the normal sequence of events for cells to proliferate to form junctional nests in the epidermis and then for these nests to migrate through the epidermal basement membrane into the dermis. Three morphological variants of melanocytes in benign naevi have been defined.

The first of these, Type A, describes cells like those found in the junctional nests. These are relatively large groups of cells, with the whole group surrounded by basement membrane material. This can be demonstrated by, for instance, staining with an antibody to type IV collagen. Type B melanocytes are an intermediate form which are aggregated in smaller groups but are still surrounded by basement membrane material. These are typically found in the upper dermal component of a compound or intradermal cellular naevus. Type C melanocytes represent the 'mature' melanocyte that occurs singly, with its own rim of basement membrane material. These are the single cells found in the deeper part of a cellular naevus.

In benign naevi differing proportions of Type A, B and C cells are present. Type A cells are in the junctional component, Type B cells typically predominate in the majority of cellular naevi and Type C cells are found in the more mature and less cellular lesions. These variations in melanocytic differentiation are recapitulated to some extent in melanomas. The typical melanoma probably shows Type C differentiation but there are smaller numbers of tumours that show Type B differentiation. These have been described as 'minimal deviation' or 'variant vertical growth phase' melanomas. There are two possible reasons for identifying them as a special sub-group within melanoma. Firstly, they may be associated with a more favourable prognosis. Secondly, and perhaps more importantly, they may be mistaken for benign cellular dermal naevi.

This confusion can arise because of the similarity of appearance of the two alternatives. The melanoma may look distinctly naevoid, with cells arranged in nests and aggregates within the dermis in a manner that can easily look benign at first glance. The diagnosis of malignancy can be made by more careful scrutiny of the sections. The cells will have definitely atypical nuclei and nucleoli. The nuclei will be enlarged by comparison with those in an unequivocally benign naevus. They may show some irregularity of the nuclear contour. The nucleoli are a particularly useful clue to the diagnosis. In naevi they will be small, round and regular. In the melanoma they will be larger and will show variation in size and shape with a tendency for the majority to be irregular to point of having a recognisably polygonal outline.

Although the cytological appearance and the architecture of the lesion is important in making a diagnosis of malignancy, of more importance is the presence of mitoses and especially the presence of unequivocally abnormal mitoses. It is most unusual to see mitoses in the dermal component of a benign naevus. Occasionally, a naevus may contain a mitosis, but if it does the mitosis is likely to look normal and to be present in the upper part of the dermal component. When multiple mitoses are present, or when the mitoses are in the deep dermal component and especially when they look atypical it is highly likely that the lesion in consideration is a melanoma and not a naevus. One should be extremely circumspect in making a benign diagnosis in the presence of any of these features.

DESMOPLASTIC OR NEUROTROPHIC MELANOMA

The desmoplastic melanoma is a difficult area for diagnosis for a number of reasons. First of all this variant of melanoma is uncommon and does not usually present as such an obvious tumour as other melanomas. It typically occurs on the face of an older person. There may or may not be an overlying lentiginous element producing obvious pigmentation of the skin. The involved skin may merely appear thickened to produce a rather indeterminate plaque.

An initial biopsy may often be a punch or incisional biopsy. In the biopsy the diagnostic features are likely to be subtle. The epidermis is unlikely to show obvious melanoma, although there may be lentiginous hyperplasia of melanocytes. More often the epidermis will appear hyperplastic leading to the potential pitfall of a mistaken diagnosis of squamous cell carcinoma. To be useful the biopsy must include a deep sample of dermis. The tumour cells are spindle-shaped and infiltrate the dermis in a subtle way that may be easily overlooked. A clue to the diagnosis is the presence of a lymphocytic host response to the tumour cells. Apparently unexplained spotty collections of lymphocytes in the dermis indicates the need for a detailed search of the dermis for a spindle cell infiltrate that may or may not be neurotrophic. An S100-stained section is invaluable in this search. In the normal dermis only the dermal nerves and parts of the sweat gland coils are usually S100-positive. The finding of S100-positive spindle cells or larger than normal cells in the dermal nerves, often with an associated lymphocytic response, should be a strong clue to the diagnosis. The S100 staining may also serve to emphasise any epidermal component of abnormal melanocytes that may be masked by the epidermal hyperplasia.

There may be residual uncertainty about the diagnosis after the most exhaustive examination of a small biopsy. In these circumstances the way forward may be to advise a formal excision biopsy, possibly followed by a further excision to ensure clearance. The problem with these tumours of course is their subtly infiltrative and neurotrophic growth pattern. Wide and complete sampling of the margins of the specimen will be needed to see if the tumour has been completely excised. The surgeon can assist in this by marking any cutaneous nerves that are identified during the excision procedure with marker suture, so that these can be sampled specifically to look for involvement of the margins by tumour cells. This is a rare problem in practice and so each case has to be approached on its merits. There is no clear evidence available to give guidance on the most satisfactory extent of any excision that may be undertaken.

DIFFERENTIAL DIAGNOSIS

MELANOMA OR NOT MELANOMA?

Even the most obvious melanoma may turn out in due course of time to be something else. This is perhaps most true of the so-called 'amelanotic melanoma'. When the tumour has everything in favour of a diagnosis of melanoma, including the clinical appearance, the architectural and cytological features of a tumour composed of large malignant cells with predominantly large single nucleoli in the nuclei and with unequivocal melanin in tumour cells then there may not be much room for doubt.

When the tumour is not obviously pigmented or when other features of the classic case are missing, then the diagnosis must be confirmed. The first and most reliable step to take is to have a section stained for S100. Although S100 is not specific for melanoma it is highly sensitive. Virtually every melanoma is strongly S100-positive. If the S100 is negative then a panel of alternative markers should clarify the situation. The differential diagnosis includes a variety of anaplastic tumours amongst which the CD30-positive anaplastic non-Hodgkin's lymphoma must be considered high on the list. This will always be CD30-positive and may or may not also show positive staining with markers of B or T cell differentiation.

It would be unusual, although not impossible, for poorly differentiated or anaplastic squamous cell carcinomas, sarcomas and even atypical fibrous histiocytomas to be confused with melanoma. These distinctions should be resolved relatively readily by staining for S100 and for epithelial cytokeratin and for markers of soft tissue differentiation.

MELANOMA OR NAEVUS?

The distinction between melanoma and naevus is not usually a problem, but, when it is, the problem can be a very difficult one. As described above the main features in differential diagnosis between benign and malignant lesions are those used in virtually every field of tumour pathology and depend upon careful scrutiny of the architectural and cytological features including the presence or absence of mitoses.

The archetype for a benign lesion is one in which there is radial symmetry at scanning magnification. In the epidermis melanocytic proliferation is limited to the lower third and may be nested or lentiginous. Individual cell 'buck shot' spread into the upper layers of the epidermis is not seen. In the dermis, maturation or differentiation from Type A to Type B and Type C melanocytes is present. Mitoses are not a feature, especially in the deeper part of the lesion.

An exception to be aware of is the spindle and epithelioid cell naevus of Reed which typically occurs as a darkly pigmented, radially symmetrical, raised nodular lesion on the leg of a young woman. These naevi can be extremely confusing. A point in favour of the diagnosis is the presence of large nests of melanocytes rather than single cells extending into the upper epidermis and even showing an appearance of transepidermal elimination of the large groups of prominently pigmented cells. The cells will be predominantly junctional although and intradermal component is sometimes seen. They show spindle and epithelioid shapes and have nuclei that are not greatly enlarged. Nucleoli are predominantly round with an absence of large and polygonal forms. Mitoses are not a prominent feature.

MELANOCYTIC TUMOURS OF UNCERTAIN MALIGNANT POTENTIAL

After the most careful, detailed and thorough analysis there will remain a small number of tumours in which it is difficult to be sure about the diagnosis: the lesion sits on the borderline between benign and malignant with features of both possible diagnoses and no overwhelming case for either one to be made with complete confidence. In these circumstances it is not unreasonable to admit to uncertainty and to adopt as fail safe an approach as possible. For the first part a diagnosis of 'melanocytic tumour of uncertain malignant potential' can be given, stating that it is not possible to be completely sure that the tumour is malignant, but that, at the same time, it does not have definite features of a benign tumour. Secondly, in circumstances such as these it would be usual to recommend a re-excision of the biopsy site if the lesion had had a simple punch or excision biopsy performed. This re-excision is done to reduce the possibility of local recurrence, on the pragmatic basis that if diagnosis of the primary is difficult then diagnosis of any recurrent lesion is likely to be even more difficult. Furthermore there is anecdotal evidence to suggest that recurrent lesions may have an increased malignant potential over the primary tumour. In summary, the advice is 'if in doubt re-excise' and re-excise early.

PROGNOSTIC FACTORS

In making a diagnosis of a melanoma there are a number of variables that can be used to add to the blunt diagnosis. There are two problems to be considered. Firstly, there do seem to be a group of melanomas that are not truly malignant in the sense that, although they show features of a malignant neoplasm down the microscope, they do not behave malignantly. Following an excision biopsy they do not recur locally and, after prolonged follow-up, they do not progress to metastasis and do not cause the death of the patient. One challenge facing the diagnostician is to recognise these lesions and to distinguish them from melanomas that behave in the expected way.[9,10] The diagnosis of these radial growth phase melanomas has been described above.

At least 70% of melanomas have progressed to vertical growth phase at the time of diagnosis.[11] A variety of attempts have been made to stratify these tumours further to give a guide to prognosis, since Clark first described a staging system based on levels of invasion and Breslow demonstrated that tumour thickness measured in mm could be even more predictive of tumour behaviour. Subsequently, there have been several reports that have examined databases to identify tumour-related variables holding independent prognostic significance, on the basis that several variables might offer more prognostic information than tumour thickness alone, although tumour thickness is clearly a very strong predictor of prognosis.[12,13]

The first large model was reported by Clark et al in 1989 and included tumour thickness, sex, site, mitotic counts, tumour regression and tumour infiltrating lymphocytes as independently acting prognostic variables that could be combined in tables that allowed 8-year probabilities of tumour-free survival to be stated for any melanoma, within the context of 95% confidence intervals.[14]

A subsequent large study of databases in Alabama and Sydney, involving 4568 patients, largely confirmed this approach and confirmed that tumour thickness was the most significant prognostic factor in predicting survival after disease free intervals of 2 years, 5 years and 10 years. Tumour ulceration and site were the other two most significant predictors of survival. The importance of tumour thickness at the time of diagnosis did not diminish with the length of disease-free survival. After a 5 year disease-free interval, ulceration ceased to have significance and, after 10 years, only tumour thickness emerged as a predictor of tumour recurrence or death in years 11–20 after diagnosis.[15]

The Clark model has subsequently been simplified by the Philadelphia Pigmented Lesion Group to include just four variables compared to the six in the original model.[16] The relative predictive power of the variables is indicated by their odds ratios: tumour thickness (odds ratio, 50.8), site (odds ratio, 4.4), age of the patient at diagnosis (odds ratio, 3.0) and the sex of the patient (odds ratio, 2.0). This model was significantly more accurate than tumour thickness alone, particularly for predicting death: the overall error rate for predicting death was reduced by 50%. The four-variable model has the advantage that the variables used are most likely to be present in non-specialist histopathology reports. This study was largely confirmed in a report from New York, although in this latter analysis the sex of the patient was not independently significant.[17] Sex was of course the weakest of the four variables in the Philadelphia model.

Thus we can conclude that important prognostic information can be derived from tumour thickness, tumour site, age and sex, but that more detailed reporting of tumours to include mitotic count, regression, ulceration, tumour infiltrating lymphocytes and possible other emerging markers are likely to be even more accurately predictive of disease-free intervals and of overall survival.[11]

RE-EXCISION

The solid information available to give guidance on how wide a re-excision should be taken is still short of that needed to be certain that we know that re-excision is being performed appropriately. It is important to remember that re-excision of a tumour site is performed to reduce the possibility of local recurrence by removing any residual primary disease and by removing any immediately adjacent local metastases. Re-excision itself has no direct bearing on the possibility of the development of metastatic disease in the patient at some future time.

At present the best available advice suggests that excision should never be less than 5 mm and never more than 30 mm. There is no place for excisions with a margin of more than 30 mm. A trial is underway in the UK, organised by the Melanoma Study Group and the British Association of Plastic Surgeons, that aims to discover whether a 10 mm or 30 mm margin is appropriate for tumours with a Breslow thickness of more than 2 mm. Recommendations for excision margins are given in the Table 1.

EXAMINATION OF THE RE-EXCISION SPECIMEN

Irrespective of the policy of any particular unit re-excisions are received in the laboratory on a fairly regular basis and the question arises about what should be done with them. It is important to know what margin of excision was reported on the primary excision specimen.

The re-excision specimen should be given a careful macroscopic examination. If the first tumour was completely excised and no macroscopic abnormality is

Table 1.1 Recommendations for excision margins.

Breslow tumour thickness	TNM stage	Minimum margin recommended	Maximum margin recommended
Melanoma *in situ*	Tis	5 mm	10 mm
< 0.76 mm	T1	5 mm	10 mm
> 0.76 – < 2.00 mm	T2 (0.76–1.5 mm) T3 < 2.0 mm	10 mm	20 mm[18]
> 2.00 mm	T3 > 2.0 mm T4a	Enter into MSG/BAPS trial, randomised between 10 and 30 mm	
> 2.00 mm not entered into MSG/BAPS trial	T3 > 2.0 mm T4a	20 mm	30 mm

seen in the re-excision specimen then it is most unlikely that any tumour will be found. In these circumstances it is adequate to take one transverse block from the centre of the previous biopsy site.

If the original tumour excision was reported as likely to be incomplete then further sampling should reflect the nature and extent of that tumour. Similarly if a macroscopic abnormality is seen in the re-excision specimen then it too should be sampled.[19]

FURTHER STAGING PROCEDURES

There is increasing clinical interest in the development of more accurate staging procedures. At the present time, there does not appear to any place for elective lymph node dissection. The procedure of sentinel node biopsy in which the node draining the immediate tumour field is identified by a dye injection or other marker procedure is of interest. In the absence of more compelling evidence, its role at the present time is limited to clinical trials that are being performed with ethical committee approval.

The sentinel node biopsy may only contain a small amount of tumour. Careful sectioning of the whole node, possibly supplemented by S100 staining may be necessary to identify tumour cells. Even more sensitive methods are being developed, such as the use of reverse transcriptase polymerase chain reaction (RT-PCR) methods to look for evidence of tyrosinase in the nodes, whose presence is indicative of the presence of melanocytes within the node.

MELANOMA IN LITIGATION

The diagnosis of melanoma, fraught as it is with difficulties, may lead to litigation when errors occur. As far as the pathologist is concerned it is the under diagnosis of malignancy rather than its over diagnosis that leads to litigation. Careful attention to the clinical history is an important factor to take into account, especially if the clinical diagnosis is a malignant one and the

BIOPSY REPORT CHECKLIST

Site of the lesion, age and sex of patient:

• Procedure:	Excision/incision or punch/ shave biopsy / other
• Lesion confirmed as primary:	yes/no ?
• Ulceration:	Present/absent
• Clark level:	I/II/III/IV/V
• Breslow tumour thickness	mm
• Mitotic count:	/sq. mm
• Regression:	Present/absent
• Excision:	Complete/incomplete-state where
• Vascular invasion:	Absent/present – blood vessel &/ or lymphatic?
• Microsatellites:	Present/absent
• Neurotrophism:	Present/absent

patient presents with a history of an enlarging lesion that has been bleeding. In a recent review of 75 malpractice cases in Canada, a pathological mistake was the basis of the case in 18; of which, 7 were where melanomas were initially diagnosed as naevi, 4 where initially diagnosis was as Spitz naevi and a further 5 miscellaneous cases also had an essentially benign first pathological diagnosis.[20] It was notable that this study looked for, but did not find, cases relating to a lack of care when moles had been described as 'dysplastic' or 'atypical'.

Overall, melanoma does not appear to cause too many cases in litigation, except when a biopsy of a suspicious lesion has either not been taken, or not submitted for histopathological examination. When a biopsy is sent to the laboratory the reporting pathologist must always pay attention to the clinical details of the case and exercise caution when proposing to give a benign diagnosis in the face of a clinically malignant lesion.

SUMMARY AND CHECKLIST

Reporting melanomas in a reliable way is an achievable prospect and depends upon a careful structured approach to the examination of all of the tissue submitted for examination, including accurate measurement of tumour thickness.[21]

The biopsy report should include details of the age and sex of the patient. As a minimum the report should attempt to comment on the details given in the box 'Biopsy report checklist' above:[3,4]

The majority of tumours will be in vertical growth phase, but up to 30% may show radial growth phase only. The growth phase should be described. Subclassification of vertical growth phase into lentigo maligna type, acral lentiginous type, desmoplastic, minimal deviation and other types may be considered but is of less importance than recording the details listed above.

REFERENCES

1. Cook MG. Diagnostic discord with melanoma. J Pathol 1997; 182: 247–249
2. Veenhuizen KCW, De Wit PEJ, Mooi WJ et al. Quality assessment by expert opinion in melanoma pathology: experience of the pathology panel of the Dutch melanoma working party. J Pathol 1997; 182: 266–272
3. Association of Directors of Anatomic and Surgical Pathology. Recommendations for the reporting of tissues removed as part of the surgical treatment of cutaneous malanoma. Hum Pathol 1997; 28: 1123–1125
4. Association of Directors of Anatomic and Surgical Pathology. Recommendations for the reporting of tissues removed as part of the surgical treatment of cutaneous malanoma. Virchows Arch 1997; 431: 79-81
5. Newton Bishop JA. The atypical naevus: a clinician's viewpoint. In: Kirkham N, Hall PA. (eds) Progress in Pathology Vol 1. Edinburgh: Churchill Livingstone, 1995; 179–189
6. Kirkham N. The atypical naevus: a histopathologist's viewpoint. In: Kirkham N, Hall PA. (eds) Progress in Pathology Vol 1. Edinburgh: Churchill Livingstone, 1995; 191–199
7. Clemente C, Cochran AJ, Elder DE et al. Histopathologic diagnosis of dysplastic nevi: concordance among pathologists convened by the World Health Organization Melanoma Programme. Hum Pathol 1991; 22: 313–319
8. Carey Jr WP., Thompson CJ, Synnestvedt M et al. Dysplastic nevi as a melanoma risk factor in patients with familial melanoma. Cancer 1994; 74: 3118–3125
9. Guerry 4th D, Synnestvedt M, Elder DE, Schultz D. Lessons from tumour progression: the invasive radial growth phase of melanoma is common, is incapable of metastasis, and indolent. J Invest Dermatol 1993; 100: 342S–345S
10. Elder DE. Skin cancer. Melanoma and other specific nonmelanoma skin cancers. Cancer 1995; 75 (Suppl 1): 245–256
11. Elder DE, Van Belle P, Elentitsas R, Halpern A, Guerry D. Neoplastic progression and prognosis in melanoma. Semin Cutan Med Surg 1996; 15: 336–348
12. Barnhill RL, Fine JA, Roush GC, Berwick M. Predicting five-year outcome for patients with cutaneous melanoma in a population-based study. Cancer 1996; 78: 427–432
13. Pritchard ML, Woosley JT. Comparison of two prognostic models predicting survival in patients with malignant melanoma. Hum Pathol 1995; 26: 1028–1031
14. Clark Jr WH, Elder DE, Guerry 4th D et al. Model predicting survival in stage 1 melanoma based on tumour progression. J Natl Cancer Inst 1989; 81: 1893–1904
15. Soong S-J, Shaw HM, Balch MD et al. Predicting survival and recurrence in localized melanoma: a multivariate approach. World J Surg 1992; 16: 191–195
16. Schuchter L, Schultz DJ, Synnestvedt BS et al. a prognostic model for predicting 10-year survival in patients with primary melanoma. Ann Intern Med 1996; 125: 369–375
17. Sahin S, Rao B, Kopf AW et al. Predicting ten-year survival of patients with primary cutaneous melanoma. Corroboration of a prognostic model. Cancer 1997; 80: 1426–1431
18. Balch CM, Urist MM, Karakousis CP et al. Efficacy of 2 cm surgical margins for intermediate thickness melanomas 1–4 mm – results of a multi-institutional randomised surgical trial. Ann Surg 1993; 218: 262–269
19. Martin HM, Birkin AJ, Theaker JM. Malignant melanoma re-excision specimens – how many blocks? Histopathology 1998; 32: In press
20. Jackson R. Malignant melanoma: a review of 75 malpractice cases. Int J Dermatol 1997; 36: 497–498
21. Kirkham N, Cotton DW. Measuring melanomas: the Vernier method. J Clin Pathol 1984; 37: 229–230

Index

A

B

C

D

E

F

G

H

I

J

K

L

M

N

O

P

R

S

T

V

W

X

Y